SpringerWienNewYork

Josef Thalhamer • Richard Weiss
Sandra Scheiblhofer
Editors

Gene Vaccines

SpringerWienNewYork

Editors
Prof. Dr. Josef Thalhamer
University of Salzburg
Department of Molecular Biology
Hellbrunnerstrasse 34
5020 Salzburg
Austria
e-mail: josef.thalhamer@sbg.ac.at

Prof. Richard Weiss
University of Salzburg
Department of Molecular Biology
Hellbrunnerstrasse 34
5020 Salzburg
Austria
e-mail: richard.weiss@sbg.ac.at

Dr. Sandra Scheiblhofer, PhD
University of Salzburg
Department of Molecular Biology
Division of Allergy & Immunology
Hellbrunnerstrasse 34
5020 Salzburg
Austria
e-mail: sandra.scheiblhofer@sbg.ac.at

All rights are reserved, whether the whole or part of the material is concerned, specifically those of translation, reprinting, re-use of illustrations, broadcasting, reproduction by photocopying machines or similar means, and storage in data banks.

Product Liability: The publisher can give no guarantee for all the information contained in this book. This does also refer to information about drug dosage and application thereof. In every individual case the respective user must check its accuracy by consulting other pharmaceutical literature.

The use of registered names, trademarks, etc. in this publication does not imply, even in the absence of a specific statement, that such names are exempt from the relevant protective laws and regulations and therefore free for general use.

© 2012 Springer-Verlag/Wien

SpringerWienNewYork is part of Springer Science+Business Media
springer.at

Typesetting: SPi-Global, Pondicherry, India
Cover design: WMXDesign, GmbH, Heidelberg, Germany

Printed on acid-free and chlorine-free bleached paper
SPIN: 80013623

With 49 (partly coloured) Figures

Library of Congress Control Number: 2011936887

ISBN 978-3-7091-0438-5   e-ISBN 978-3-7091-0439-2
DOI 10.1007/978-3-7091-0439-2
SpringerWienNewYork

Preface

In the early nineties, the induction of a specific immune response by injecting a eukaryotic expression vector into the skin or muscle appeared somewhat "magic". However, the basic mechanisms underlying "genetic immunization" could be explained by simple rules of text book immunology, i.e. transcription of the gene, translation of the gene product, processing and presentation on MHC, and induction of the immune reaction. The simplicity of using a genetic "sentence" and thus talk to the immune system inspired the imagination of scientists, and the approach was appraised as a revolution in modern vaccine design. Obviously, a dialog with the immune system was possible – you talk, using the genetic code, and the system responds. This analogy still holds true, and from my point of view, is the major cause of fascination for gene vaccines. As scientists gained a deeper understanding of the language of the immune system, they were able to extend their vocabulary and improved the dialog with the system. Elucidation of the manifold regulatory pathways and mechanisms of activating or inhibitory immune mediators enabled to command the immune system and to trigger desired immune responses.

Another intriguing aspect of genetic immunization is the quick and easy implementation of the latest knowledge into application. Within several days, a novel gene of interest can be inserted into vectors, or any steering sequence can be added to the basic vaccine constructs, and within weeks, the resulting effects can be evaluated in animal models. Logically, the vast potential of this novel approach stimulated the creativity of researchers worldwide, with the result of a "DNA vaccine hype" in the late nineties.

As often happens with highly praised new developments, the peak of popularity and excessive hopes was followed by disillusion, which in the case of gene vaccines was triggered by the results of the first clinical trials. Yet again, their outcome confirmed the well-known and dreaded "mice to men" barrier, and seemed to prove the common proverb "mice lie and monkeys exaggerate". Barely any of the striking successes observed in animal models could be validated in humans. The consequence was a drastic drop of acceptance, the so-called "gene vaccine hangover" (as termed by David Weiner) during the first years of the new century.

Fortunately, many scientists distinguish themselves by thirst for knowledge paired with a certain stubbornness. The authors of the present book belong to this category and their work reversed the disparaging attitude towards gene vaccines. In the past years, they elucidated hitherto unknown mechanisms underlying genetic immunization and improved existing, or developed novel application modes and techniques. Thus, they could overcome the hurdles of impaired immunogenicity in humans and initiated a new era of gene vaccines.

Many of the chapters of this book focus on human vaccine approaches and describe recent progress and current strategies. Leading companies in the field were invited to present their vaccine platforms and clinical research. This application-oriented view is complemented with up-to-date scientific knowledge of the mechanisms underlying gene-based vaccines.

I hope, "gene vaccines" will both, provide insight into a still young and exciting field of immunological research and its applications, as well as transfer a portion of our enthusiasm and curiosity to the reader.

Salzburg, August 2011   Josef Thalhamer

Contents

1 General Mechanisms of Gene Vaccines 1
Richard Weiss, Viggo Van Tendeloo, Sandra Scheiblhofer,
and Josef Thalhamer

**2 Strategies to Improve DNA Vaccine Potency: HPV-Associated
Cervical Cancer as a Model System** 27
Chien-Fu Hung, Barbara Ma, Yijie Xu, and T.-C. Wu

**3 Immune-Activating Mechanisms of Replicase-Based DNA
and RNA Vaccines and Their Role in Immune-Apoptosis** 67
Wolfgang W. Leitner

4 Cytokine Genes as Molecular Adjuvants for DNA Vaccines 89
Bin Wang, Youmin Kang, and Richard Ascione

5 Pharmaceutical Non-Viral Formulations for Gene Vaccines 109
Glen Perera and Andreas Bernkop-Schnürch

**6 Rational Design of Formulated DNA Vaccines:
The DermaVir Approach**. 127
Eszter Nátz and Julianna Lisziewicz

7 Improvement of DNA Vaccines by Electroporation 145
Arielle A. Ginsberg, Xuefei Shen, Natalie A. Hutnick,
and David B. Weiner

**8 Electroporation Based TriGrid™ Delivery System (TDS)
for DNA Vaccine Administration** 163
Drew Hannaman

**9 Prime Boost Regimens for Enhancing Immunity: Magnitude,
Quality of Mucosal and Systemic Gene Vaccines** 183
Danushka K. Wijesundara and Charani Ranasinghe

10 Intralymphatic Vaccination. 205
Thomas M. Kündig, Adrian Bot, and Gabriela Senti

11 Messenger RNA Vaccines 223
Jochen Probst, Mariola Fotin-Mleczek, Thomas Schlake,
Andreas Thess, Thomas Kramp, and Karl-Josef Kallen

**12 DNA and RNA Vaccines for Prophylactic and Therapeutic
Treatment of Type I Allergy** 247
Richard Weiss, Sandra Scheiblhofer, Elisabeth Rösler,
and Josef Thalhamer

**13 Approved Veterinary Vaccines: Paving the Way to Products
for Human Health** 265
Matthias Giese

14 Current Status of Regulations for DNA Vaccines 285
Bettina Klug, Jens Reinhardt, and James Robertson

15 Minicircle DNA 297
Peter Mayrhofer and Michaela Iro

**16 Industrial Manufacturing of Plasmid-DNA Products
for Gene Vaccination and Therapy** 311
Jochen Urthaler, Hermann Schuchnigg, Patrick Garidel,
and Hans Huber

Contributors

Andreas Bernkop-Schnürch Department of Pharmaceutical Technology, Institute of Pharmacy, University of Innsbruck, Innsbruck, Austria

Adrian Bot Research & Development, MannKind Corp., Paine Valencia, CA, USA

Mariola Fotin-Mleczek CureVac GmbH, Tübingen, Germany

Patrick Garidel Boehringer Ingelheim Pharma GmbH & Co. KG, Biberach an der Riss, Germany

Matthias Giese Institute for Molecular Vaccines (IMV) Heidelberg, Heidelberg, Germany

Arielle A. Ginsberg Department of Pathology and Laboratory Medicine, University of Pennsylvania, Philadelphia, PA, USA

Drew Hannaman Ichor Medical Systems, Inc., San Diego, CA, USA

Hans Huber Biomay AG, Vienna, Austria

Chien-Fu Hung Departments of Pathology and Oncology, The Johns Hopkins Medical Institutions, Baltimore, MD, USA

Natalie A. Hutnick Department of Pathology and Laboratory Medicine, University of Pennsylvania, Philadelphia, PA, USA

Michaela Iro RBPS-Technologies e.U, Vienna, Austria

Thomas M. Kündig Department of Dermatology, University Hospital of Zurich, Zurich, Switzerland

Karl-Josef Kallen CureVac GmbH, Tübingen, Germany

Youmin Kang State Key Laboratory for Agro-Biotechnology, College of Biological Science, China Agricultural University, Beijing, China

Bettina Klug, Paul-Ehrlich Institut, Langen, Germany

Thomas Kramp CureVac GmbH, Tübingen, Germany

Wolfgang W. Leitner, National Institute of Allergy and Infectious Diseases, NIH, Basic Immunology Branch, Bethesda, MD, USA

Julianna Lisziewicz Genetic Immunity, Budapest, Hungary

Barbara Ma Department of Pathology, The Johns Hopkins Medical Institutions, Baltimore, MD, USA

Peter Mayrhofer RBPS-Technologies e.U, Vienna, Austria
Department of Pathobiology, Institute of Bacteriology, Mycology and Hygiene, University of Veterinary Medicine Vienna, Vienna, Austria

Eszter Nátz Genetic Immunity, Budapest, Hungary

Glen Perera Department of Pharmaceutical Technology, Institute of Pharmacy, University of Innsbruck, Innsbruck, Austria

Jochen Probst CureVac GmbH, Tübingen, Germany

Elisabeth Rösler Department of Molecular Biology, Division of Allergy and Immunology, University of Salzburg, Salzburg, Austria

Charani Ranasinghe Department of Emerging Pathogens and Vaccines, Molecular Mucosal Vaccine Immunology Group, The John Curtin School of Medical Research, The Australian National University, Canberra, ACT, Australia

Jens Reinhardt Paul-Ehrlich Institut, Langen, Germany

James Robertson NIBSC, Blanche Lane, South Mimms, Potters Bar, Herts, UK

Sandra Scheiblhofer Department of Molecular Biology, Division of Allergy and Immunology, University of Salzburg, Salzburg, Austria

Thomas Schlake CureVac GmbH, Tübingen, Germany

Hermann Schuchnigg Boehringer Ingelheim RCV GmbH & Co KG, Vienna, Austria

Gabriela Senti Clinical Trials Center, Center for Clinical Research, University and University Hospital of Zurich, Zurich, Switzerland

Xuefei Shen Inovio Pharmaceuticals Inc., San Diego CA, USA

ViggoVanTendeloo Faculty of Medicine Vaccine & Infectious Disease Institute (Vaxinfectio), University of Antwerp, & Center for Cellular Therapy and Regenerative Medicine, Antwerp University Hospital, Antwerp, Belgium

Josef Thalhamer Department of Molecular Biology, Division of Allergy and Immunology, University of Salzburg, Salzburg, Austria

Andreas Thess CureVac GmbH, Tübingen, Germany

Jochen Urthaler Boehringer Ingelheim RCV GmbH & Co KG, Vienna, Austria

Contributors

Bin Wang Key Lab for Medical Molecular Virology of MOE & MOH, Fudan University Shanghai Medical College, Shanghai, China

David B. Weiner Department of Pathology and Laboratory Medicine, University of Pennsylvania, Philadelphia, PA, USA

Richard Weiss Department of Molecular Biology, Division of Allergy and Immunology, University of Salzburg, Salzburg, Austria

Danushka K. Wijesundara Department of Emerging Pathogens and Vaccines, Molecular Mucosal Vaccine Immunology Group, The John Curtin School of Medical Research, The Australian National University, Canberra, ACT, Australia

T.-C. Wu Departments of Pathology, Obstetrics and Gynecology, Molecular Microbiology and Immunology, and Oncology, The Johns Hopkins University School of Medicine, Baltimore, MD, USA

Yijie Xu Department of Pathology, The Johns Hopkins Medical Institutions, Baltimore, MD, USA

General Mechanisms of Gene Vaccines

1

Richard Weiss, Viggo Van Tendeloo,
Sandra Scheiblhofer, and Josef Thalhamer

Gene vaccines have emerged as attractive alternative to conventional vaccines as they have the potential to activate both branches of the immune system, similar to live attenuated vaccines, but at a higher safety profile and with superior efficacy in production and costs. After impressive performance in small animal models, gene vaccines were quickly transferred into the clinics without detailed knowledge of the underlying molecular and immunological mechanisms. As a result, these early clinical trials led to disappointing results, nearly terminating the "DNA vaccine revolution." Today, we know a lot more about vector design, uptake and processing of gene vaccines, immunostimulatory properties of DNA and RNA, and about numerous ways to modulate immune responses. Utilizing this knowledge has led to a new generation of improved vaccines and delivery modalities, and progress in the clinics is emerging. This introductory chapter will give a broad overview on the current status of gene vaccine design, their delivery and fate after introduction into the body, their immunostimulatory capacities, and finally, the processing and presentation of vaccine-encoded antigen to the immune system.

Introduction

Gene vaccines, consisting of either DNA or RNA, represent a fairly new field in vaccine research. A considerable number of publications demonstrated their broad range of application, including vaccines against viruses (Beckett et al. 2011; Asmuth et al. 2010; Mancini-Bourgine et al. 2006; Martin et al. 2007; Jones et al. 2009;

J. Thalhamer (✉)
Department of Molecular Biology, Division of Allergy and Immunology,
University of Salzburg, Salzburg, Austria
e-mail: Josef.Thalhamer@sbg.ac.at

J. Thalhamer et al. (eds.), *Gene Vaccines*,
DOI 10.1007/978-3-7091-0439-2_1, © Springer-Verlag/Wien, 2012

Cattamanchi et al. 2008; Lin et al. 2010), bacteria (Okada and Kita 2010; Yamanaka et al. 2010; Martin et al. 2001; Li et al. 2006), and parasites (Wang et al. 2005b; Ramos et al. 2009; Gupta and Garg 2010). Furthermore, gene vaccines opened up new perspectives for the treatment of cancer (van den Berg et al. 2010; Stevenson et al. 2010; Signori et al. 2010) and also allergic diseases (Weiss et al. 2010, 2006).

This chapter summarizes the basic properties of gene-based vaccines and the underlying immunological principles.

General Properties of Naked DNA Vaccines

Basically, DNA vaccines consist of circular plasmid DNA containing a eukaryotic promoter (e.g. the CMV promoter), which ensures the expression of the encoded antigen. A polyadenylation site downstream and/or an intron upstream of the antigen sequence serve to increase the stability of the transcribed mRNA, and thus the amount of protein expressed. Additional elements such as a bacterial origin of replication and an antibiotic resistance gene are integrated for plasmid propagation in bacteria. This first generation of DNA vaccines induced powerful immune responses in rodent models, but did not come up to expectations in primates and humans. A deeper understanding of the mechanisms underlying the immunogenicity of DNA vaccines, and novel technologies optimizing the vector and improving the gene design as well as novel adjuvants and delivery methods, have led to the development of next-generation gene-based vaccines.

Vector Design

Vector design of DNA vaccines basically has to address two important aspects, i.e. the avoidance of prokaryotic elements such as antibiotic resistance genes, as recommended by regulatory agencies (for details see Chap. 14 in this book), and the requirement of strong immunogenicity, which primarily correlates with antigen expression (Manoj et al. 2004).

Removal of Prokaryotic Vector Elements

Antibiotic resistance genes have commonly been used as selectable markers for propagation of plasmid DNA in bacteria. However, several concerns associated with the use of these markers, such as dissemination of resistances to enteric bacteria and suppression of gene expression have initiated the development of alternative selection methods, e.g. by using the natural RNA I from the plasmid replication origin to silence a host-encoded repressor gene. This approach is discussed in Chap. 16 of this book. A drawback of this selection system is the still remaining prokaryotic origin of replication, which was overcome by a strategy employing so-called DNA minicircles. By using site specific recombination (see Chap. 15 of this book), these constructs are completely devoid of prokaryotic elements. A third approach utilizes linear double-stranded DNA, end-protected by hairpin oligodeoxynucleotides

1 General Mechanisms of Gene Vaccines

(known as MIDGE – minimalistic immunogenic defined gene expression vector), which can be additionally coupled to ligands such as a nuclear localization signal peptide (Zheng et al. 2006).

Besides enhancing the safety profile, removal of prokaryotic vector elements is considered to increase bioavailability, as well as cellular uptake and nuclear entry due to reduced plasmid size (Molnar et al. 2004).

Transcriptional Elements

In order to ensure high gene expression in vivo, DNA vaccines utilize strong and ubiquitous viral promoters, of which the CMV immediate early enhancer-promoter is most prominent. Concerning the expression levels, this promoter is superior to other viral promoters such as SV40 or RSV (Lee et al. 1997) or cellular promoters, including the strong human ubiquitin C promoter (Garapin et al. 2001). However, its expression capacity can be further improved by using modified or hybrid promoters (Xu et al. 2001; Li et al. 2001) or the incorporation of introns downstream of the promoter sequence, which enhance the rate of polyadenlyation and facilitate nuclear export of the transcribed mRNA (Huang and Gorman 1990).

Stability of the transcribed mRNA and efficient translation is not only important for DNA-based vaccines, but also critical for the efficacy of mRNA vaccines. Incorporation of 5′ and 3′ untranslated regions, which form complex interactions with RNA-binding proteins, can strongly influence the stability and translation efficacy of mRNA (Grillo et al. 2010; Holtkamp et al. 2006). Furthermore, utilization of a Kozaks consensus sequence (Kozak 1997), avoidance of secondary structures at the 5′ end of the mRNA (Zhang et al. 2006), removal of inhibitory cryptic sequences (Zhou et al. 2002), and a poly(A) tail of at least 30 residues are essential for efficient translation. In DNA vaccines, poly(A) tails are generated by incorporation of terminator/polyadenylation signals such as the SV40, bovine growth hormone, or rabbit β-globin poly(A) signal (Xu et al. 2001).

Antigen Design

The general mechanisms described above are responsible for stabilizing mRNA, ensure optimal antigen expression, and thus are an important first step to an effective immune response. Further optimization of the encoded antigen itself can enhance its expression and modulate the induced immune response by guiding its translation to specialized cellular compartments.

Codon Optimization

Besides the stability of the antigen-encoding mRNA, the codon usage of the gene of interest has gained much attention (Gustafsson et al. 2004). The pattern of codon usage differs between genes and organisms and has been correlated with gene expression levels, tissue-specific patterns of expression, the degree of evolutionary conservation of proteins, and the overall or regional nucleotide composition of the genome. Because the codon usage of taxonomically-remote organisms (such as plants) is usually suboptimal with regards to the codon usage of mammalian cells, these genes are frequently poorly expressed in the mammalian host (also see Chap. 12). The first attempts to overcome this problem used algorithms which simply exchanged each codon for the codon most frequently used in eukaryotes. Novel codon adaption utilizes complex algorithms including factors such as tRNA depletion, CpG content, RNA structure, and inhibitory motifs. In general, codon optimization can lead to an increase in protein expression of about 10–100-fold. Surprisingly, recent empirical data provide evidence that favorable codons are predominantly those read by tRNAs that are most highly charged during amino acid starvation, but not codons that are most abundant in highly expressed *E. coli* proteins (Welch et al. 2009). It was also shown that stability of mRNA folding near the ribosomal binding site is responsible for high expression, rather than the codon bias (Kudla et al. 2009). These findings question the validity of frequently used algorithms, and it remains to be determined whether foreign gene expression in mammalian cells follows the rules found for *E. coli*.

Guided Translation

The specific features of genetic immunization opened the possibility to direct translation of the gene products and to target different cellular compartments by adding, removing or combining specific signal sequences, thus determining the fate of translated antigen.

1. Secretion: Addition of an ER-targeting signal peptide to the coding sequence results in secretion of the antigen, usually correlating with higher levels of humoral immune responses, and a bias towards TH2 type immune responses (Haddad et al. 1998; Weiss et al. 1999).
2. Proteasomal degradation: By attachment of ubiquitin to the encoded antigen (Rodriguez et al. 1998) or the use of a PEST signal sequence (Starodubova et al. 2008), the translated protein undergoes proteasomal degradation into peptides, which subsequently are presented on MHC class I. A considerable amount of proteasome-derived peptides is also presented on MHC class II, probably by autophagy-mediated mechanisms (Schmid et al. 2007). These strategies are usually employed with the goal to enhance CTL responses (Wu and Kipps 1997), but can also be used to generate hypoallergenic DNA vaccines (see Chap. 12).
3. Targeting the endosome: Similarly, by fusion to the lysosomal membrane proteins LIMP-II, LAMP, or peptides thereof, proteins can be targeted into the endosomal pathway in order to facilitate access to MHC class II (Ji et al. 1999; Rodriguez et al. 2001). Such strategies usually favor Th1-biased immune responses.
4. Cytoplasmic expression: Deletion of the signal sequence leads to expression of the antigen into the cytoplasm of the cell and, by default, the antigen follows the MHC class I pathway via proteasomal degradation. However, it also can gain access to different cellular compartments via autophagy (Nimmerjahn et al. 2003), or give rise to antibody production due to cellular leakage or release from disintegrated cells.
5. Membrane-bound expression: Insertion of a hydrophobic membrane anchor, or a signal sequence responsible for attachment of a GPI anchor, can target antigens to cell surface expression (Boyle et al. 1997; Johansson et al. 2007; Wang et al. 2005a).

1 General Mechanisms of Gene Vaccines

Besides targeting antigen to subcellular compartments, modifications of the antigen can also be used to specifically address cell types such as dendritic cells (DCs), or to enhance antigen spread between cells. These strategies are described in more detail in Chap. 2 of this book.

Delivery Modalities

Traditionally, intramuscular (i.m.) injection is the most commonly used route for DNA based vaccination. However, the number of transfected cells after i.m. injection of gene vaccines in saline solution is relatively low and depends on plasmid size, buffer composition, and used volume. For example, buffers containing $CaCl_2$ (e.g. Ringer solution), induce higher transfection rates for DNA (unpublished data) and mRNA (Probst et al. 2007) compared to PBS, probably because Ca^{++} acts as a bridging ion between the negatively charged phosphate backbone and the negatively charged cell surface. Also the hydrostatic pressure induced by injecting large volumes of DNA solution into a small muscle (Dupuis et al. 2000), or in case of intradermal (i.d.) injection into a small blister (Gonzalez-Gonzalez et al. 2010), seems to affect transfection efficacy, and may be one of the reasons for the observed discrepancy between small animal models and studies in humans. This suboptimal transfection efficiency has fueled large efforts to develop improved delivery modalities.

In Vivo Electroporation

One method that has recently gained much attention is in vivo electroporation for the delivery of DNA vaccines, which has been shown to increase antigen expression up to 1000-fold and thereby enhance the immune reactions. Increased uptake of plasmid DNA is usually attributed to current-induced electropermeabilization of the cell membrane, and the formation of temporal hydrophobic pores (Andre and Mir 2004). However, the detailed mechanisms are still controversially discussed (Liu et al. 2006). Immunogenicity seems to be increased not only due to enhanced protein expression, but also by the physical injury associated with delivery. This injury is assumed to augment immunity by activation of immune receptors via damage associated danger signals (DAMPs) (Chiarella et al. 2008). Furthermore, in vivo electroporation fulfills the criterion of triggering the Th1 type of immunity that is usually observed with injection of naked DNA or RNA (see section "Adjuvanticity of Nucleic Acids: Immunostimulatory Properties of DNA and RNA" in this chapter), and represents a major prerequisite for many applications of gene vaccines.

In vivo electroporation has greatly spurred the field of DNA vaccines as first clinical trials indicate that this approach represents an important step towards breaking the so-called primate barrier, i.e. the lack of immunogenicity in primates and humans in contrast to small animal models. In vivo electroporation is discussed in more detail in Chaps. 7 and 8 of this book.

Gene Gun Immunization

A different physical method that results in highly efficient in vivo transfection is the biolistic delivery of DNA-coated micro particles, made of gold or other materials (e.g. tungsten). Using helium discharge pressure, particles are propelled into the upper layers of the skin. Depending on the applied pressure, either primarily keratinocytes and Langerhans cells of the epidermis, or predominantly fibroblasts, smooth muscles cells and DCs of the underlying dermal layers of the skin are transfected.

Gene gun vaccination has turned out to be an extremely efficient way of DNA or RNA vaccine delivery. In contrast to other methods, it directly delivers its cargo into the target cell, partly even into the nucleus. Therefore, low doses in the nanogram range lead to efficient in vivo transfection and induce strong immunogenicity (Pertmer et al. 1995). It is tempting to speculate, that targeting the vaccine to an organ rich in antigen presenting cells (APCs), such as the skin, and thereby directly transfecting high numbers of APCs, may account for the high efficacy of gene gun vaccination. However, it has been shown that restricting the antigen expression to keratinocytes, using a tissue specific promoter, is sufficient to induce potent immune responses (Hon et al. 2005). Furthermore, epidermal Langerhans cells are dispensable for the induction of immunogenicity by gene gun vaccination (Stoecklinger et al. 2007), but dermal langerin-positive cells are required for activation of CD8+ T cell and antibody responses (Stoecklinger et al. 2011). Together, these data imply that direct transfection of APCs, and more precisely, epidermal Langerhans cells, does not represent the main mechanism underlying gene gun-induced immune responses.

Gene gun vaccination has been demonstrated to induce both, high levels of antibody titers as well as CTLs, making it an interesting application technique for anti-viral vaccines and cancer immunotherapy. Indeed, gene gun vaccination has been used to generate cross-protecting influenza vaccines (Chen et al. 2000; Kodihalli et al. 1997), could trigger seroconversion in hepatitis B vaccine non-responders (Rottinghaus et al. 2003), and has been used to treat established melanomas (Ginsberg et al. 2010). Interestingly, gene gun immunization triggers a different immune response type compared to saline injections with or without electroporation, or other delivery modalities. Whereas these application modes induce a Th1-biased response with IFN-γ-producing CD4+ and CD8+ T cells and a corresponding "Th-1 type" of the antibody response, as indicated by the production of IgG2a antibodies (in mice), gene gun immunization in general does not induce IgG2a antibodies, but only IgG1. It even leads to high levels of IgE, and T cells of spleen and lymph nodes express the typical pattern of Th2 type cytokines, i.e. IL-4, 5, 10, and 13 (Alvarez et al. 2005). Obviously, the mechanisms of this Th2-polarization correlate with the bombardment itself. A gene gun shot using naked gold bullets alone was sufficient to induce a Th2-stimulating skin milieu that even counteracted the Th1 bias of i.d. injected plasmid DNA, applied at the same site (Weiss et al. 2002). A possible explanation for these observations is, that superficial skin damage and disruption of the skin barrier function can polarize immune responses towards the Th2 type, as has been demonstrated by epicutaneous antigen application after removal of the stratum corneum by tape stripping (Strid et al. 2004). Similarly, introducing Leishmania antigen into the epidermis of naturally resistant C57BL/6 mice modulated the immune response towards a Th2 type, resulting in loss of protection from infection (Weiss et al. 2007). In an evolutionary context it seems "reasonable and useful" to induce rather immune-dampening (Th2/Treg) than inflammatory (Th1/Th17) signals at superficial skin sites. This helps to protect skin and hair derivatives such as horns and hooves (Paus et al. 2005), which are in constant contact to environmental antigens, from damage by inflammatory immune responses. Only when pathogens overcome the barrier of the basal lamina and gain access to the blood system and lymph, a full inflammatory response is necessary and appropriate.

In addition to these poorly understood mechanisms underlying the particle bombardment effects on immunity, gene gun immunization represents a true immunological paradox. Induction of a Th2 type immune response, including its typical cytokine expression patterns and the production of the serological Th2 counterpart IgG1, is only one side of the coin. There is also strong evidence for gene gun immunization as a superior method to induce CD8+ IFN-γ-producing cytotoxic T cells (Yoshida et al. 2000; Cho et al. 2001; Lindinger et al. 2003). These data indicate that gene gun immunization can induce two types of immune responses, which as a rule are mutually exclusive, against one antigen, in one organism at the same time. It seems obvious, that these adversatively polarized processes must be tightly controlled and kept separate, probably by compartmentalization within the lymphatic tissues, in order to avoid interference.

Investigations of the underlying mechanisms will not only help to elucidate the gene gun paradox, but contribute to the understanding how to run several immune response types in parallel, which may be an everyday challenge for the immune system.

Biojector 2000™

Another immunization device that is sometimes mistaken for the gene gun is the Biojector 2000™. In contrast to gene gun, this device uses a needle-free jet injection stream. The strength and distribution of the stream can be modulated thus targeting the skin, the subjacent muscle or a mixture of both. Although the Biojector induced superior immune responses compared to i.m. injection in animal models (Aguiar et al. 2001), this benefit could not be confirmed in models of non-human primates (Rao et al. 2006), or in healthy human volunteers (Epstein et al. 2002). Nevertheless, as needle-free vaccination systems are of great importance, especially with respect to mass vaccinations in developing countries, the Biojector 2000™ is extensively used in a large number of finished and still ongoing clinical trials focused on HIV, influenza and dengue fever.

Other Delivery Methods

Various different delivery modalities for DNA vaccines have been investigated over the past years, including the vast field of using specific formulations for vaccine delivery (described in Chap. 2) but also exotic ones such as sonoporation with ultrasound, or the use of lasers, which are in part described in the next chapter of this book.

Recently, delivery of vaccines via the skin has attracted attention and propelled intense research. Vaccination via skin is considered a potent modality not only due to the richness of APCs in this tissue, but it could also help to increase patient compliance, which is a major obstacle of needle vaccination. In Chap. 6 one of the most advanced DNA vaccines administered via skin patches, the so-called Dermavir approach will be discussed.

Other approaches targeting the skin for gene vaccination include various types of microneedles (Gill and Prausnitz 2007; Lee et al. 2008), and even tattooing devices have been investigated for their potential to deliver DNA vaccines (van den Berg et al. 2009).

Mechanisms of In Vivo Uptake of Naked Gene Vaccines

In vivo expression of naked gene vaccines requires their uptake by cells followed by the transport into the cytoplasm and, in the case of DNA vaccines, the intracellular transfer into the nucleus for transcription. Uptake, intracellular trafficking, and pharmacokinetics of plasmid DNA have largely been investigated for nucleic acids complexed with cationic lipids or polymers into nano- or microparticles of various sizes and characteristics. These strategies are discussed in detail in Chaps. 2, 5, and 6 of this book. In contrast, for naked DNA and mRNA, the individual steps of this process are only poorly understood. After injection, gene vaccines are quickly degraded by mucosal, skin derived, or plasma nucleases (Nishikawa et al. 2005; Barry et al. 1999; Probst et al. 2006) and only a minute amount of the initially applied nucleic acids is taken up by cells present at the injection site. These cells include immunocompetent macrophages and DCs, and also somatic bystander cells such as fibroblasts and keratinocytes in the skin (i.d., epidermal application) or myocytes (i.m. application) (Fig. 1.1).

Several mechanisms for cellular uptake of macromolecules have been described including phagocytosis and pinocytosis. While phagocytic activity is mainly restricted to granulocytes, macrophages and DCs, different forms of pinocytosis are employed by essentially all mammalian cell types and have been associated with the uptake of nucleic acids: clathrin-mediated endocytosis by macrophages and DCs (Trombone et al. 2007; Latz et al. 2004) as well as caveolin-mediated endocytosis in muscle cells (Wolff et al. 1992a; Budker et al. 2000) have been demonstrated, while macropinocytosis seems to be the main mechanism for the uptake of DNA by keratinocytes (Basner-Tschakarjan et al. 2004). In contrast, inhibitors blocking macropinocytosis, clathrin-coated pits, or caveolae showed no effect on the uptake

1 General Mechanisms of Gene Vaccines

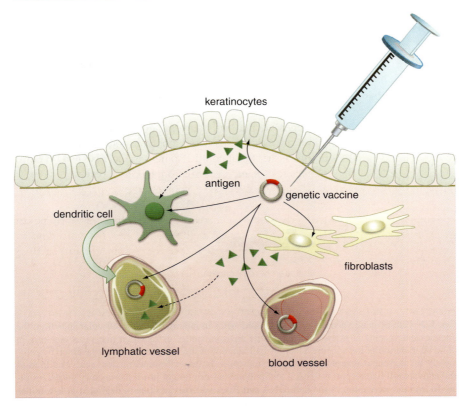

Fig. 1.1 Naked gene vaccines in saline solution can be applied by direct injection into the skin. After injection, in situ transfection of somatic cells such as keratinocytes or fibroblasts takes place, which serve as factories of antigen production. Soluble antigen can then be taken up by antigen presenting cells or directly reach lymphatic vessels. In parallel, antigen presenting cells may be directly transfected and activated by the immunostimulatory properties of nucleic acid, and travel to draining lymph nodes via lymphatic vessels. Gene vaccines predominantly transfect cells at the site of injection, however, small amounts of the vaccine enter the lymph and blood system and are distributed over the whole body

of extracellular mRNA (Probst et al. 2007). Additionally, receptor mediated uptake of nucleic acids could be demonstrated for different receptors. For instance, in mammals intravenously injected DNA is rapidly cleared from circulation and degraded by sinusoidal liver cells via a scavenger receptor mediated mechanism (Hisazumi et al. 2004; Kawabata et al. 1995). In contrast, in cod fish, scavenger receptor mediated clearance is mainly accomplished by heart endothelial cells rather than liver cells, and DNA is rapidly degraded without detectable expression (Seternes et al. 2007). Polyanion-specific scavenger receptors are also involved in the uptake of plasmid DNA by murine and human macrophages (Takagi et al. 1998; Yamane et al. 2005) and DCs (Yoshinaga et al. 2002) as well as in the uptake of mRNA

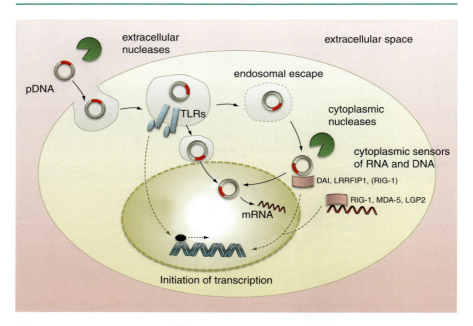

Fig. 1.2 Fate of gene vaccines after injection. After intradermal or intramuscular injection, the nucleic acid vaccine is exposed to the hostile environment of extracelluar nucleases resulting in rapid degradation of the vaccine. Only a small amount of the injected vaccine is taken up by cells, mostly by scavenger receptor mediated endocytosis. In the endosome, nucleic acids can bind to and activate toll like receptors (TLRs) and initiate transcription of pro-inflammatory genes, resulting in immune activation of the cell. DNA and RNA vaccines are finally degraded in lysosomes and only a small fraction of the molecules escape from the endosome into the cytoplasm where they can activate cytoplasmic sensors of nucleic acids that in turn stimulate induction of inflammation. The persistence of gene vaccines in the cytoplasm is low, due to degradation by cytoplasmic nucleases. Finally, DNA vaccines (but not mRNA vaccines) have to overcome the nuclear membrane to be transcribed into mRNA. Alternatively, plasmid DNA vaccines may directly travel in vesicles from endosomes to the nucleus, while being protected from cellular nucleases

(Probst et al. 2007) and dsRNA. The latter is dependent on the length of the RNA and much faster, compared to DNA of the same length (Saleh et al. 2006). In general, it seems most likely that uptake of nucleic acids includes several receptors simultaneously, and may also be sequence-specific (Lehmann and Sczakiel 2005; Wheeler et al. 2006).

Pharmacokinetics and Nuclear Import of Plasmid DNA

Endocytosis and subsequent transport to lysosomes usually leads to total degradation of nucleic acids. However, a small proportion of the gene vaccine escapes from endocytic compartments by still unknown mechanisms (Fig. 1.2). While RNA based vaccines can be translated into their respective gene product within the cytoplasm of the cell, DNA vaccines have to traverse the nuclear membrane to enter the nucleus, where they can be transcribed into mRNA. In replicating cells, nuclear entry is achieved in the course of reorganization of the nuclear membrane during mitosis (Dean et al. 2005), however, active transport across nuclear pores has to take place in non-dividing cells. Early studies indicated that DNA itself can pass through the nuclear pore complex in a semi-active manner, which can be prevented by the nuclear transport inhibitor wheat germ agglutinin (Salman et al. 2001). Furthermore, the import into the nucleus emerged to be sequence dependent (Dean 1997). Recently, a range of cytoplasmic shuttle proteins (importins) have been identified that bind exogenous plasmid DNA in a sequence specific manner, and then translocate it to the nucleus using the minimal import machinery (Munkonge et al. 2009). The half-life of DNA in the cytoplasm of the cell amounts to approximately 90 min. Exposure to cytosolic nuclease activity and a markedly decreased diffusion capacity may explain why the amount of intact plasmid in the nucleus is 1000-fold less when DNA is microinjected into the cytoplasm compared to direct microinjection into the nucleus (Lukacs et al. 2000; Lechardeur et al. 1999).

A recent study suggests that the majority of naked plasmid DNA is not released into the cytoplasm but travels in vesicles from early endosomes to the nucleus, protected from cytoplasmic nucleases. Plasmid DNA displayed inhibition of lysosome acidification, thereby preventing its own degradation by lysosomal nucleases (Trombone et al. 2007). Such mechanisms could explain the unexpectedly high in vivo transfection capacity of naked gene vaccines.

Adjuvanticity of Nucleic Acids: Immunostimulatory Properties of DNA and RNA

It is now well accepted that microbial genomes contain specific DNA or RNA signatures that can be recognized by mammalian cells through their expression of specific pattern-recognition receptors (PRRs) able to discriminate foreign from self nucleic acids and to engage a set of innate immune responses upon recognition of microbial DNA and/or RNA. This PRR system constitutes a family of evolutionarily highly conserved receptors in mammals and is designed to detect highly conserved structural motifs called pathogen-associated molecular patterns (PAMPs) derived from microbial pathogens (Brennan and Bowie 2010; Kawai and Akira 2010; Palm and Medzhitov 2009). Examples of such PAMPs include various bacterial cell wall components such as lipopolysaccharide (LPS), peptidoglycan (PGN) and lipopeptides, as well as flagellin, but also bacterial and viral nucleic acids.

For sensing non-self nucleic acids during natural microbial infection or upon genetic vaccination, several PRRs exist in mammalian cells which can be discriminated either by their differential recognition of nucleic acid ligands (DNA or RNA moieties) or by their different subcellular localization (cytosolic or endosomal compartment) (Ranjan et al. 2009).

Toll-like Receptors (TLRs): Endosomal Sensors of RNA and DNA

In Drosophila melanogaster, the Toll receptor controls anti-bacterial and anti-fungal responses and induces strong and rapid expression of genes, such as the nuclear factor-κB family of transcription factors (Medzhitov et al. 1997). In humans, the Toll-like receptor (TLR) family consists of ten conserved membrane-spanning molecules each containing an ectodomain of leucine-rich repeats, a transmembrane domain and a cytoplasmic domain known as the TIR (Toll/IL-1 receptor) domain (Kawai and Akira 2010). TLRs play a pivotal role in the early innate immune response to invading pathogens by sensing microorganisms. TLR activation by their cognate agonists leads to the recruitment of cellular adaptor molecules including myeloid differentiation primary-response gene 88 (MyD88), TIR-domain-containing adaptor protein (TIRAP), TIRAP-inducing IFN (TRIF) and TRIF-related adaptor molecule (TRAM), which directly bind to TLRs in various combinations. These signaling cascades lead to the activation of transcription factors, such as AP-1, NF-κB, and IFN-regulatory factors (IRFs), and initiate the transcription of genes encoding pro-inflammatory cytokines, chemokines and co-stimulatory molecules that direct the adaptive immune response (Hoshino and Kaisho 2008). While membrane-bound TLRs are able to immediately sense extracellular microbial pathogens through recognition of LPS (TLR4 ligand), bacterial flagellin (TLR5 ligand), and lipoprotein and peptidoglycan (by TLR2 complexed with TLR1 or TLR6), TLRs involved in the detection of intracellular nucleic acids, i.e. TLR3, TLR7, TLR8 and TLR9, are located in the endosomal compartment (Hoshino and Kaisho 2008; Kawai and Akira 2010).

TLR9 can recognize DNA molecules containing unmethylated CpG-containing motifs commonly found in the genomes of bacteria and viruses, as well as in plasmid DNA (Hemmi et al. 2000). TLR9 is expressed by numerous cells of the immune system such as DCs, B lymphocytes and natural killer (NK) cells and functions to alarm the immune system of viral and bacterial infections by binding to DNA rich in CpG motifs (Krieg 2006). CpG sequences are relatively (~1%) scarce in mammalian genomes as compared to bacterial or viral genomes. The adjuvanticity of CpG motifs has already been translated into immunotherapeutic applications by designing synthetic oligonucleotides (ODNs) containing CpG motifs that can interact directly with the ectodomain of TLR9 and induce conformational changes that lead to downstream immune signalling activation (Latz et al. 2007). Depending on the primary structure of the ODN, different types of immune activation can be detected, including induction of B-cell proliferation and immunoglobulin production, as well as secretion of pro-inflammatory cytokines (type I IFN, IL-12, TNF, IL-6) (Krieg 2006).

Following the discovery by Akira and colleagues that bacterial DNA showed immunostimulatory effects through TLR9 (Hemmi et al. 2000), two closely related endosomal TLRs namely TLR7 and TLR8, sharing a high sequence homology, were revealed (Heil et al. 2004). In contrast to TLR9 which detects DNA sequences, TLR7 and TLR8 respond to guanosine- or uridine-rich single-stranded RNA (ssRNA) from viruses but also to synthetic imidazoquinoline compounds imiquimod and

1 General Mechanisms of Gene Vaccines

R-848, as well as to guanosine analogues. Recently, TLR7/8 have been ascribed a key role for sensing 21-bp small interfering RNA (siRNA) but the effect depends on the variation in siRNA sequences and presence of secondary structures (Heil et al. 2004; Diebold et al. 2004).

Despite their difference in nucleic acid detection, TLR7, TLR8 and TLR9 share a similar signalling cascade pathway. After ligand engagement, they interact solely with the MyD88 adaptor molecule, that functions to recruit IL-1-receptor-associated kinases (IRAKs), leading to activation of NF-κB and IRFs (Sasai et al. 2010).

Another endosomally located TLR, known as TLR3, recognizes viral double-stranded RNA (dsRNA) signatures – present as replication intermediates during the replication cycle of RNA viruses – and its synthetic mimic products such as polyinosinic-polycytidylic acid (polyI:C) (Alexopoulou et al. 2001). TLR3 has also been shown to be involved in the detection of hairpin dsRNA structures sometimes present in viral RNAs, in siRNA duplexes or in long in vitro transcribed mRNAs (Kariko et al. 2005). However, unlike the other endosomal TLRs, TLR3 seems to transduce its signals predominantly through a MyD88-independent pathway, as stimulation with polyI:C in MyD88-deficient cells does not affect the production of pro-inflammatory cytokines and co-stimulatory molecules. Indeed, TLR3 was shown to associate with TRIF and signals through IRF3, a key factor involved in type I IFN production (Yamamoto et al. 2002).

RIG-I-like Receptors (RLRs): Cytosolic Sensors of RNA

Because the ligand-binding domains of TLR3, TLR7 and TLR8 are topologically endosomal, pathogens that manage to infiltrate into the cytosol will evade detection by TLRs. The finding that nearly all nucleated cells can produce IFNα/β after viral infection or in response to dsRNA in the cytosol, even in the absence of endosomal TLRs and their adaptors, pointed to the existence of an TLR-independent PRR system that detects nucleic acids in the cytosol. Indeed, three genes have been identified in humans and mice that encode a group of proteins known as the RIG-I-like receptors (RLRs) or RIG-I-like helicases (RLHs) including retinoic-acid-inducible gene I (RIG-I), melanoma differentiation-associated antigen 5 (MDA5) and laboratory of genetics and physiology 2 (LGP2). They constitute a family of cytoplasmic RNA helicases that are critical for host antiviral innate immune responses (Yoneyama and Fujita 2008; Rehwinkel and Reis e Sousa 2010; Nakhaei et al. 2009; Barral et al. 2009).

At first, it was believed that both RIG-I (retinoic-acid-inducible protein 1, also known as DDX58) and MDA-5 (melanoma-differentiation-associated gene 5, also known as IFIH1 or Helicard) were dsRNA sensors, leading to production of type I interferons (IFNs) in infected cells. Later, in a set of elegant experiments, it was demonstrated that RIG-I, next to dsRNA, also recognizes uncapped 5′-triphosphate RNA present in viral genomes or replication intermediates, the latter ligand being responsible to activate the translocase activity of RIG-I (Hornung et al. 2006). Notably, mammalian RNA is either capped or contains base modifications suggesting a mechanism whereby RIG-I is able to discriminate between self and non-self RNA.

Despite the overall structural similarity between these two RNA sensors, they detect distinct viral species. RIG-I enables the recognition of Paramyxoviruses (Newcastle disease virus (NDV), Sendai virus), Rhabdoviruses (vesicular stomatitis virus), Flaviviruses (hepatitis C) and Orthomyxoviruses (Influenza), whereas MDA-5 plays a key role in the recognition of Picornaviruses (encephalo-myocarditis virus) and poly(I:C), a synthetic mimic of viral dsRNA (Loo et al. 2008). In addition, in a set of experiments where poly(I:C) was treated with RNase III, it was shown that RIG-I binds preferentially to short dsRNA while MDA-5 recognizes preferentially long dsRNA (Kato et al. 2008).

Although RIG-I and MDA-5 recognize different ligands, they share common signalling features. Upon recognition of dsRNA, they are recruited by the adaptor IPS-1 (also known as MAVS, CARDIF or VISA) to the outer membrane of the mitochondria leading to the activation of several transcription factors including IRF3, IRF7 and NF-κB. IRF3 and IRF7 control the expression of type I IFNs, while NF-κB regulates the production of inflammatory cytokines. IRF3 and IRF7 activation involves TNF (tumor necrosis factor) receptor-associated factor 3 (TRAF3), NAK-associated protein 1 (NAP1), TANK and the protein kinase TANK-binding kinase 1 (TBK1) or IκB kinase epsilon (IKKε) (Yoneyama and Fujita 2009).

A third RLR has recently been described: laboratory of genetics and physiology 2 (LGP2) is believed to act as a negative feedback regulator of RIG-I and MDA-5 through sequestration of dsRNA or binding directly to RIG-I through a repressor domain (Satoh et al. 2010). Many other molecules such as A20, ring-finger protein 125 (RNF125), suppressor of IKKε (SIKE), and peptidyl-propyl isomerase 1 (Pin1) seem to be involved in the negative control of RIG-I/MDA-5-induced IFN production (Komuro et al. 2008). Furthermore, some viral proteases such as NS3/NS4A of the hepatitis C virus can inactivate RIG-I/MDA-5 signaling by targeting IPS-1 as a means to evade innate immunity (Johnson et al. 2007).

Finally, other RNA-sensing cytosolic receptors not belonging to the TLR or RLR family can be found in mammalian cells, especially in response to autocrine or paracrine type I IFN production. For example, RNAs with short stem-loops can activate IFN-inducible dsRNA-dependent protein kinase R (PKR) in a 5′-triphosphate-dependent manner, independent of RIG-I. In addition, activation of the ribonuclease L by 2′,5′-linked oligoadenylate leads to the production of small RNA cleavage products from self RNA, which then function to amplify antiviral IFN responses and to induce apoptosis (Schlee et al. 2007) (see also Chap. 3).

Cytosolic Sensors of DNA

While the recognition of extra-cellular DNA involves mainly Toll-like receptor 9, recognition of cytosolic DNA appears to involve several sensors. The first identified cytosolic DNA sensor, named DNA-dependent activator of IFN-regulatory factors (DAI), binds cytosolic dsDNA (Takaoka et al. 2007). DAI signalling occurs through

1 General Mechanisms of Gene Vaccines

TBK1 and IRF3 to activate NF-κB and leads to the production of type I IFNs. However, DAI deficiency does not affect the induction of type I IFNs in response to poly(dA:dT), a synthetic analog of B-DNA, suggesting that redundant cytosolic DNA sensors exist (Takeshita and Ishii 2008).

RIG-I, known as an RNA-binding and not DNA-binding protein, was also postulated as a second candidate DNA sensor based on the observation that a human cell line deficient for RIG-I had lost the ability to recognize poly(dA:dT) (Cheng et al. 2007). Two independent teams confirmed the involvement of RIG-I in the response to dsDNA but demonstrated that rather than the cytosolic DNA, a double-stranded RNA intermediate containing a 5′-triphosphate moiety was responsible for RIG-I activation. They found that transfected poly(dA:dT) is transcribed by RNA polymerase III giving rise to dsRNA intermediates (Chiu et al. 2009; Ablasser et al. 2009). Both DAI and RIG-I induce the production of type I IFNs through the TBK1/IRF3 pathway.

Recently, another cytosolic dsDNA sensor has been identified. This sensor, termed LRRFIP1, can recognize AT-rich B-form dsDNA as well as GC-rich Z-form dsDNA. With the use of LRRFIP1-specific siRNA, Yang et al. demonstrated that LRRFIP1 triggers the production of IFN-β in a β-catenin-dependent manner. β-Catenin binds to the C-terminal domain of IRF3 inducing an increase in IFN-β expression (Yang et al. 2010). Furthermore, the so-called absent in melanoma 2 (AIM2), a member of the hematopoietic interferon-inducible nuclear protein HIN-200 family, was identified as a cytosolic dsDNA sensor that upon activation promotes the assembly of an inflammasome (Fernandes-Alnemri et al. 2009). DNA of various origins, such as poly(dA:dT), plasmid DNA and DNA from the bacterium *L. monocytogenes* have been shown to activate AIM2. Upon activation, AIM2 interacts with ASC, a common adapter of the inflammasomes, leading to the cleavage of caspase-1 and the secretion of IL-1β and IL-18 (Hornung et al. 2009). Even though several studies clearly indicate that AIM2 is a potential sensor of cytosolic DNA, the precise role of AIM2 in innate responses against DNA viruses has yet to be explored.

Impact on Immunogenicity of DNA and RNA Vaccines

Gene-based vaccines capitalize on the fact that in vivo introduction of antigen-encoding DNA or RNA, whether or not encapsulated in liposomes or cloned into recombinant viral vectors, are able to elicit an effective and protective antigen-specific immune response against infectious pathogens, tumors or, conversely, to induce tolerance towards auto-immune or allergic reactions, or organ rejection (Ferrera et al. 2007). While the former strategy favors the adjuvanticity of nucleic acids to render the gene-based vaccine more immunogenic, the latter approach (also known as "negative" vaccination (Hill and Cuturi 2010)) will have to circumvent or abolish these undesirable innate immunostimulatory properties. Indeed, nowadays, plasmid DNA vectors can be modified to augment their unmethylated CpG content for enhanced immunogenicity or be engineered to have a minimal amount of CpG motifs to avoid TLR9-mediated innate immune reactions (Klinman et al. 2000; Jiang et al. 2006). To date, also mRNA-based vaccines are being designed with an enhanced self-adjuvanting activity through complexing with protamine or incorporation of synthetic oligoribonucleotides (ORNs) with a phosphorothioate backbone (Pascolo 2008) (see also Chap. 11). It was postulated that these modifications could be sensed by DCs as a strong danger signal depending on MyD88 signalling likely through TLR7/8 (Scheel et al. 2005), although involvement of other TLRs such as TLR3 cannot be excluded, as suggested in an earlier report (Kariko et al. 2004). However, with respect to naked DNA and RNA vaccines, TLR recognition does not seem to play a dominant role with respect to immunogenicity. Two independent groups demonstrated that CpG-DNA/TLR9 interactions were not essential for the induction of immune responses in long-term DNA vaccination protocols by using MyD88−/− and/or TLR−/− deficient mice (Spies et al. 2003; Babiuk et al. 2004). Furthermore, cytotoxic T cell responses to a self-replicating DNA vaccine were found not to be diminished in the absence of TLR3 (Diebold et al. 2009). We could also show that naked mRNA vaccines largely maintain their immunogenicity in MyD88 knockout mice (Roesler et al. 2009). Together, these data underscore the existence of redundant pathways and that other (cytosolic) sensors of DNA/RNA may be of greater importance for in vivo immunogenicity.

Altogether, it will be of utmost importance to understand the interactions of gene-based vaccines with the farrago of PRR systems linked to the innate immune system present in virtually all cells. First, the outcome and magnitude of the innate defense reactions against the transfected/transduced nucleic acids will be cell-type dependent given the fact that each cell type exhibits a unique array of cytosolic and endosomal nucleic acid sensors. For instance, recognition of dsRNA by RIG-I/MDA-5 or TLR3 was shown to be cell-type dependent. Studies of RIG-I- and MDA-5-deficient mice have revealed that conventional myeloid dendritic cells (cDCs), macrophages and fibroblasts isolated from these mice have impaired IFN induction after RNA virus infection, while production of IFN is still observed in plasmacytoid DCs (pDCs). Thus in cDCs, macrophages and fibroblasts, RLRs are the major sensors for viral infection, while in pDCs, TLRs play a dominant role (Kato et al. 2005). On the same note, pDCs have the unique capacity to respond to CpG motifs, e.g. in plasmid DNA, as evident from their marked amount of type I IFN production, thanks to their expression of TLR9 which is absent in monocytes and cDC (Gilliet et al. 2008).

Secondly, another determinant that will likely influence the outcome of the immune responses towards the non-self nucleic acids is the route of introduction because of the topologically different intracellular location of the various PRR systems. For example, in vivo electroporation of naked plasmid DNA or mRNA is believed to result in cytosolic localisation of the nucleic acids, whereas DNA or RNA lipoplexes can be ingested via endocytosis and will hence end up in the endosomal/lysosomal compartment (Van Tendeloo et al. 2007). Also, when professional antigen-presenting cells such as DCs are residing at the site of vaccination, they can phagocytose transfected or infected (dying) cells and process their nucleic acid content using their endosomal TLRs, whilst processing simultaneously the vaccine-encoded antigens (Smits et al. 2007).

1 General Mechanisms of Gene Vaccines

Thirdly, the signalling cascade pathways of nucleic acid receptors potently induce the production of high levels of type I IFNs and pro-inflammatory cytokines (IL-6, IL-1, TNF-α, IL-12) creating a cytokine milieu that will affect the outcome of the adaptive immune response against the encoded antigens. Moreover, in cDC and pDC, these pathways have also been shown to induce upregulation of costimulatory molecules (e.g. CD80, CD86) and the production of cytokines, resulting in DC maturation and activation, respectively (Gilliet et al. 2008; Hoshino and Kaisho 2008). In turn, these activated mature DCs will be quintessential for the correct presentation of the introduced vaccine-associated antigens to (naive) T cells for the generation of protective T cell immunity. Indeed, immunogenicity of DNA vaccines proved to be highly dependent on the activation of TBK-1 (Ishii et al. 2008) and the induction of type I interferons (Leitner et al. 2006), underscoring the importance of this pathway.

Lastly, we have only begun to understand the complexity of the different nucleic acid sensor systems and their mode of action, let alone the complexity of their interactions and potential synergy and/or negative feedback loops. Increased knowledge into their signalling pathways and subsequent immune responses will undoubtly have an impact on the design of future gene-based vaccines.

Distribution and Presentation of Antigens Encoded by Gene Vaccines

T cell responses induced upon vaccination with DNA greatly depend on the distribution of the plasmid DNA, the different types and localizations of cells presenting the encoded antigen, as well as on the amount and persistence of the gene product. Conventional, i.e. non self-replicating DNA vaccines, have been shown to produce antigen in vivo only in the nanogram range (Chastain et al. 2001), hence primary immune responses may be difficult to detect in contrast to memory responses, which seem to be favored by DNA immunization (Laylor et al. 1999). This may be explained by the fact that unlike most other vaccine types, DNA vaccines constantly produce small amounts of the encoded antigen over a prolonged period of time (Chastain et al. 2001).

Free, as well as cell-associated plasmid DNA has been found in muscle, peripheral blood, draining lymph nodes and bone marrow, minutes to months after i.m. injection (Coelho-Castelo et al. 2003; Dupuis et al. 2000; Ledwith et al. 2000; Manam et al. 2000; Manthorpe et al. 1993; Winegar et al. 1996). The fact that cell-associated plasmid DNA can be found in peripheral blood within 1 h after DNA injection and within cells of distal lymph nodes, spleen and bone marrow after 24 h, suggests that plasmid is rather carried as free DNA than transported by cells (Rush et al. 2010).

Antigen Persistence

Gene expression after delivery of plasmid DNA is characterized by a peak of expression for a few days followed by sustained low level expression. In most cases, the delivered DNA molecules will stay episomal in the nucleus, and are diluted with cell replication (Al-Dosari and Gao 2009). Transfected cells can also be killed by the transfection process itself, or undergo programmed cell death due to exposure to DNA degradation products (Nguyen et al. 2007). Furthermore, inflammatory reactions might contribute to the rapid decline of expression, either by promoting clearance of injured cells or by promoter downregulation (Yew et al. 1999). Immune responses directed against cells presenting encoded (foreign) protein may also shorten the duration of expression.

On the other hand, plasmids can persist for extended periods of time in the absence of gene expression after i.m. injection or hydrodynamic delivery of DNA into the liver (Al-Dosari et al. 2005; Wolff et al. 1992b). This loss of expression has been attributed to promoter shutdown, promoter methylation (Newell-Price et al. 2000), and lack of essential transcription factors under non-inflammatory conditions (Loser et al. 1998). Prolonged expression duration has also been reported for large sized plasmids (Hibbitt et al. 2007), linearized short DNA fragments (Chen et al. 2001), plasmids deplete of CpG sequences (Hodges et al. 2004) or minicircles (Chen et al. 2003) and for the use of tissue-specific promoters in addition to native or viral scaffold/matrix attachment region (Argyros et al. 2008).

In principle, the duration of antigen expression after gene vaccination seems to be a result of a complex balance between mechanisms resulting in degradation and those leading to plasmid survival. In most animal models, expression of the encoded antigen could be detected up to 12 months after immunization (Doh et al. 1997; Kessler et al. 1996; Wolff and Budker 2005; Wolff et al. 1992b; Zi et al. 2006).

Antigen Distribution

Somatic cells at the site of vaccine application, e.g. myocytes or keratinocytes, are assumed to be the "factories" of antigens, which are delivered to secondary lymphoid tissues, in a hitherto unknown way. Expression of antigen in somatic cells surrounding the injection site has been demonstrated to occur within 24 h after immunization (Rush et al. 2010). The role of transfected somatic cells seems to be pivotal as restricting antigen expression to somatic cells was sufficient to induce protection against influenza, but the same vaccine expressing the antigen exclusively in CD11c+ cells failed to induce protective immunity (Hon et al. 2005). Similarly, increasing transfection efficacy of muscle cells more than 100-fold by in vivo electroporation markedly enhances the immunogenicity of gene vaccines (described in detail in Chaps. 2, 7, and 8 of this book).

Nevertheless, also direct transfection of immunocompetent cells is assumed to be involved in successful induction of immunity via genetic vaccination, which has been demonstrated for haematopoietic cells, including CD11b+ cells at the site of injection (Akbari et al. 1999; Condon et al. 1996; Gronevik et al. 2003).

Furthermore, low numbers of cells in draining lymph nodes, which contained antigen as early as 48 h after injection, have been found. Due to their location within the paracortex, and their dendritic appearance, they were assumed to be DCs. However, it remains to be elucidated whether these cells had acquired the antigen

1 General Mechanisms of Gene Vaccines

from other cells or expressed the protein themselves (Rush et al. 2010). Another hint, indicating the requirement of both, directly transfected APCs as well as antigen transfer from somatic cells to APCs (Bot et al. 2000; Casares et al. 1997; Corr et al. 1999), comes from a study demonstrating that limiting antigen expression to DCs reduces the quality of CD4+ as well as CD8+ T cell responses (Lauterbach et al. 2006).

Under certain conditions, somatic cells may present endogenously produced antigen to immune cells, e.g. myocytes can upregulate expression of MHC class I, costimulatory molecules, chemokines, and adhesion molecules upon transfection with plasmid DNA (Shirota et al. 2007). Type I interferon induction, which can be induced in many types of nonimmune cells by cytoplasmic sensors of dsDNA, including myocytes, fibroblasts, hepatocytes, and pancreatic cells, plays a key role in these mechanisms (Shirota et al. 2006; Li et al. 2005). Type I interferons can convert numerous cell types into facultative APCs with the ability to present antigens and activate T cells. Such inducible cells are fibroblasts, keratinocytes and epithelial cells (Jamaluddin et al. 2001; Kundig et al. 1995; Fan et al. 2003), but also endothelial cells and vascular smooth muscle cells (Fabry et al. 1990). Thus, somatic cells have the potential to contribute to the overall immunogenicity of DNA vaccines besides their role as antigen "factories"; however, their overall contribution and the underlying detailed mechanisms remain to be determined yet.

Antigen Kinetics

A complex correlation seems to exist between the antigen expression and the time course of the immunization. Whereas sustained exposure to low amounts of antigen has been associated with the induction of high numbers of central memory cells, short-term exposure to high amounts of antigen seems to favor expansion of CD8+ effector cells rather than long-lived memory cells (Bachmann et al. 2006; Stock et al. 2004; Williams and Bevan 2004). As a result of exposure to low amounts of antigen, precursors of long-lived CD4+ memory cells undergo weak activation upon first antigen contact, but strongly respond to subsequent antigen challenge, a process which may reflect some basic features of DNA vaccination (Catron et al. 2006).

In an elegant experiment, Rush et al. shed light on the kinetics of appearance and the anatomical distribution of antigen presented on MHC class II after plasmid DNA injection versus protein immunization. Three days after both vaccination modalities similar numbers of CD11c+ DCs presented the antigen in peripheral lymph nodes. However, only after protein immunization large numbers of CD11c negative cells were found to display antigenic peptide on MHC class II. CD11c+ APCs carrying the antigen after plasmid immunization were mainly found in the subcapsular sinus of draining lymph nodes and may have migrated to the lymph nodes via afferent lymphatics or were subcapsular sinus resident macrophages (Gretz et al. 2000; Hume et al. 1983). Presentation of antigenic peptides coincided with the accumulation and blastogenesis of antigen specific T cells in peripheral

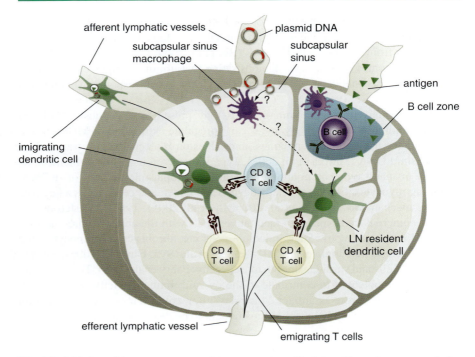

Fig. 1.3 Initiation of immune responses by gene vaccines. Nucleic acid vaccines can reach the draining lymph nodes (DLNs) via different routes. Antigen presenting cells that have been directly transfected in the periphery, or have taken up antigen translated by somatic cells, enter the DLNs via afferent lymphatic vessels and present endogenously produced antigen to CD8+ T cells, or exogenously acquired antigen to CD4+ T cells. Both pathways can also lead to alternative presentation via cross-priming (presentation of exogenous antigen on MHC I) or autophagy (presentation of endogenous antigen on MHC II). Alternatively, antigen translated in the periphery may enter the subcapsular sinus (SCS) of the lymph node and is then channeled into follicles via conduits secreted by fibroblastic reticular cells. Alternatively, particulate antigen or large immune complexes can be sampled from the SCS by SCS macrophages and transferred to B-cells as intact antigen (Gonzalez et al. 2009). Due to its high molecular weight, plasmid DNA might also be acquired by SCS macrophages which then could serve as antigen factories, present antigen to T cells, or transfer antigen and/or plasmid DNA to LN resident dendritic cells (Rush et al. 2010). Once activated, effector CD4+ and CD8+ T cells leave the LN via efferent lymphatic vessels

lymph nodes and spleen 3 days after immunization. However, also empty control vectors induced enlarged, hypercellular peripheral lymph nodes between 24 and 48 h after injection, thus indicating CpG-driven non-specific inflammation. Although simultaneous T cell accumulation was observed also in distal secondary lymphatic organs, T cell division in draining lymph nodes clearly preceded that in distal lymph nodes and spleen. This implies that although T cells are activated at sites distal to the injection site, they might receive unsufficient stimulus, antigen dose or inflammation-driven co-stimulation at this early time point to divide (Rush et al. 2010).

The early events of antigen transport and presentation in a draining lymph node following gene vaccination are depicted in Fig. 1.3.

Processing of Antigens Encoded by DNA Vaccines

The efficacy of DNA vaccines depends on their ability to stimulate both, CD4+ and CD8+ cells. Among APCs, DCs are by far the most potent inducers of these priming events; hence detailed knowledge about the processing of the gene products encoded by DNA vaccines is crucial. DCs gain access to antigen either via direct transfection with the gene vaccine or via uptake of antigen synthesized by bystander cells.

The two major antigen-processing pathways in DCs are processing of endogenous antigen for presentation on MHC class I and processing of exogenous antigen for presentation on MHC class II. These default pathways are complemented by processing of endogenous antigen for presentation by MHC class II via autophagy-related mechanisms, and processing of exogenous antigen for presentation by MHC I via processes termed as cross-presentation.

MHC Class I Presentation

Any type of DNA vaccination, regardless of whether the constructs are delivered i.m. by needle injection, i.d. following scarification of the skin, or by gene gun, leads to direct transfection of DCs, and there is evidence for the importance of CD8+ DEC-205+ DCs concerning CTL priming (Akbari et al. 1999; Bouloc et al. 1999; Porgador et al. 1998).

Generally, endogenous antigens are degraded in the cytosol by proteases and the generated peptides are transported into the endoplasmatic reticulum by the transporter associated with antigen processing (TAP), are loaded onto class I molecules, and migrate to the cell surface. Surprisingly, 50% of the translated proteins are ubiquitinated and targeted for degradation before their synthesis has been completed (Turner and Varshavsky 2000). Additionally, one third of proteins undergo degradation within 10 min of their synthesis. Thus, defective ribosomal products and those from early ubiquitination comprise a major proportion of the substrates for proteasomal degradation (Reits et al. 2000; Schubert et al. 2000). These facts are highly relevant for the design of DNA vaccines, because they imply that MHC class I presentation rather reflects protein synthesis than protein concentration.

In order to optimize cellular immune responses by targeting DNA vaccines into the MHC class I pathway, various strategies have been employed. These include covalent attachment of ER-targeting sequences to plasmid encoded peptides (Ciernik et al. 1996), fusion of antigen to molecules known to serve as substrates for the proteasome (Dantuma et al. 2000; Xu et al. 2005), and the use of constructs encoding ubiquitin-fusion molecules (Rodriguez et al. 1997). These approaches generally enhance CTL production but diminish humoral responses. Both outcomes are in accordance with the expectation that removal of native antigen by proteasomal degradation should abolish activation of B cells, but enhance the delivery of antigenic peptides into the ER.

Another strategy to target the endogenous processing pathway is the use of cytosolic (hsp90, hsp70) as well as ER (calreticulin) chaperones which act as vehicles for the delivery of partially processed peptides but also excert adjuvant activity by activation of DCs. DCs express several receptors for internalization of chaperone-peptide complexes, opening the possibility to target vaccines for cross-priming.

Indeed, improved anti-tumor cytotoxicity was observed following immunization with a fusion construct of the human papillomavirus oncoprotein antigen E7 with calreticulin, a chaperon involved in the assembly of MHC class I molecules (Cheng et al. 2001). Both, targeting peptide to freshly synthesized class I molecules as well as enhanced cross-priming contributed to enhanced immunogenicity. However, calreticulin also owns anti-angiogenic properties which have contributed to the antitumor effect of this fusion DNA vaccine.

The situation becomes more complicated as the ability of chaperons to facilitate cross-priming may be highly dependend on minor changes of the bound peptide. Castellino et al. have shown that loading a hybrid peptide consisting of a hydrophobic anchor peptide, and the major CTL epitope of ovalbumine (SIINFEKL) on hsp70, results in delivery to the cytosol (followed by MHC I loading via TAP), or to endosomes, depending on N- or C-terminal attachment of the anchor peptide (Castellino et al. 2000).

Although the canonic pathway for presenting cytosolic antigen is the enogenous MHC I pathway, also extracellular antigen can be targeted to the MHC class I pathway, a process termed cross-presentation. Evidence that cross-presentation could be the primary route for priming class I-restricted CTLs following DNA immunization origins from experimental setups with differential expression of the encoded antigen in APCs vs. non-APCs. Corr et al. demonstrated only weak T cell responses after direct transfection of APCs, compared to strong responses resulting from a combination of direct transfection and cross-presentation (Corr et al. 1999). However, results from Freigang et al. question the importance of cross-presentation and cross-priming for antiviral CTL responses, in cases where APCs are not directly infected by the virus. The authors provide evidence, that APCs rather take up viral RNA, and translate viral antigen themselves, than cross-present antigen acquired from infected bystander cells (Freigang et al. 2003).

An important question in the context of cross-priming is whether exogenously acquired antigens prime CTLs to the same epitopes as endogenously synthesized antigens do. Irrespective of the mechanism of shuttling exogenous antigens into the endogenous processing pathway in DCs, the antigen will differ from that produced endogenously. Whereas the majority of endogenously synthesized antigens enter the endogenous pathway as defective ribosomal products, antigens taken up by DCs and entering the endogenous pathway via phagolysosome-to-ER transfer originate from native, folded proteins and may have acquired some resistance to proteolysis (Schirmbeck and Reimann 2002). Wolkers et al. have shown a marked divergence in the efficiency of endogenous and exogenous antigen presentation of an influenza nucleoprotein epitope and postulate that especially peptides that assemble with cellular factors, such as signal peptides, may display reduced access to the exogenous presentation pathway (Wolkers et al. 2004).

MHC Class II Presentation

Usually, antigens from outside the cell gain access to the MHC class II compartment via receptor-mediated endocytosis, phagocytosis, or macropinocytosis. Therefore, antigens encoded by DNA vaccines, which should stimulate CD4+ T cells, will

1 General Mechanisms of Gene Vaccines

most likely have to be synthesized by "bystander" cells first, and then taken up by APCs.

Depending on the form of the antigen, different receptor systems will be used for uptake by DCs. After apoptosis of gene vaccine transfected cells, apoptotic bodies containing translated antigen can be taken up by the avb5 integrin/CD36 complex via thrombospondin (Albert et al. 1998), by the scavenger receptor LOX-1, by the receptor tyrosine kinase MER (Scott et al. 2001), or by the $\alpha 1$ macroglobulin receptor CD91, which recognizes surface-bound C1q/mannose-binding lectin via a calreticulin bridge (Ogden et al. 2001). In contrast, soluble antigens can be taken up as immune complexes via Fc receptors given that specific antibodies exist, or via C-type lectin receptors when antigens are appropriately glycosylated. Glycosylation will also affect the processing of a secreted antigen, which is of special importance for the design of gene vaccines, as depending on the source of the antigen, the glycosylation pattern of the translated protein may not resemble that of the wild type molecule (Howarth and Elliott 2004).

Several strategies facilitating class II presentation of antigens from an endogenous source after direct transfection of DCs with DNA-based vaccines have been developed. One approach utilizes a specific feature of the MHC II pathway: The invariant chain complexed with MHC class II during assembly is proteolytically cleaved in the endosome, leaving the class II-associated invariant chain peptide (CLIP) bound to the major groove. This mechanism prevents pre-mature loading of antigenic peptides onto the MHC class II complex. By replacing CLIP with a known class II epitope, DNA vaccines encoding a mutated invariant chain can be designed to directly target MHC class II. Originally invented for screening of cDNA libraries for class II restricted tumor antigens (Wang et al. 1999), this technology has been used for electroporation of DCs with mRNA encoding an invariant chain with an incorporated MAGE-3 epitope and found to be superior to peptide-pulsed DCs concerning their immunostimulatory capacity (Bonehill et al. 2003). Also, fusion to the phagolysosome-targeted protein LAMP-1 has been shown to elicit enhanced CD4+ T cell and B cell induction (Arruda et al. 2006; Ruff et al. 1997). Alternatively, by using the CD1 endosomal targeting sequence, antigens can be directed to discrete endosomal sites depending on the CD1 isotype from which the targeting sequence is derived. There is increasing evidence, that processing of MHC II epitopes is more likely to occur in early/recycling endosomes, and thus addressing this specific compartment may enhance vaccine efficacy (Dutronc and Porcelli 2002; Niazi et al. 2007).

An important fact for presentation of endogenous antigens by MHC class II is the capacity of DCs for autophagy, a process for normal turnover of some cellular proteins. It was recently demonstrated that a cytosolic antigen can be transported to phagolysosomes for processing, followed by uptake into autophagosomes and finally by presentation on MHC class II (Nimmerjahn et al. 2003). Interestingly, naturally processed peptides bound to MHC II are predominantly self peptides, indicating that presentation of enogenous antigen on MHC II may not be an exception, but a very general pathway (Rudensky et al. 1991).

Taken together, we have acquired a detailed knowledge how antigen is taken up, processed and presented after immunization with nucleic acid based vaccines.

Exploiting this knowledge to specifically address distinct processing pathways enables us to induce tailor made immune responses for different applications and generating more powerful vaccines for the clinics.

Conclusions

Gene vaccines have become a promising alternative to conventional vaccine approaches. Our increasing understanding of the fundamental mechanisms involved in vector uptake, immune activation by innate immune receptors, and translation and presentation of encoded antigen has opened a wide field for vaccine optimization and enables the design of specialized vaccines for a broad range of applications. While the main focus today lies on intervention against infectious diseases such as HIV and the treatment of tumors, many other fields may benefit from the development of more immunogenic, precisely targeted, and safety optimized gene vaccines, including treatment of autoimmune diseases and allergic disorders. The following chapters in this book will give insight into recent advances in the field, the status of licensed veterinary DNA vaccines, and highlight the most promising applications that are currently under evaluation in the clinics. Finally, regulatory questions and industrial production processes of state of the art GMP plasmid DNA are discussed.

References

Ablasser A, Bauernfeind F, Hartmann G, Latz E, Fitzgerald KA, Hornung V (2009) RIG-I-dependent sensing of poly(dA:dT) through the induction of an RNA polymerase III-transcribed RNA intermediate. Nat Immunol 10(10):1065–1072

Aguiar JC, Hedstrom RC, Rogers WO, Charoenvit Y, Sacci JB Jr, Lanar DE, Majam VF, Stout RR, Hoffman SL (2001) Enhancement of the immune response in rabbits to a malaria DNA vaccine by immunization with a needle-free jet device. Vaccine 20(1–2):275–280

Akbari O, Panjwani N, Garcia S, Tascon R, Lowrie D, Stockinger B (1999) DNA vaccination: transfection and activation of dendritic cells as key events for immunity. J Exp Med 189(1):169–178

Albert ML, Pearce SF, Francisco LM, Sauter B, Roy P, Silverstein RL, Bhardwaj N (1998) Immature dendritic cells phagocytose apoptotic cells via alphavbeta5 and CD36, and cross-present antigens to cytotoxic T lymphocytes. J Exp Med 188(7):1359–1368

Al-Dosari MS, Gao X (2009) Nonviral gene delivery: principle, limitations, and recent progress. AAPS J 11(4):671–681

Al-Dosari MS, Knapp JE, Liu D (2005) Hydrodynamic delivery. Adv Genet 54:65–82

Alexopoulou L, Holt AC, Medzhitov R, Flavell RA (2001) Recognition of double-stranded RNA and activation of NF-κB by Toll-like receptor 3. Nature 413(6857):732–738

Alvarez D, Harder G, Fattouh R, Sun J, Goncharova S, Stampfli MR, Coyle AJ, Bramson JL, Jordana M (2005) Cutaneous antigen priming via gene gun leads to skin-selective Th2 immune-inflammatory responses. J Immunol 174(3):1664–1674

Andre F, Mir LM (2004) DNA electrotransfer: its principles and an updated review of its therapeutic applications. Gene Ther 11(Suppl 1):S33–S42

Argyros O, Wong SP, Niceta M, Waddington SN, Howe SJ, Coutelle C, Miller AD, Harbottle RP (2008) Persistent episomal transgene expression in liver following delivery of a scaffold/matrix attachment region containing non-viral vector. Gene Ther 15(24):1593–1605

Arruda LB, Sim D, Chikhlikar PR, Maciel M Jr, Akasaki K, August JT, Marques ET (2006) Dendritic cell-lysosomal-associated membrane protein (LAMP) and LAMP-1-HIV-1 gag chimeras have distinct cellular trafficking pathways and prime T and B cell responses to a diverse repertoire of epitopes. J Immunol 177(4):2265–2275

Asmuth DM, Brown EL, DiNubile MJ, Sun X, del Rio C, Harro C, Keefer MC, Kublin JG, Dubey SA, Kierstead LS, Casimiro DR, Shiver JW, Robertson MN, Quirk EK, Mehrotra DV (2010) Comparative cell-mediated immunogenicity of DNA/DNA, DNA/adenovirus type 5 (Ad5), or Ad5/Ad5 HIV-1 clade B gag vaccine prime-boost regimens. J Infect Dis 201(1):132–141

Babiuk S, Mookherjee N, Pontarollo R, Griebel P, van Drunen Littel-van den Hurk S, Hecker R, Babiuk L (2004) TLR9–/– and TLR9+/+ mice display similar immune responses to a DNA vaccine. Immunology 113(1):114–120

Bachmann MF, Beerli RR, Agnellini P, Wolint P, Schwarz K, Oxenius A (2006) Long-lived memory CD8+ T cells are programmed by prolonged antigen exposure and low levels of cellular activation. Eur J Immunol 36(4):842–854

Barral PM, Sarkar D, Su ZZ, Barber GN, DeSalle R, Racaniello VR, Fisher PB (2009) Functions of the cytoplasmic RNA sensors RIG-I and MDA-5: key regulators of innate immunity. Pharmacol Ther 124(2):219–234

Barry ME, Pinto-Gonzalez D, Orson FM, McKenzie GJ, Petry GR, Barry MA (1999) Role of endogenous endonucleases and tissue site in transfection and CpG-mediated immune activation after naked DNA injection. Hum Gene Ther 10(15):2461–2480

Basner-Tschakarjan E, Mirmohammadsadegh A, Baer A, Hengge UR (2004) Uptake and trafficking of DNA in keratinocytes: evidence for DNA-binding proteins. Gene Ther 11(9):765–774

Beckett CG, Tjaden J, Burgess T, Danko JR, Tamminga C, Simmons M, Wu SJ, Sun P, Kochel T, Raviprakash K, Hayes CG, Porter KR (2011) Evaluation of a prototype dengue-1 DNA vaccine in a phase 1 clinical trial. Vaccine 29(5):960–968

Bonehill A, Heirman C, Tuyaerts S, Michiels A, Zhang Y, van der Bruggen P, Thielemans K (2003) Efficient presentation of known HLA class II-restricted MAGE-A3 epitopes by dendritic cells electroporated with messenger RNA encoding an invariant chain with genetic exchange of class II-associated invariant chain peptide. Cancer Res 63(17):5587–5594

Bot A, Stan AC, Inaba K, Steinman R, Bona C (2000) Dendritic cells at a DNA vaccination site express the encoded influenza nucleoprotein and prime MHC class I-restricted cytolytic lymphocytes upon adoptive transfer. Int Immunol 12(6):825–832

Bouloc A, Walker P, Grivel JC, Vogel JC, Katz SI (1999) Immunization through dermal delivery of protein-encoding DNA: a role for migratory dendritic cells. Eur J Immunol 29(2):446–454

Boyle JS, Koniaras C, Lew AM (1997) Influence of cellular location of expressed antigen on the efficacy of DNA vaccination: cytotoxic T lymphocyte and antibody responses are suboptimal when antigen is cytoplasmic after intramuscular DNA immunization. Int Immunol 9(12):1897–1906

Brennan K, Bowie AG (2010) Activation of host pattern recognition receptors by viruses. Curr Opin Microbiol 13(4):503–507

Budker V, Budker T, Zhang G, Subbotin V, Loomis A, Wolff JA (2000) Hypothesis: naked plasmid DNA is taken up by cells in vivo by a receptor-mediated process. J Gene Med 2(2):76–88

Casares S, Inaba K, Brumeanu TD, Steinman RM, Bona CA (1997) Antigen presentation by dendritic cells after immunization with DNA encoding a major histocompatibility complex class II-restricted viral epitope. J Exp Med 186(9):1481–1486

Castellino F, Boucher PE, Eichelberg K, Mayhew M, Rothman JE, Houghton AN, Germain RN (2000) Receptor-mediated uptake of antigen/heat shock protein complexes results in major histocompatibility complex class I antigen presentation via two distinct processing pathways. J Exp Med 191(11):1957–1964

Catron DM, Rusch LK, Hataye J, Itano AA, Jenkins MK (2006) CD4+ T cells that enter the draining lymph nodes after antigen injection participate in the primary response and become central-memory cells. J Exp Med 203(4):1045–1054

Cattamanchi A, Posavad CM, Wald A, Baine Y, Moses J, Higgins TJ, Ginsberg R, Ciccarelli R, Corey L, Koelle DM (2008) Phase I study of a herpes simplex virus type 2 (HSV-2) DNA vaccine administered to healthy, HSV-2-seronegative adults by a needle-free injection system. Clin Vaccine Immunol 15(11):1638–1643

Chastain M, Simon AJ, Soper KA, Holder DJ, Montgomery DL, Sagar SL, Casimiro DR, Middaugh CR (2001) Antigen levels and antibody titers after DNA vaccination. J Pharm Sci 90(4):474–484

Chen Z, Kadowaki S, Hagiwara Y, Yoshikawa T, Matsuo K, Kurata T, Tamura S (2000) Cross-protection against a lethal influenza virus infection by DNA vaccine to neuraminidase. Vaccine 18(28):3214–3222

Chen ZY, Yant SR, He CY, Meuse L, Shen S, Kay MA (2001) Linear DNAs concatemerize in vivo and result in sustained transgene expression in mouse liver. Mol Ther 3(3):403–410

Chen ZY, He CY, Ehrhardt A, Kay MA (2003) Minicircle DNA vectors devoid of bacterial DNA result in persistent and high-level transgene expression in vivo. Mol Ther 8(3):495–500

Cheng WF, Hung CF, Chai CY, Hsu KF, He L, Ling M, Wu TC (2001) Tumor-specific immunity and antiangiogenesis generated by a DNA vaccine encoding calreticulin linked to a tumor antigen. J Clin Invest 108(5):669–678

Cheng G, Zhong J, Chung J, Chisari FV (2007) Double-stranded DNA and double-stranded RNA induce a common antiviral signaling pathway in human cells. Proc Natl Acad Sci USA 104(21):9035–9040

Chiarella P, Massi E, De Robertis M, Sibilio A, Parrella P, Fazio VM, Signori E (2008) Electroporation of skeletal muscle induces danger signal release and antigen-presenting cell recruitment independently of DNA vaccine administration. Expert Opin Biol Ther 8(11):1645–1657

Chiu YH, Macmillan JB, Chen ZJ (2009) RNA polymerase III detects cytosolic DNA and induces type I interferons through the RIG-I pathway. Cell 138(3):576–591

Cho JH, Youn JW, Sung YC (2001) Cross-priming as a predominant mechanism for inducing CD8(+) T cell responses in gene gun DNA immunization. J Immunol 167(10):5549–5557

Ciernik IF, Berzofsky JA, Carbone DP (1996) Induction of cytotoxic T lymphocytes and antitumor immunity with DNA vaccines expressing single T cell epitopes. J Immunol 156(7):2369–2375

Coelho-Castelo AA, Santos Junior RR, Bonato VL, Jamur MC, Oliver C, Silva CL (2003) B-lymphocytes in bone marrow or lymph nodes can take up plasmid DNA after intramuscular delivery. Hum Gene Ther 14(13):1279–1285

Condon C, Watkins SC, Celluzzi CM, Thompson K, Falo LD Jr (1996) DNA-based immunization by in vivo transfection of dendritic cells. Nat Med 2(10):1122–1128

Corr M, von Damm A, Lee DJ, Tighe H (1999) In vivo priming by DNA injection occurs predominantly by antigen transfer. J Immunol 163(9):4721–4727

Dantuma NP, Lindsten K, Glas R, Jellne M, Masucci MG (2000) Short-lived green fluorescent proteins for quantifying ubiquitin/proteasome-dependent proteolysis in living cells. Nat Biotechnol 18(5):538–543

Dean DA (1997) Import of plasmid DNA into the nucleus is sequence specific. Exp Cell Res 230(2):293–302

Dean DA, Strong DD, Zimmer WE (2005) Nuclear entry of nonviral vectors. Gene Ther 12(11):881–890

Diebold SS, Kaisho T, Hemmi H, Akira S, Reis e Sousa C (2004) Innate antiviral responses by means of TLR7-mediated recognition of single-stranded RNA. Science 303(5663):1529–1531

Diebold SS, Schulz O, Alexopoulou L, Leitner WW, Flavell RA, Reis e Sousa C (2009) Role of TLR3 in the immunogenicity of replicon plasmid-based vaccines. Gene Ther 16(3):359–366

Doh SG, Vahlsing HL, Hartikka J, Liang X, Manthorpe M (1997) Spatial-temporal patterns of gene expression in mouse skeletal muscle after injection of lacZ plasmid DNA. Gene Ther 4(7):648–663

Dupuis M, Denis-Mize K, Woo C, Goldbeck C, Selby MJ, Chen M, Otten GR, Ulmer JB, Donnelly JJ, Ott G, McDonald DM (2000) Distribution of DNA vaccines determines their immunogenicity after intramuscular injection in mice. J Immunol 165(5):2850–2858

Dutronc Y, Porcelli SA (2002) The CD1 family and T cell recognition of lipid antigens. Tissue Antigens 60(5):337–353

Epstein JE, Gorak EJ, Charoenvit Y, Wang R, Freydberg N, Osinowo O, Richie TL, Stoltz EL, Trespalacios F, Nerges J, Ng J, Fallarme-Majam V, Abot E, Goh L, Parker S, Kumar S, Hedstrom RC, Norman J, Stout R, Hoffman SL (2002) Safety, tolerability, and lack of antibody responses after administration of a PfCSP DNA malaria vaccine via needle or needle-free jet injection, and comparison of intramuscular and combination intramuscular/intradermal routes. Hum Gene Ther 13(13):1551–1560

Fabry Z, Waldschmidt MM, Moore SA, Hart MN (1990) Antigen presentation by brain microvessel smooth muscle and endothelium. J Neuroimmunol 28(1):63–71

Fan L, Busser BW, Lifsted TQ, Oukka M, Lo D, Laufer TM (2003) Antigen presentation by keratinocytes directs autoimmune skin disease. Proc Natl Acad Sci USA 100(6):3386–3391

Fernandes-Alnemri T, Yu JW, Datta P, Wu J, Alnemri ES (2009) AIM2 activates the inflammasome and cell death in response to cytoplasmic DNA. Nature 458(7237):509–513

Ferrera F, La Cava A, Rizzi M, Hahn BH, Indiveri F, Filaci G (2007) Gene vaccination for the induction of immune tolerance. Ann NY Acad Sci 1110:99–111

Freigang S, Egger D, Bienz K, Hengartner H, Zinkernagel RM (2003) Endogenous neosynthesis vs. cross-presentation of viral antigens for cytotoxic T cell priming. Proc Natl Acad Sci USA 100(23):13477–13482

Garapin A, Ma L, Pescher P, Lagranderie M, Marchal G (2001) Mixed immune response induced in rodents by two naked DNA genes coding for mycobacterial glycosylated proteins. Vaccine 19(20–22):2830–2841

Gill HS, Prausnitz MR (2007) Coated microneedles for transdermal delivery. J Control Release 117(2):227–237

Gilliet M, Cao W, Liu YJ (2008) Plasmacytoid dendritic cells: sensing nucleic acids in viral infection and autoimmune diseases. Nat Rev Immunol 8(8):594–606

Ginsberg BA, Gallardo HF, Rasalan TS, Adamow M, Mu Z, Tandon S, Bewkes BB, Roman RA, Chapman PB, Schwartz GK, Carvajal RD, Panageas KS, Terzulli SL, Houghton AN, Yuan JD, Wolchok JD (2010) Immunologic response to xenogeneic gp100 DNA in melanoma patients: comparison of particle-mediated epidermal delivery with intramuscular injection. Clin Cancer Res 16(15):4057–4065

Gonzalez SF, Pitcher LA, Mempel T, Schuerpf F, Carroll MC (2009) B cell acquisition of antigen in vivo. Curr Opin Immunol 21(3):251–257

Gonzalez-Gonzalez E, Ra H, Spitler R, Hickerson RP, Contag CH, Kaspar RL (2010) Increased interstitial pressure improves nucleic acid delivery to skin enabling a comparative analysis of constitutive promoters. Gene Ther 17(10):1270–1278

Gretz JE, Norbury CC, Anderson AO, Proudfoot AE, Shaw S (2000) Lymph-borne chemokines and other low molecular weight molecules reach high endothelial venules via specialized conduits while a functional barrier limits access to the lymphocyte microenvironments in lymph node cortex. J Exp Med 192(10):1425–1440

Grillo G, Turi A, Licciulli F, Mignone F, Liuni S, Banfi S, Gennarino VA, Horner DS, Pavesi G, Picardi E, Pesole G (2010) UTRdb and UTRsite (RELEASE 2010): a collection of sequences and regulatory motifs of the untranslated regions of eukaryotic mRNAs. Nucleic Acids Res 38(Database issue):D75–D80

Gronevik E, Tollefsen S, Sikkeland LI, Haug T, Tjelle TE, Mathiesen I (2003) DNA transfection of mononuclear cells in muscle tissue. J Gene Med 5(10):909–917

Gupta S, Garg NJ (2010) Prophylactic efficacy of TcVac2 against *Trypanosoma cruzi* in mice. PLoS Negl Trop Dis 4(8):e797

Gustafsson C, Govindarajan S, Minshull J (2004) Codon bias and heterologous protein expression. Trends Biotechnol 22(7):346–353

Haddad D, Liljeqvist S, Stahl S, Perlmann P, Berzins K, Ahlborg N (1998) Differential induction of immunoglobulin G subclasses by immunization with DNA vectors containing or lacking a signal sequence. Immunol Lett 61(2–3):201–204

Heil F, Hemmi H, Hochrein H, Ampenberger F, Kirschning C, Akira S, Lipford G, Wagner H, Bauer S (2004) Species-specific recognition of single-stranded RNA via toll-like receptor 7 and 8. Science 303(5663):1526–1529

Hemmi H, Takeuchi O, Kawai T, Kaisho T, Sato S, Sanjo H, Matsumoto M, Hoshino K, Wagner H, Takeda K, Akira S (2000) A Toll-like receptor recognizes bacterial DNA. Nature 408(6813): 740–745

Hibbitt OC, Harbottle RP, Waddington SN, Bursill CA, Coutelle C, Channon KM, Wade-Martins R (2007) Delivery and long-term expression of a 135 kb LDLR genomic DNA locus in vivo by hydrodynamic tail vein injection. J Gene Med 9(6):488–497

Hill M, Cuturi MC (2010) Negative vaccination by tolerogenic dendritic cells in organ transplantation. Curr Opin Organ Transplant 15(6):738–743

Hisazumi J, Kobayashi N, Nishikawa M, Takakura Y (2004) Significant role of liver sinusoidal endothelial cells in hepatic uptake and degradation of naked plasmid DNA after intravenous injection. Pharm Res 21(7):1223–1228

Hodges BL, Taylor KM, Joseph MF, Bourgeois SA, Scheule RK (2004) Long-term transgene expression from plasmid DNA gene therapy vectors is negatively affected by CpG dinucleotides. Mol Ther 10(2):269–278

Holtkamp S, Kreiter S, Selmi A, Simon P, Koslowski M, Huber C, Tureci O, Sahin U (2006) Modification of antigen-encoding RNA increases stability, translational efficacy, and T-cell stimulatory capacity of dendritic cells. Blood 108(13):4009–4017

Hon H, Oran A, Brocker T, Jacob J (2005) B lymphocytes participate in cross-presentation of antigen following gene gun vaccination. J Immunol 174(9):5233–5242

Hornung V, Ellegast J, Kim S, Brzozka K, Jung A, Kato H, Poeck H, Akira S, Conzelmann KK, Schlee M, Endres S, Hartmann G (2006) 5′-Triphosphate RNA is the ligand for RIG-I. Science 314(5801):994–997

Hornung V, Ablasser A, Charrel-Dennis M, Bauernfeind F, Horvath G, Caffrey DR, Latz E, Fitzgerald KA (2009) AIM2 recognizes cytosolic dsDNA and forms a caspase-1-activating inflammasome with ASC. Nature 458(7237):514–518

Hoshino K, Kaisho T (2008) Nucleic acid sensing Toll-like receptors in dendritic cells. Curr Opin Immunol 20(4):408–413

Howarth M, Elliott T (2004) The processing of antigens delivered as DNA vaccines. Immunol Rev 199:27–39

Huang MT, Gorman CM (1990) Intervening sequences increase efficiency of RNA 3′ processing and accumulation of cytoplasmic RNA. Nucleic Acids Res 18(4):937–947

Hume DA, Robinson AP, MacPherson GG, Gordon S (1983) The mononuclear phagocyte system of the mouse defined by immunohistochemical localization of antigen F4/80. Relationship between macrophages, Langerhans cells, reticular cells, and dendritic cells in lymphoid and hematopoietic organs. J Exp Med 158(5):1522–1536

Ishii KJ, Kawagoe T, Koyama S, Matsui K, Kumar H, Kawai T, Uematsu S, Takeuchi O, Takeshita F, Coban C, Akira S (2008) TANK-binding kinase-1 delineates innate and adaptive immune responses to DNA vaccines. Nature 451(7179):725–729

Jamaluddin M, Wang S, Garofalo RP, Elliott T, Casola A, Baron S, Brasier AR (2001) IFN-beta mediates coordinate expression of antigen-processing genes in RSV-infected pulmonary epithelial cells. Am J Physiol Lung Cell Mol Physiol 280(2):L248–L257

Ji H, Wang TL, Chen CH, Pai SI, Hung CF, Lin KY, Kurman RJ, Pardoll DM, Wu TC (1999) Targeting human papillomavirus type 16 E7 to the endosomal/lysosomal compartment enhances the antitumor immunity of DNA vaccines against murine human papillomavirus type 16 E7-expressing tumors. Hum Gene Ther 10(17):2727–2740

Jiang W, Reich CF, Pisetsky DS (2006) In vitro assay of immunostimulatory activities of plasmid vectors. Meth Mol Med 127:55–70

Johansson S, Ek M, Wahren B, Stout R, Liu M, Hallermalm K (2007) Intracellular targeting of CEA results in Th1-type antibody responses following intradermal genetic vaccination by a needle-free jet injection device. Sci World J 7:987–999

Johnson CL, Owen DM, Gale M Jr (2007) Functional and therapeutic analysis of hepatitis C virus NS3.4A protease control of antiviral immune defense. J Biol Chem 282(14): 10792–10803

Jones S, Evans K, McElwaine-Johnn H, Sharpe M, Oxford J, Lambkin-Williams R, Mant T, Nolan A, Zambon M, Ellis J, Beadle J, Loudon PT (2009) DNA vaccination protects against an influenza challenge in a double-blind randomised placebo-controlled phase 1b clinical trial. Vaccine 27(18):2506–2512

Kariko K, Ni H, Capodici J, Lamphier M, Weissman D (2004) mRNA is an endogenous ligand for Toll-like receptor 3. J Biol Chem 279(13):12542–12550

Kariko K, Buckstein M, Ni H, Weissman D (2005) Suppression of RNA recognition by Toll-like receptors: the impact of nucleoside modification and the evolutionary origin of RNA. Immunity 23(2):165–175

Kato H, Sato S, Yoneyama M, Yamamoto M, Uematsu S, Matsui K, Tsujimura T, Takeda K, Fujita T, Takeuchi O, Akira S (2005) Cell type-specific involvement of RIG-I in antiviral response. Immunity 23(1):19–28

Kato H, Takeuchi O, Mikamo-Satoh E, Hirai R, Kawai T, Matsushita K, Hiiragi A, Dermody TS, Fujita T, Akira S (2008) Length-dependent recognition of double-stranded ribonucleic acids by retinoic acid-inducible gene-I and melanoma differentiation-associated gene 5. J Exp Med 205(7):1601–1610

Kawabata K, Takakura Y, Hashida M (1995) The fate of plasmid DNA after intravenous injection in mice: involvement of scavenger receptors in its hepatic uptake. Pharm Res 12(6):825–830

Kawai T, Akira S (2010) The role of pattern-recognition receptors in innate immunity: update on Toll-like receptors. Nat Immunol 11(5):373–384

Kessler PD, Podsakoff GM, Chen X, McQuiston SA, Colosi PC, Matelis LA, Kurtzman GJ, Byrne BJ (1996) Gene delivery to skeletal muscle results in sustained expression and systemic delivery of a therapeutic protein. Proc Natl Acad Sci USA 93(24):14082–14087

Klinman DM, Ishii KJ, Verthelyi D (2000) CpG DNA augments the immunogenicity of plasmid DNA vaccines. Curr Top Microbiol Immunol 247:131–142

Kodihalli S, Haynes JR, Robinson HL, Webster RG (1997) Cross-protection among lethal H5N2 influenza viruses induced by DNA vaccine to the hemagglutinin. J Virol 71(5):3391–3396

Komuro A, Bamming D, Horvath CM (2008) Negative regulation of cytoplasmic RNA-mediated antiviral signaling. Cytokine 43(3):350–358

Kozak M (1997) Recognition of AUG and alternative initiator codons is augmented by G in position +4 but is not generally affected by the nucleotides in positions +5 and +6. EMBO J 16(9):2482–2492

Krieg AM (2006) Therapeutic potential of Toll-like receptor 9 activation. Nat Rev Drug Discov 5(6):471–484

Kudla G, Murray AW, Tollervey D, Plotkin JB (2009) Coding-sequence determinants of gene expression in *Escherichia coli*. Science 324(5924):255–258

Kundig TM, Bachmann MF, DiPaolo C, Simard JJ, Battegay M, Lother H, Gessner A, Kuhlcke K, Ohashi PS, Hengartner H et al (1995) Fibroblasts as efficient antigen-presenting cells in lymphoid organs. Science 268(5215):1343–1347

Latz E, Schoenemeyer A, Visintin A, Fitzgerald KA, Monks BG, Knetter CF, Lien E, Nilsen NJ, Espevik T, Golenbock DT (2004) TLR9 signals after translocating from the ER to CpG DNA in the lysosome. Nat Immunol 5(2):190–198

Latz E, Verma A, Visintin A, Gong M, Sirois CM, Klein DC, Monks BG, McKnight CJ, Lamphier MS, Duprex WP, Espevik T, Golenbock DT (2007) Ligand-induced conformational changes allosterically activate Toll-like receptor 9. Nat Immunol 8(7):772–779

Lauterbach H, Gruber A, Ried C, Cheminay C, Brocker T (2006) Insufficient APC capacities of dendritic cells in gene gun-mediated DNA vaccination. J Immunol 176(8):4600–4607

Laylor R, Porakishvili N, De Souza JB, Playfair JH, Delves PJ, Lund T (1999) DNA vaccination favours memory rather than effector B cell responses. Clin Exp Immunol 117(1): 106–112

Lechardeur D, Sohn KJ, Haardt M, Joshi PB, Monck M, Graham RW, Beatty B, Squire J, O'Brodovich H, Lukacs GL (1999) Metabolic instability of plasmid DNA in the cytosol: a potential barrier to gene transfer. Gene Ther 6(4):482–497

Ledwith BJ, Manam S, Troilo PJ, Barnum AB, Pauley CJ, Griffiths TG 2nd, Harper LB, Beare CM, Bagdon WJ, Nichols WW (2000) Plasmid DNA vaccines: investigation of integration into host cellular DNA following intramuscular injection in mice. Intervirology 43(4–6):258–272

Lee AH, Suh YS, Sung JH, Yang SH, Sung YC (1997) Comparison of various expression plasmids for the induction of immune response by DNA immunization. Mol Cells 7(4):495–501

Lee JW, Park JH, Prausnitz MR (2008) Dissolving microneedles for transdermal drug delivery. Biomaterials 29(13):2113–2124

Lehmann MJ, Sczakiel G (2005) Spontaneous uptake of biologically active recombinant DNA by mammalian cells via a selected DNA segment. Gene Ther 12(5):446–451

Leitner WW, Bergmann-Leitner ES, Hwang LN, Restifo NP (2006) Type I Interferons are essential for the efficacy of replicase-based DNA vaccines. Vaccine 24(24):5110–5118

Li S, MacLaughlin FC, Fewell JG, Gondo M, Wang J, Nicol F, Dean DA, Smith LC (2001) Muscle-specific enhancement of gene expression by incorporation of SV40 enhancer in the expression plasmid. Gene Ther 8(6):494–497

Li S, Wilkinson M, Xia X, David M, Xu L, Purkel-Sutton A, Bhardwaj A (2005) Induction of IFN-regulated factors and antitumoral surveillance by transfected placebo plasmid DNA. Mol Ther 11(1):112–119

Li Q, Zhu Y, Chu J, Wang Y, Xu Y, Hou Q, Zhang S, Guo X (2006) Protective immunity against *Bordetella pertussis* by a recombinant DNA vaccine and the effect of coinjection with a granulocyte-macrophage colony stimulating factor gene. Microbiol Immunol 50(12):929–936

Lin K, Roosinovich E, Ma B, Hung CF, Wu TC (2010) Therapeutic HPV DNA vaccines. Immunol Res 47(1–3):86–112

Lindinger P, Mostbock S, Hammerl P, Hartl A, Thalhamer J, Abrams SI (2003) Induction of murine ras oncogene peptide-specific T cell responses by immunization with plasmid DNA-based minigene vectors. Vaccine 21(27–30):4285–4296

Liu F, Heston S, Shollenberger LM, Sun B, Mickle M, Lovell M, Huang L (2006) Mechanism of in vivo DNA transport into cells by electroporation: electrophoresis across the plasma membrane may not be involved. J Gene Med 8(3):353–361

Loo YM, Fornek J, Crochet N, Bajwa G, Perwitasari O, Martinez-Sobrido L, Akira S, Gill MA, Garcia-Sastre A, Katze MG, Gale M Jr (2008) Distinct RIG-I and MDA5 signaling by RNA viruses in innate immunity. J Virol 82(1):335–345

Loser P, Jennings GS, Strauss M, Sandig V (1998) Reactivation of the previously silenced cytomegalovirus major immediate-early promoter in the mouse liver: involvement of NFκB. J Virol 72(1):180–190

Lukacs GL, Haggie P, Seksek O, Lechardeur D, Freedman N, Verkman AS (2000) Size-dependent DNA mobility in cytoplasm and nucleus. J Biol Chem 275(3):1625–1629

Manam S, Ledwith BJ, Barnum AB, Troilo PJ, Pauley CJ, Harper LB, Griffiths TG 2nd, Niu Z, Denisova L, Follmer TT, Pacchione SJ, Wang Z, Beare CM, Bagdon WJ, Nichols WW (2000) Plasmid DNA vaccines: tissue distribution and effects of DNA sequence, adjuvants and delivery method on integration into host DNA. Intervirology 43(4–6):273–281

Mancini-Bourgine M, Fontaine H, Brechot C, Pol S, Michel ML (2006) Immunogenicity of a hepatitis B DNA vaccine administered to chronic HBV carriers. Vaccine 24(21):4482–4489

Manoj S, Babiuk LA, van Drunen Littel-van den Hurk S (2004) Approaches to enhance the efficacy of DNA vaccines. Crit Rev Clin Lab Sci 41(1):1–39

Manthorpe M, Cornefert-Jensen F, Hartikka J, Felgner J, Rundell A, Margalith M, Dwarki V (1993) Gene therapy by intramuscular injection of plasmid DNA: studies on firefly luciferase gene expression in mice. Hum Gene Ther 4(4):419–431

Martin E, Roche PW, Triccas JA, Britton WJ (2001) DNA encoding a single mycobacterial antigen protects against leprosy infection. Vaccine 19(11–12):1391–1396

Martin JE, Pierson TC, Hubka S, Rucker S, Gordon IJ, Enama ME, Andrews CA, Xu Q, Davis BS, Nason M, Fay M, Koup RA, Roederer M, Bailer RT, Gomez PL, Mascola JR, Chang GJ,

1 General Mechanisms of Gene Vaccines

Nabel GJ, Graham BS (2007) A West Nile virus DNA vaccine induces neutralizing antibody in healthy adults during a phase 1 clinical trial. J Infect Dis 196(12):1732–1740

Medzhitov R, Preston-Hurlburt P, Janeway CA Jr (1997) A human homologue of the Drosophila Toll protein signals activation of adaptive immunity. Nature 388(6640):394–397

Molnar MJ, Gilbert R, Lu Y, Liu AB, Guo A, Larochelle N, Orlopp K, Lochmuller H, Petrof BJ, Nalbantoglu J, Karpati G (2004) Factors influencing the efficacy, longevity, and safety of electroporation-assisted plasmid-based gene transfer into mouse muscles. Mol Ther 10(3):447–455

Munkonge FM, Amin V, Hyde SC, Green AM, Pringle IA, Gill DR, Smith JW, Hooley RP, Xenariou S, Ward MA, Leeds N, Leung KY, Chan M, Hillery E, Geddes DM, Griesenbach U, Postel EH, Dean DA, Dunn MJ, Alton EW (2009) Identification and functional characterization of cytoplasmic determinants of plasmid DNA nuclear import. J Biol Chem 284(39): 26978–26987

Nakhaei P, Genin P, Civas A, Hiscott J (2009) RIG-I-like receptors: sensing and responding to RNA virus infection. Semin Immunol 21(4):215–222

Newell-Price J, Clark AJ, King P (2000) DNA methylation and silencing of gene expression. Trends Endocrinol Metab 11(4):142–148

Nguyen LT, Atobe K, Barichello JM, Ishida T, Kiwada H (2007) Complex formation with plasmid DNA increases the cytotoxicity of cationic liposomes. Biol Pharm Bull 30(4):751–757

Niazi KR, Ochoa MT, Sieling PA, Rooke NE, Peter AK, Mollahan P, Dickey M, Rabizadeh S, Rea TH, Modlin RL (2007) Activation of human CD4+ T cells by targeting MHC class II epitopes to endosomal compartments using human CD1 tail sequences. Immunology 122(4): 522–531

Nimmerjahn F, Milosevic S, Behrends U, Jaffee EM, Pardoll DM, Bornkamm GW, Mautner J (2003) Major histocompatibility complex class II-restricted presentation of a cytosolic antigen by autophagy. Eur J Immunol 33(5):1250–1259

Nishikawa M, Takakura Y, Hashida M (2005) Pharmacokinetics of plasmid DNA-based non-viral gene medicine. Adv Genet 53:47–68

Ogden CA, deCathelineau A, Hoffmann PR, Bratton D, Ghebrehiwet B, Fadok VA, Henson PM (2001) C1q and mannose binding lectin engagement of cell surface calreticulin and CD91 initiates macropinocytosis and uptake of apoptotic cells. J Exp Med 194(6):781–795

Okada M, Kita Y (2010) Tuberculosis vaccine development: The development of novel (preclinical) DNA vaccine. Hum Vaccin 6(4):297–308

Palm NW, Medzhitov R (2009) Pattern recognition receptors and control of adaptive immunity. Immunol Rev 227(1):221–233

Pascolo S (2008) Vaccination with messenger RNA (mRNA). Handb Exp Pharmacol 183:221–235

Paus R, Nickoloff BJ, Ito T (2005) A 'hairy' privilege. Trends Immunol 26(1):32–40

Pertmer TM, Eisenbraun MD, McCabe D, Prayaga SK, Fuller DH, Haynes JR (1995) Gene gun-based nucleic acid immunization: elicitation of humoral and cytotoxic T lymphocyte responses following epidermal delivery of nanogram quantities of DNA. Vaccine 13(15):1427–1430

Porgador A, Irvine KR, Iwasaki A, Barber BH, Restifo NP, Germain RN (1998) Predominant role for directly transfected dendritic cells in antigen presentation to CD8+ T cells after gene gun immunization. J Exp Med 188(6):1075–1082

Probst J, Brechtel S, Scheel B, Hoerr I, Jung G, Rammensee HG, Pascolo S (2006) Characterization of the ribonuclease activity on the skin surface. Genet Vaccines Ther 4:4

Probst J, Weide B, Scheel B, Pichler BJ, Hoerr I, Rammensee HG, Pascolo S (2007) Spontaneous cellular uptake of exogenous messenger RNA in vivo is nucleic acid-specific, saturable and ion dependent. Gene Ther 14(15):1175–1180

Ramos I, Alonso A, Peris A, Marcen JM, Abengozar MA, Alcolea PJ, Castillo JA, Larraga V (2009) Antibiotic resistance free plasmid DNA expressing LACK protein leads towards a protective Th1 response against Leishmania infantum infection. Vaccine 27(48): 6695–6703

Ranjan P, Bowzard JB, Schwerzmann JW, Jeisy-Scott V, Fujita T, Sambhara S (2009) Cytoplasmic nucleic acid sensors in antiviral immunity. Trends Mol Med 15(8):359–368

Rao SS, Gomez P, Mascola JR, Dang V, Krivulka GR, Yu F, Lord CI, Shen L, Bailer R, Nabel GJ, Letvin NL (2006) Comparative evaluation of three different intramuscular delivery methods for DNA immunization in a nonhuman primate animal model. Vaccine 24(3):367–373

Rehwinkel J, Reis e Sousa C (2010) RIGorous detection: exposing virus through RNA sensing. Science 327(5963):284–286

Reits EA, Vos JC, Gromme M, Neefjes J (2000) The major substrates for TAP in vivo are derived from newly synthesized proteins. Nature 404(6779):774–778

Rodriguez F, Zhang J, Whitton JL (1997) DNA immunization: ubiquitination of a viral protein enhances cytotoxic T-lymphocyte induction and antiviral protection but abrogates antibody induction. J Virol 71(11):8497–8503

Rodriguez F, An LL, Harkins S, Zhang J, Yokoyama M, Widera G, Fuller JT, Kincaid C, Campbell IL, Whitton JL (1998) DNA immunization with minigenes: low frequency of memory cytotoxic T lymphocytes and inefficient antiviral protection are rectified by ubiquitination. J Virol 72(6):5174–5181

Rodriguez F, Harkins S, Redwine JM, de Pereda JM, Whitton JL (2001) CD4(+) T cells induced by a DNA vaccine: immunological consequences of epitope-specific lysosomal targeting. J Virol 75(21):10421–10430

Roesler E, Weiss R, Weinberger EE, Fruehwirth A, Stoecklinger A, Mostbock S, Ferreira F, Thalhamer J, Scheiblhofer S (2009) Immunize and disappear-safety-optimized mRNA vaccination with a panel of 29 allergens. J Allergy Clin Immunol 124(5):1070–1077, e1071–1011

Rottinghaus ST, Poland GA, Jacobson RM, Barr LJ, Roy MJ (2003) Hepatitis B DNA vaccine induces protective antibody responses in human non-responders to conventional vaccination. Vaccine 21(31):4604–4608

Rudensky A, Preston-Hurlburt P, Hong SC, Barlow A, Janeway CA Jr (1991) Sequence analysis of peptides bound to MHC class II molecules. Nature 353(6345):622–627

Ruff AL, Guarnieri FG, Staveley-O'Carroll K, Siliciano RF, August JT (1997) The enhanced immune response to the HIV gp160/LAMP chimeric gene product targeted to the lysosome membrane protein trafficking pathway. J Biol Chem 272(13):8671–8678

Rush CM, Mitchell TJ, Garside P (2010) A detailed characterisation of the distribution and presentation of DNA vaccine encoded antigen. Vaccine 28(6):1620–1634

Saleh MC, van Rij RP, Hekele A, Gillis A, Foley E, O'Farrell PH, Andino R (2006) The endocytic pathway mediates cell entry of dsRNA to induce RNAi silencing. Nat Cell Biol 8(8):793–802

Salman H, Zbaida D, Rabin Y, Chatenay D, Elbaum M (2001) Kinetics and mechanism of DNA uptake into the cell nucleus. Proc Natl Acad Sci USA 98(13):7247–7252

Sasai M, Linehan MM, Iwasaki A (2010) Bifurcation of Toll-like receptor 9 signaling by adaptor protein 3. Science 329(5998):1530–1534

Satoh T, Kato H, Kumagai Y, Yoneyama M, Sato S, Matsushita K, Tsujimura T, Fujita T, Akira S, Takeuchi O (2010) LGP2 is a positive regulator of RIG-I- and MDA5-mediated antiviral responses. Proc Natl Acad Sci USA 107(4):1512–1517

Scheel B, Teufel R, Probst J, Carralot JP, Geginat J, Radsak M, Jarrossay D, Wagner H, Jung G, Rammensee HG, Hoerr I, Pascolo S (2005) Toll-like receptor-dependent activation of several human blood cell types by protamine-condensed mRNA. Eur J Immunol 35(5):1557–1566

Schirmbeck R, Reimann J (2002) Alternative processing of endogenous or exogenous antigens extends the immunogenic, H-2 class I-restricted peptide repertoire. Mol Immunol 39(3–4): 249–259

Schlee M, Barchet W, Hornung V, Hartmann G (2007) Beyond double-stranded RNA-type I IFN induction by 3pRNA and other viral nucleic acids. Curr Top Microbiol Immunol 316:207–230

Schmid D, Pypaert M, Munz C (2007) Antigen-loading compartments for major histocompatibility complex class II molecules continuously receive input from autophagosomes. Immunity 26(1):79–92

Schubert U, Anton LC, Gibbs J, Norbury CC, Yewdell JW, Bennink JR (2000) Rapid degradation of a large fraction of newly synthesized proteins by proteasomes. Nature 404(6779):770–774

1 General Mechanisms of Gene Vaccines

Scott RS, McMahon EJ, Pop SM, Reap EA, Caricchio R, Cohen PL, Earp HS, Matsushima GK (2001) Phagocytosis and clearance of apoptotic cells is mediated by MER. Nature 411(6834):207–211

Seternes T, Tonheim TC, Lovoll M, Bogwald J, Dalmo RA (2007) Specific endocytosis and degradation of naked DNA in the endocardial cells of cod (Gadus morhua L.). J Exp Biol 210(Pt 12):2091–2103

Shirota H, Ishii KJ, Takakuwa H, Klinman DM (2006) Contribution of interferon-beta to the immune activation induced by double-stranded DNA. Immunology 118(3):302–310

Shirota H, Petrenko L, Hong C, Klinman DM (2007) Potential of transfected muscle cells to contribute to DNA vaccine immunogenicity. J Immunol 179(1):329–336

Signori E, Iurescia S, Massi E, Fioretti D, Chiarella P, De Robertis M, Rinaldi M, Tonon G, Fazio VM (2010) DNA vaccination strategies for anti-tumour effective gene therapy protocols. Cancer Immunol Immunother 59(10):1583–1591

Smits EL, Ponsaerts P, Van de Velde AL, Van Driessche A, Cools N, Lenjou M, Nijs G, Van Bockstaele DR, Berneman ZN, Van Tendeloo VF (2007) Proinflammatory response of human leukemic cells to dsRNA transfection linked to activation of dendritic cells. Leukemia 21(8):1691–1699

Spies B, Hochrein H, Vabulas M, Huster K, Busch DH, Schmitz F, Heit A, Wagner H (2003) Vaccination with plasmid DNA activates dendritic cells via Toll-like receptor 9 (TLR9) but functions in TLR9-deficient mice. J Immunol 171(11):5908–5912

Starodubova ES, Boberg A, Litvina M, Morozov A, Petrakova NV, Timofeev A, Latyshev O, Tunitskaya V, Wahren B, Isaguliants MG, Karpov VL (2008) HIV-1 reverse transcriptase artificially targeted for proteasomal degradation induces a mixed Th1/Th2-type immune response. Vaccine 26(40):5170–5176

Stevenson FK, Ottensmeier CH, Rice J (2010) DNA vaccines against cancer come of age. Curr Opin Immunol 22(2):264–270

Stock AT, Mueller SN, van Lint AL, Heath WR, Carbone FR (2004) Cutting edge: prolonged antigen presentation after herpes simplex virus-1 skin infection. J Immunol 173(4):2241–2244

Stoecklinger A, Grieshuber I, Scheiblhofer S, Weiss R, Ritter U, Kissenpfennig A, Malissen B, Romani N, Koch F, Ferreira F, Thalhamer J, Hammerl P (2007) Epidermal langerhans cells are dispensable for humoral and cell-mediated immunity elicited by gene gun immunization. J Immunol 179(2):886–893

Stoecklinger A, Eticha TD, Mesdaghi M, Kissenpfennig A, Malissen B, Thalhamer J, Hammerl P (2011) Langerin+dermal dendritic cells are critical for CD8+ T cell activation and IgH gamma-1 class switching in response to gene gun vaccines. J Immunol 186(3):1377–1383

Strid J, Hourihane J, Kimber I, Callard R, Strobel S (2004) Disruption of the stratum corneum allows potent epicutaneous immunization with protein antigens resulting in a dominant systemic Th2 response. Eur J Immunol 34(8):2100–2109

Takagi T, Hashiguchi M, Mahato RI, Tokuda H, Takakura Y, Hashida M (1998) Involvement of specific mechanism in plasmid DNA uptake by mouse peritoneal macrophages. Biochem Biophys Res Commun 245(3):729–733

Takaoka A, Wang Z, Choi MK, Yanai H, Negishi H, Ban T, Lu Y, Miyagishi M, Kodama T, Honda K, Ohba Y, Taniguchi T (2007) DAI (DLM-1/ZBP1) is a cytosolic DNA sensor and an activator of innate immune response. Nature 448(7152):501–505

Takeshita F, Ishii KJ (2008) Intracellular DNA sensors in immunity. Curr Opin Immunol 20(4):383–388

Trombone AP, Silva CL, Lima KM, Oliver C, Jamur MC, Prescott AR, Coelho-Castelo AA (2007) Endocytosis of DNA-Hsp65 alters the pH of the late endosome/lysosome and interferes with antigen presentation. PLoS ONE 2(9):e923

Turner GC, Varshavsky A (2000) Detecting and measuring cotranslational protein degradation in vivo. Science 289(5487):2117–2120

van den Berg JH, Nuijen B, Beijnen JH, Vincent A, van Tinteren H, Kluge J, Woerdeman LA, Hennink WE, Storm G, Schumacher T, Haanen JB (2009) Optimization of intradermal vaccination by DNA tattooing in human skin. Hum Gene Ther 20(3):181–189 van den Berg JH, Oosterhuis K, Beijnen JH, Nuijen B, Haanen JB (2010) DNA vaccination in oncology: current status, opportunities and perspectives. Curr Clin Pharmacol 5(3):218–225

Van Tendeloo VF, Ponsaerts P, Berneman ZN (2007) mRNA-based gene transfer as a tool for gene and cell therapy. Curr Opin Mol Ther 9(5):423–431

Wang RF, Wang X, Atwood AC, Topalian SL, Rosenberg SA (1999) Cloning genes encoding MHC class II-restricted antigens: mutated CDC27 as a tumor antigen. Science 284(5418):1351–1354

Wang L, Kedzierski L, Schofield L, Coppel RL (2005a) Influence of glycosylphosphatidylinositol anchorage on the efficacy of DNA vaccines encoding *Plasmodium yoelii* merozoite surface protein 4/5. Vaccine 23(32):4120–4127

Wang R, Richie TL, Baraceros MF, Rahardjo N, Gay T, Banania JG, Charoenvit Y, Epstein JE, Luke T, Freilich DA, Norman J, Hoffman SL (2005b) Boosting of DNA vaccine-elicited gamma interferon responses in humans by exposure to malaria parasites. Infect Immun 73(5):2863–2872

Weiss R, Durnberger J, Mostbock S, Scheiblhofer S, Hartl A, Breitenbach M, Strasser P, Dorner F, Livey I, Crowe B, Thalhamer J (1999) Improvement of the immune response against plasmid DNA encoding OspC of Borrelia by an ER-targeting leader sequence. Vaccine 18(9–10):815–824

Weiss R, Scheiblhofer S, Freund J, Ferreira F, Livey I, Thalhamer J (2002) Gene gun bombardment with gold particles displays a particular Th2-promoting signal that over-rules the Th1-inducing effect of immunostimulatory CpG motifs in DNA vaccines. Vaccine 20(25–26):3148–3154

Weiss R, Scheiblhofer S, Gabler M, Ferreira F, Leitner WW, Thalhamer J (2006) Is genetic vaccination against allergy possible? Int Arch Allergy Immunol 139(4):332–345

Weiss R, Scheiblhofer S, Thalhamer J, Bickert T, Richardt U, Fleischer B, Ritter U (2007) Epidermal inoculation of Leishmania-antigen by gold bombardment results in a chronic form of leishmaniasis. Vaccine 25(1):25–33

Weiss R, Scheiblhofer S, Roesler E, Ferreira F, Thalhamer J (2010) Prophylactic mRNA vaccination against allergy. Curr Opin Allergy Clin Immunol 10(6):567–574

Welch M, Govindarajan S, Ness JE, Villalobos A, Gurney A, Minshull J, Gustafsson C (2009) Design parameters to control synthetic gene expression in *Escherichia coli*. PLoS ONE 4(9):e7002

Wheeler M, Cortez-Gonzalez X, Frazzi R, Zanetti M (2006) Ex vivo programming of antigen-presenting B lymphocytes: considerations on DNA uptake and cell activation. Int Rev Immunol 25(3–4):83–97

Williams MA, Bevan MJ (2004) Shortening the infectious period does not alter expansion of CD8 T cells but diminishes their capacity to differentiate into memory cells. J Immunol 173(11):6694–6702

Winegar RA, Monforte JA, Suing KD, O'Loughlin KG, Rudd CJ, Macgregor JT (1996) Determination of tissue distribution of an intramuscular plasmid vaccine using PCR and in situ DNA hybridization. Hum Gene Ther 7(17):2185–2194

Wolff JA, Budker V (2005) The mechanism of naked DNA uptake and expression. Adv Genet 54:3–20

Wolff JA, Dowty ME, Jiao S, Repetto G, Berg RK, Ludtke JJ, Williams P, Slautterback DB (1992a) Expression of naked plasmids by cultured myotubes and entry of plasmids into T tubules and caveolae of mammalian skeletal muscle. J Cell Sci 103(Pt 4):1249–1259

Wolff JA, Ludtke JJ, Acsadi G, Williams P, Jani A (1992b) Long-term persistence of plasmid DNA and foreign gene expression in mouse muscle. Hum Mol Genet 1(6):363–369

Wolkers MC, Brouwenstijn N, Bakker AH, Toebes M, Schumacher TN (2004) Antigen bias in T cell cross-priming. Science 304(5675):1314–1317

Wu Y, Kipps TJ (1997) Deoxyribonucleic acid vaccines encoding antigens with rapid proteasome-dependent degradation are highly efficient inducers of cytolytic T lymphocytes. J Immunol 159(12):6037–6043

Xu ZL, Mizuguchi H, Ishii-Watabe A, Uchida E, Mayumi T, Hayakawa T (2001) Optimization of transcriptional regulatory elements for constructing plasmid vectors. Gene 272(1–2):149–156

Xu W, Chu Y, Zhang R, Xu H, Wang Y, Xiong S (2005) Endoplasmic reticulum targeting sequence enhances HBV-specific cytotoxic T lymphocytes induced by a CTL epitope-based DNA vaccine. Virology 334(2):255–263

Yamamoto M, Sato S, Mori K, Hoshino K, Takeuchi O, Takeda K, Akira S (2002) Cutting edge: a novel Toll/IL-1 receptor domain-containing adapter that preferentially activates the IFN-beta promoter in the Toll-like receptor signaling. J Immunol 169(12):6668–6672

Yamanaka H, Hoyt T, Yang X, Bowen R, Golden S, Crist K, Becker T, Maddaloni M, Pascual DW (2010) A parenteral DNA vaccine protects against pneumonic plague. Vaccine 28(18):3219–3230

Yamane I, Nishikawa M, Takakura Y (2005) Cellular uptake and activation characteristics of naked plasmid DNA and its cationic liposome complex in human macrophages. Int J Pharm 305(1–2):145–153

Yang P, An H, Liu X, Wen M, Zheng Y, Rui Y, Cao X (2010) The cytosolic nucleic acid sensor LRRFIP1 mediates the production of type I interferon via a beta-catenin-dependent pathway. Nat Immunol 11(6):487–494

Yew NS, Wang KX, Przybylska M, Bagley RG, Stedman M, Marshall J, Scheule RK, Cheng SH (1999) Contribution of plasmid DNA to inflammation in the lung after administration of cationic lipid:pDNA complexes. Hum Gene Ther 10(2):223–234

Yoneyama M, Fujita T (2008) Structural mechanism of RNA recognition by the RIG-I-like receptors. Immunity 29(2):178–181

Yoneyama M, Fujita T (2009) RNA recognition and signal transduction by RIG-I-like receptors. Immunol Rev 227(1):54–65

Yoshida A, Nagata T, Uchijima M, Higashi T, Koide Y (2000) Advantage of gene gun-mediated over intramuscular inoculation of plasmid DNA vaccine in reproducible induction of specific immune responses. Vaccine 18(17):1725–1729

Yoshinaga T, Yasuda K, Ogawa Y, Takakura Y (2002) Efficient uptake and rapid degradation of plasmid DNA by murine dendritic cells via a specific mechanism. Biochem Biophys Res Commun 299(3):389–394

Zhang W, Xiao W, Wei H, Zhang J, Tian Z (2006) mRNA secondary structure at start AUG codon is a key limiting factor for human protein expression in *Escherichia coli*. Biochem Biophys Res Commun 349(1):69–78

Zheng C, Juhls C, Oswald D, Sack F, Westfehling I, Wittig B, Babiuk LA, van Drunen Littel-van den Hurk S (2006) Effect of different nuclear localization sequences on the immune responses induced by a MIDGE vector encoding bovine herpesvirus-1 glycoprotein D. Vaccine 24(21):4625–4629

Zhou W, Cook RF, Cook SJ, Hammond SA, Rushlow K, Ghabrial NN, Berger SL, Montelaro RC, Issel CJ (2002) Multiple RNA splicing and the presence of cryptic RNA splice donor and acceptor sites may contribute to low expression levels and poor immunogenicity of potential DNA vaccines containing the env gene of equine infectious anemia virus (EIAV). Vet Microbiol 88(2):127–151

Zi XY, Yao YC, Zhu HY, Xiong J, Wu XJ, Zhang N, Ba Y, Li WL, Wang XM, Li JX, Yu HY, Ye XT, Lau JT, Hu YP (2006) Long-term persistence of hepatitis B surface antigen and antibody induced by DNA-mediated immunization results in liver and kidney lesions in mice. Eur J Immunol 36(4):875–886

Strategies to Improve DNA Vaccine Potency: HPV-Associated Cervical Cancer as a Model System

2

Chien-Fu Hung, Barbara Ma, Yijie Xu, and T.-C. Wu

Cancer immunotherapy, particularly antigen-specific immunotherapy, has become a potentially promising approach for control of cancer due to its ability to kill tumor cells without harming normal cells. Among different forms of antigen-specific immunotherapy, DNA vaccines are an attractive approach because of their safety, simplicity and ease of mass production. However, they suffer from low immunogenicity due to their inability to amplify and spread in vivo and therefore require innovative strategies to enhance the immune response stimulated by DNA vaccines. Strategies to improve DNA vaccine efficacy should focus on dendritic cells (DCs) because they are the most potent activators of an antigen-specific T cell response, which is crucial in the control of tumors. Increased understanding of DC biology has created opportunities to improve DNA vaccine potency through the applications of strategies that modify the function of DCs. In this review, we use human papillomavirus (HPV)-associated cervical cancer as a model system to illustrate the various strategies that improve DNA vaccine potency. Specifically, we will discuss the various strategies to improve targeting of DNA to DCs, antigen processing and presentation by DCs and DC interactions with T cells in this book chapter.

Introduction

Antigen-specific Immunotherapy for the Treatment of Cancers

Over the past decade, progress in the understanding of tumor biology and immunology has led to the development of cancer immunotherapy, which induces potent tumor-specific T cell-mediated or antibody-mediated immune responses. The field of cancer immunotherapy has progressed towards antigen-specific immunotherapy

---

T.-C. Wu (✉)
Department of Pathology, The Johns Hopkins University School of Medicine,
Baltimore, MD, USA
e-mail: wutc@jhmi.edu

J. Thalhamer et al. (eds.), *Gene Vaccines*,
DOI 10.1007/978-3-7091-0439-2_2, © Springer-Verlag/Wien, 2012

for the treatment of malignant disease for the following reasons. First, compared to other forms of cancer immunotherapy, antigen-specific immunotherapy has improved safety due to a decreased likelihood of non-specific autoimmunity. Second, it has more flexibility with antigen dosage and method of antigen presentation to the immune system. Third, the results of antigen-specific cancer immunotherapy may be more reproducible from patient to patient. Fourth, the use of specific antigens in this approach permits a correlation of clinical outcome to a specific immune response. Therefore, antigen-specific cancer immunotherapy is a potent approach for the control of tumors. The development of antigen-specific immunotherapy requires the identification of tumor-associated antigens, which are present on normal cells but overexpressed on tumor cells, or tumor-specific antigens, which are solely expressed by tumor cells. Identification of tumor-associated antigens and tumor-specific antigens in various cancers has spurred the development of several antigen-specific cancer vaccines.

HPV-associated Cervical Cancer as a Model for Antigen-specific Cancer Immunotherapy

Human papillomavirus (HPV)-associated cervical cancer represents one of the best model systems for the development of antigen-specific immunotherapy. HPV, classified into low- and high-risk types according to carcinogenicity, is a key etiological agent for cervical cancer and is present in 99.7% of all cervical cancers and their precursor lesions (Walboomers et al. 1999). Among the high-risk types, HPV-16 is most commonly present in cervical cancer, identified in nearly 60% of all tumors, while HPV-18 accounts for an additional 15% (Munoz et al. 2003). In cervical cancer and its precursor lesions, upregulation of the two viral oncogenic proteins, E6 and E7, which inactivate tumor suppressors p53 and Rb respectively, contribute to the tumor progression of HPV-associated malignancies [for review, see zur Hausen (2002)]. E6 and E7 are constitutively expressed in cervical cancer cells but not in normal cells and they play an essential role in cellular transformation of the malignant cell. Furthermore, E6 and E7 are foreign antigens and thus do not face the issue of tolerance. Thus, HPV E6 and E7 represent ideal targets for antigen-specific immunotherapy. Cervical cancer vaccines targeting HPV E6 and/or E7 antigens have been explored in several platforms such as live vector, protein, peptide, DNA, RNA, whole cell, or combinational treatments [for review, see Hung et al. (2008)].

DNA Vaccines as an Attractive Vaccination Approach

Among the different forms of antigen-specific cancer vaccines, DNA vaccines have emerged as an attractive approach for antigen-specific cancer immunotherapy due to their safety, simplicity and capacity for repeated administration. DNA immunization involves directly injecting plasmid DNA encoding the antigenic protein of interest into host cells, thereby causing the expression and presentation of the

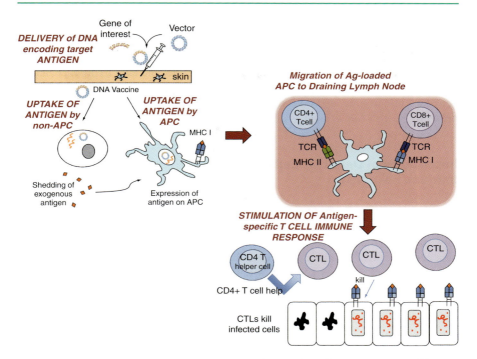

Fig. 2.1 Mechanism of DNA vaccine. A DNA vaccine consists of a gene sequence of interest inserted into a plasmid DNA vector. Conventionally, the vaccine is delivered intramuscularly via a microneedle. After cells uptake the plasmid DNA, the antigenic protein of interest is processed into peptides and presented by major histocompatibility (MHC) molecules on the cell surface. The plasmid can enter the nucleus of transfected muscle cells and resident antigen-presenting cells (APCs), such as dendritic cells. All nucleated cells, such as muscle cells and DCs, can present endogenous antigen via MHC class I molecules following direct transfection by DNA vaccine. Cross-presentation of exogenous antigens may also occur in APCs. For example, APCs may engulf apoptotic transfected cells and they may also mediate display of peptides on MHC II molecules after antigenic protein has been shed from transfected cells and captured and processed within the endocytic MHC class II pathway. The MHC:peptide complex then interacts with the T-cell receptor (TCR) of naïve T cells. CD8+ T cells are activated to become cytotoxic T lymphocytes (CTLs) and participate in the cytotoxic T-cell mediated immune response, in which the antigen-specific CTLs induce apoptosis in tumor cells expressing the antigen. MHC II complexes activate naïve CD4+ T cells into CD4+ T helper cells, which can augment CD8+ T cell immune responses by CD4+ T cell help

encoded antigen by transfected cells and subsequently stimulates cell-mediated and/or humoral immune responses against the encoded antigen (Fig. 2.1). Unlike tumor cell-based or live vector-based vaccines, DNA vaccines are relatively safe and do not pose intrinsic pathogenic risks of introducing a tumor cell, bacteria, or virus into a patient. In addition, DNA vaccines do not generate neutralizing antibodies like bacterial or viral vaccines and allow for multiple administrations. Their ease of production makes them more favorable than the labor-intensive, individual-specific dendritic cell-based vaccines. Additionally, they do not have the limitation of major histocompatibility complex (MHC) restriction associated with peptide-based vaccines. Furthermore, unlike protein-based vaccines, DNA vaccines mainly generate the cellular immunity, rather than humoral immunity, necessary for a therapeutic vaccine. However, while DNA vaccines are safe, stable, and easy to produce, naked DNA suffers from low immunogenicity, has limited capacity to amplify and spread between cells in vivo, and does not have specificity to directly target key antigen-presenting cells (APCs) such as dendritic cells (DCs).

Importance of Dendritic Cells for Potent Immune Responses

It is clear now that dendritic cells are the most potent activators of antigen-specific cell- and antibody-mediated immunities, which are essential for significant antitumor effects. Immature DCs located in the peripheral tissue uptake and process antigens and present the antigenic peptides on the cell surface via major histocompatibility (MHC) molecules. Transfected DCs undergo a maturation process and develop increased levels of MHC I, MHC II, and co-stimulatory molecules necessary to act as efficient professional antigen presenting cells (APCs). Mature DCs travel to lymphoid organs to activate antigen-specific naïve T cells. Through the presentation of antigens to naïve CD4+ and CD8+ T cells, DCs stimulate both cellular and humoral immune responses. Activated CD8+ T cells directly kill infected tumor cells while activated CD4+ T cells enhance the CD8+ T cell immune response and facilitate antibody-mediated immunity.

Therefore, strategies that target DNA directly to DCs or improve the uptake and presentation of DNA-encoded antigen may further augment the intrinsic advantages of DNA vaccines. In addition, strategies that are able to improve the antigen processing and presentation by the DCs will also improve the DNA vaccine potency. Furthermore, strategies that potentiate DC interaction with the T cells may also result in the enhanced priming of antigen-specific T cell immunity for boosting DNA vaccine potency. This chapter will review all these strategies to improve DNA vaccine potency for therapeutic vaccine development.

Strategies to Improve DNA Vaccine Potency Through Modification of DCs

Targeting DNA to DCs Through Different Delivery Methods

While DNA vaccines are conventionally administered intramuscularly or subcutaneously, novel modes of delivery have been developed. These methods include targeting the vaccine to DC-rich areas by gene gun, or encapsulating DNA vaccine in a microparticle or papillomavirus pseudovirion to enhance delivery of DNA to DCs while preventing DNA vaccine degradation. These DC-targeting DNA vaccine delivery approaches are summarized in Fig.2.2.

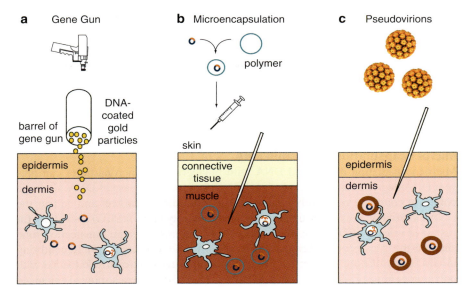

Fig. 2.2 Delivery methods to target vaccine to DCs. While DNA vaccines are traditionally delivered intramuscularly via a microneedle, novel routes of administration have focused on improving the transfection efficiency of vaccines by targeting the plasmids to DCs. (**a**) Gene gun. While the gene gun can administer DNA vaccines intramuscularly (IM), it generally delivers the vaccines intradermally. Pressurized helium delivers DNA-coated gold particles to the dermis, which contains more immature DCs than muscle tissue, to enhance the vaccine uptake. (**b**) Microencapsulation. An IM injection delivers a biodegradable polymer encapsulating the DNA plasmid of interest. The polymer prevents the degradation of the DNA by nucleases and allows for sustained release of the vaccine. (**c**) Pseudovirions. Non-replicative HPV pseudovirions containing DNA vaccine can be delivered by subcutaneous injection into the infected cell. Since HPV pseudovirions lack the viral genome, they lack many of the safety concerns associated with live viral vectors. They can efficiently infect DCs to deliver encoded gene

Gene Gun

One of the most efficient routes of administration of DNA vaccines is intradermal vaccination via the gene gun, which traditionally utilizes compressed helium to deliver DNA-coated gold particles to immature DCs (Langerhans cells) in the epidermis. After transfection, the DCs mature, travel to lymphoid organs, and prime T cells for an adaptive immune response. Compared to intramuscular injection, which targets the vaccine to muscle tissue with fewer immature DCs, the gene gun is more dose-efficient (Trimble et al. 2003). Currently, there is an ongoing clinical trial utilizing clinical grade gene gun device containing therapeutic HPV DNA vaccine to treat high-grade cervical intraepithelial neoplasia (CIN) lesions in HPV-positive patients (NCT00988559).

Recently, a low-pressured gene gun has been used to deliver non-carrier naked DNA (without coating DNA on gold particles). A DNA vaccine encoding calreticulin linked to E7 delivered by non-carrier system generated similar E7-specific immunity and antitumor effects as gold particle-mediated vaccination. More importantly, the vaccine delivered via low-pressured gene gun generated no definite skin damage after vaccination compared to significant local skin damage caused by the vaccine delivered by gold particle-mediated gene gun (Chen et al. 2009). The same gene gun device has also been used to deliver plasmid therapeutic HPV E7 DNA vaccine encapsulated into poly(methyl methacrylate) synthetic polymer, which was shown to generate better protective antitumor effects against E7-expressing tumors compared to naked DNA (Lou et al. 2009).

Microencapsulation of Plasmid DNA

Microencapsulation of plasmid DNA with biodegradable microparticles can prevent DNA degradation by nucleases and allow for gradual release of DNA. Cationic polymers condense negatively charged DNA molecules to protect and deliver the DNA effectively. Polymers such as poly(lactide-co-glycolide) (PLG) also allow for sustained release of DNA for up to a month, which increases the transfection time and thus the transfection efficiency in vivo (Storrie and Mooney 2006). Recently, an in vitro study of poly(D,L-lactide-co-glycolide) (PGLA) microparticle loaded with polyamidoamine (PAMAM)-plasmid DNA (pDNA) dendriplexes showed enhanced pDNA loading onto the microparticle, reduced particle size, and increased transfection efficiency compared to PGLA loaded with pDNA alone (Intra and Salem 2009).

Microencapsulation has been evaluated in several clinical trials (Gnjatic et al. 2009; Cassaday et al. 2007; Klencke et al. 2002; Sheets et al. 2003; Garcia et al. 2004). A plasmid encoding a HPV-16 E7 HLA-A2 restricted peptide encapsulated in 1–2 µm microparticles composed of PLG (ZYC101) has been used in a Phase I clinical trial for anal dysplasia. Ten of twelve patients generated E7-specific immune responses and three out of twelve showed histological improvements (Klencke et al. 2002). Another Phase I trial studied the effect of ZYC101 on patients with high-grade cervical intraepithelial neoplasia. Five of fifteen patients experienced complete histological regression and eleven showed significant HPV-specific T cell responses with no serious adverse effects (Sheets et al. 2003). A more recent version encoding HPV-16 and 18 E6 and E7 fragments encapsulated in PLG (ZYC101a) was used in a Phase II clinical trial involving 127 subjects with high-grade cervical intraepithelial neoplasia (CIN2/3). The vaccine was well tolerated and promoted CIN2/3 resolution in patients under 25 years of age compared to the placebo group (70% versus 23%) (Garcia et al. 2004).

An overview on non-viral pharmacological formulations of DNA and its application in the clinics can be found in Chaps. 5 and 6 of this book.

HPV Pseudovirions

HPV pseudovirions have recently emerged as an innovative mode of delivery for DNA vaccines in vivo. The latest technological advances enable the use of papillomavirus capsid proteins to package DNA plasmids to generate a "pseudovirion" that can efficiently deliver the DNA into the infected cell. The capsid proteins of HPV confer tropism for the basal epithelium. As these HPV pseudovirions lack the viral

2 Strategies to Improve DNA Vaccine Potency: HPV-Associated Cervical Cancer

genome, they are non-replicative and do not have the safety concerns associated with viral vectors. Improvements in the pseudovirion preparation methods now allow for the generation of high-titers of infectious HPV pseudovirions for cutaneous vaccination (Buck et al. 2004, 2005). It has been shown that mucosal delivery of human papillomavirus pseudovirions encapsidating DNA plasmids expressing an experimental antigen derived from M and M2 proteins of respiratory syncytial virus led to local and systemic M-M2-specific CD8+ T cell and antibody responses that were comparable to a ~10,000-fold higher dose of naked DNA in vaccinated mice (Graham et al. 2010). In addition, HPV pseudovirions carrying DNA encoding model antigen ovalbumin (OVA) were shown to generate significantly stronger antigen-specific CD8+ T cell immune responses compared with intradermal vaccination with naked OVA DNA. HPV pseudovirions can also efficiently infect bone marrow-derived DCs in vitro and can lead to the expression of the encapsulated DNA in the draining lymph nodes. Furthermore, HPV pseudovirions carrying DNA encoding OVA were able to generate strong protective antitumor effects against OVA-expressing tumors in vaccinated mice (Peng et al. 2010). Thus, HPV pseudovirions represent a highly efficient and promising method for DNA vaccine delivery in vivo.

The use of viral particles and pseudovirions as well as self-replicating viral RNAs and DNAs is also discussed in Chap. 3 of this book.

Strategies to Facilitate Uptake of Antigen Encoded by DNA Vaccine into DCs

Other important approaches for increasing the number of DCs that can present the antigen to T cells are the strategies that can lead to the increased uptake of antigen encoded by DNA into the DCs. These strategies include linking the antigen to molecules that can bind with molecules expressed on DCs or to molecules that can spread antigen to surrounding DCs. Additionally, strategies to facilitate the release of antigen from transfected cells will release more antigen into the DC milieu. Furthermore, physical methods such as electroporation and femtosecond laser can enhance the transfection efficiency of DNA vaccines to generate more antigen in transfected cells, resulting in an increase in number of antigen-loaded DCs (Fig. 2.3).

Linking Antigen to DC-Targeting Molecules

One strategy to enhance DNA vaccine potency by improving the uptake of antigens by DCs is to link the antigen with factors that target molecules on the surface of the DCs. For example, FMS-like tyrosine kinase 3 (Flt3) ligand can bind to Flt3 ligand receptors on the surface of DCs. It has been shown that a DNA vaccine of HPV-16 E7 linked to the extracellular domain of Flt3 ligand significantly enhanced E7-specific CD8+ T cell response and antitumor effects in mice compared to wild type E7 (Hung et al. 2001c). Another molecule of interest is CTLA4, which is a ligand for B7 molecules expressed on the surface of DCs. Recently, it has been

Fig. 2.3 Physical methods to increase DNA-encoded antigen uptake by DCs. (**a**) Electroporation. In electroporation, two needle electrodes carry an electrical current to the cells in the muscle layer. The current renders the cell membrane of DCs temporarily permeable, allowing DNA plasmid to enter the cell easily. (**b**) Laser treatment. Laser treatments have similar mechanistic actions as electroporation. A femtosecond laser targeted towards the muscle allows the membrane of DCs to be permeable temporarily to plasmid DNA, thus increasing the transfection efficiency

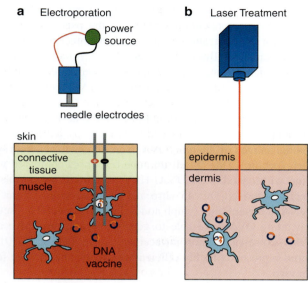

demonstrated that DNA vaccine encoding hepatitis B surface antigen fused to extracellular domain of CTLA4 elicited enhanced antigen-specific CD8+ cytotoxic T cell as well as CD4+ T cell immune responses (Zhou et al. 2010).

Heat shock protein 70 (HSP70) has also been explored extensively as a molecule of interest in targeting antigen to DCs. HSP70 is capable of binding to scavenger receptors such as CD91 on the surface of DCs. Furthermore, HSP70 can target the linked antigen to the MHC class I cross-presentation pathway of DCs for efficient antigen processing and presentation (Hauser and Chen 2003). It has been shown that a DNA vaccine of HPV-16 E7 linked to secretory HSP70 strongly enhanced E7-specific CD8+ T cell response as well as generated enhanced antibody responses (Hauser et al. 2004). This strategy has been applied to several antigenic systems including E7 linked to Mycobacterium tuberculosis HSP70 (Chen et al. 2000), E7 linked to mouse HSP70 (Li et al. 2006), malarial antigen EB200 linked to *Plasmodium falciparum* HSP70 (Qazi et al. 2005) and MAGE-1 linked to Mycobacterium tuberculosis HSP70 (Ye et al. 2004), and generated enhanced antigen-specific CD8+ T cell immune responses. Likewise, DNA encoding a fusion of heat shock protein 60 and HPV-16 E6 and E7 showed significantly enhanced E6- and E7-specific CD8+ T cell responses in mice (Huang et al. 2007b).

The Fc portion of immunoglobulin G represents another DC-targeting molecule of interest. Linkage of antigen to IgG Fc fragment can target antigen to Fc receptors on the surface of DCs. In this manner, antigen-Fc complexes can be internalized by DCs for increased vaccine immunogenicity. It has been shown that a recombinant DNA vaccine of a model hepatitis B viral antigen linked to the Fc portion of the IgG antibody generated significantly higher levels of antigen-specific CD4+ T cells as well as higher levels of antigen-specific CD8+ T cells (You et al. 2001). It has also

2 Strategies to Improve DNA Vaccine Potency: HPV-Associated Cervical Cancer 45

been shown that this strategy can be further enhanced by linkage to a secondary lymphoid tissue chemokine (SLC), which can promote co-clustering of T cells and DCs in the lymph nodes and spleen for increased potential to induce T cell immune responses. It has been shown that linking a SLC and Fc gene to each end of E7 generated much stronger E7-specific CD8+ T cell immune responses than control DNA and generated strong protective and therapeutic antitumor effects (Liu et al. 2006). This linkage of antigen to Fc and SLC has been applied to other tumor-associated antigens including PSA-PSM-PAP, Her-2/neu, p53, and hTERT. In these systems, including HPV-16 E7 antigenic system, linkage of antigen to the SLC CCR7 and the IgG Fc fragment was able to attract CCR7+ T cells, B cells, NK cells and DCs to the injection site, inhibit tumor growth and prolong survival in tumor-bearing mice (Zhang and Zhang 2008). Methods that target DCs by linking antigen to molecules on the surface of DCs represent a promising way to improve DNA vaccine potency.

Intercellular Antigen Spread

One key disadvantage of DNA vaccines is their poor ability to spread the antigen to surrounding cells in vivo. Fusion of the antigen of interest with a protein capable of intercellular spread may overcome this obstacle and improve vaccine efficacy. The herpes simplex virus type 1 (HSV-1) tegument protein, VP22, is a transport protein capable of efficient entry into the nuclei of surrounding cells (Elliott and O'Hare 1997). Linkage of HSV-1 VP22 with green fluorescent protein (Elliott and O'Hare 1997, p. 53; Phelan et al. 1998), HSV thymidine kinase (Dilber et al. 1999), and *E. coli* cytosine deaminase (Wybranietz et al. 2001) have demonstrated the potential of VP22 as a transport protein to enhance transfection rates. In all cases, the linked protein of interest was transported to the nuclei of adjacent cells. While some investigators have raised concerns on the validity of VP22's intercellular spreading effect (Lundberg and Johansson 2001), it has been demonstrated that a fusion of VP22 and HPV-16 E7 enhanced antigen spread and generated a 50-fold increase of E7-specific CD8+ T cell precursors compared to fusions of mutant nonspreading VP22 and HPV-16 E7 (Hung et al. 2001a). Kim et al. have shown that a HSV-1 VP22 and HPV-16 E7 fusion DNA vaccine increased the number of E7-expressing DCs and enhanced E7-specific CD8+ T cell response in mice due to improved MHC class I presentation. An increase in the number of E7-specific CD8+ memory T cells and enhanced E7-specific protective antitumor immunity were also observed compared to vaccination with E7 alone (Kim et al. 2004).

While most studies involving VP22 have focused on the HSV-1 derivative, analogous tegument proteins from other viruses have also been used in DNA therapeutic vaccines. VP22 derived from Marek's disease virus type 1 (MDV-1) (Hung et al. 2002) and bovine herpes virus 1 (BHV-1) (Mwangi et al. 2005; Zheng et al. 2006) have exhibited similar intercellular transport properties and enhanced immunogenicity of DNA vaccines. A fusion DNA vaccine of BHV-1 VP22 and truncated glycoprotein D (tgD) generated significantly stronger tgD-specific immune responses and improved immune protection in cattle, showing VP22's potential to help overcome the poor efficacy of DNA vaccines in large animals (Zheng et al.

2005). Since qualitative differences exist between VP22 from different viruses (Harms et al. 2000), further study is needed on the different VP22 and other potential proteins to find the optimal transporter protein to enhance DNA vaccine efficacy.

Increase Release of Tumor Antigen from Transfected Cells

The release of tumor antigen from transfected cells in the DC milieu may facilitate an increase in antigen uptake by DCs. Generally, intracellular and extracellular antigens are processed via MHC class I and class II pathways, respectively. However, extracellular antigens may be presented by MHC class I molecules to prime naïve CD8+ T cells in a mechanism known as cross-priming. During the conventional intramuscular injection of DNA vaccines, cross-priming is largely responsible for the antigen-specific immune response because myocytes generally lack MHC II molecules necessary for presentation through the MHC class II pathway. A previous study has shown that DCs recruited to local tissue can activate CD8+ T cells through cross-priming (Le Borgne et al. 2006). Therefore, strategies to facilitate increased release of tumor antigen from transfected cells may enhance DNA vaccine potency through cross priming mechanisms. Recently, Kang et al. found that intramuscular administration of calreticulin linked to HPV-16 E7 (CRT/E7) coadministered with DNA encoding human MHC class I molecules HLA-A2 generated significantly higher levels of E7-specific CD8+ T cells and better antitumor effects than CRT/E7 alone. Coadministration of DNA encoding other xenogenic MHC class I molecules yielded similarly elevated E7-specific CD8+ T cell levels (Kang et al. 2009). The use of xenogenic MHC class I molecules enhanced cross-priming by inducing local inflammation and antigen release by myocytes. In addition, it was recently found that intramuscular administration by electroporation of HPV-16 E7 DNA vaccine coadministered with DNA encoding viral fusogenic membrane glycoprotein VSV G elicited robust E7-specific CD8+ T cell responses and therapeutic antitumor effects against E7-expressing tumors (Mao et al. 2010). It was shown that VSV G could couple concentrated antigen transfer to DCs with local induction of the acute inflammatory response. Furthermore, VSV G was found to lead to increased transfected cell death through mainly nonapoptotic mechanisms, provoke leukocyte infiltration into the inoculation site, enhance cross-presentation of antigen to DCs, and stimulate DCs to mature efficiently. Thus, the promoted release of tumor antigen from transfected cells holds promise for improving DNA vaccine potency.

Physical Methods to Enhance Transfection Efficiency of DNA Vaccine

After delivery, inefficient transfection in situ may also limit vaccine efficacy. Antigen uptake by DCs may be improved by increasing the membrane permeability of DCs via electroporation, in which a small electric current at the injection site results in a temporarily more permeable membrane that allows DNA to enter the cell. In addition to increasing DNA uptake, electroporation may also cause inflammation, which augments the innate immune response for a more immunogenic DNA vaccine. In a study comparing intramuscular injection (IM), IM followed by electroporation, and intradermal gene gun delivery methods of a DNA vaccine linking calreticulin and HPV-16 E7, electroporation generated the most E7-specific CD8+ T cells and the longest sustained anti-tumor response (Best et al. 2009). Although DNA vaccines have traditionally been more effective in mice than in larger animals due to their low transfection efficiency, electroporation has improved vaccine efficacy for large animals (Babiuk et al. 2002; Otten et al. 2004; Scheerlinck et al. 2004). Current studies have also focused on intradermal electroporation, which targets DC-rich areas and is more tolerable than intramuscular delivery, to improve the method for clinical use (Roos et al. 2009). Electroporation in conjunction with intramuscular injection of DNA encoding TAA has been evaluated in several clinical trials (NCT00471133, NCT00685412, NCT00859729, NCT01064375). More details about in vivo electroporation can be found in Chaps. 7 and 8 of this book.

Likewise, laser treatments can also enhance transfection rates for effective intradermal naked DNA delivery. A laser beam delivers a focused amount of energy to a cell in order to increase membrane permeability thermally and transiently. Treatment with the femtosecond infrared titanium sapphire laser and plasmid showed stronger cellular and humoral immune responses than plasmid vaccination alone (Zeira et al. 2007). A more recent study also confirmed the femtosecond lasers' ability to significantly enhance intradermal and intratumoral transfection efficiencies of DNA vaccines. Furthermore, use of reduced laser focusing increased the transfection area as well as decreased tissue damage (Tsen et al. 2009). Despite the limited number of studies, laser treatment has a high potential in enhancing DNA vaccine efficacy due to its precise control and safety. The physical methods to enhance transfection efficiency of DNA vaccine are depicted in Fig. 2.3.

Employment of Methods to Improve Antigen Expression, Processing and Presentation in DCs

Strategies to increase the expression, processing and presentation of antigen in DCs can enhance the immunogenicity of DNA vaccines. Methods to enhance the expression of encoded antigen on DCs have involved the use of codon optimization or the use of demethylating agents. As antigen is presented on MHC molecules to activate antigen-specific T cells, a strategy to increase MHC class I and MHC class II transcription and subsequently expression on the surface of DCs may further enhance the activation of antigen-specific T cell immunity. In addition, strategies that enhance antigen processing and presentation through the MHC class I and/or MHC class II pathways can lead to the activation of larger populations of antigen-specific T cells and the generation of stronger antitumor immunity.

Enhancing Antigen Expression

Some strategies to enhance DNA vaccine potency focus on increasing levels of expression of the antigens of interest. Codon optimization replaces rare codons with ones more commonly recognized by the host without changing the amino acid sequence to enhance genetic translation. Synthetic HPV-16 E7 gene containing preferred human codons showed up to 100-fold increase in E7 protein expression than wild type E7 (Cid-Arregui et al. 2003). While the protein's half-life remained unchanged, the enhanced E7 had a more stable mRNA for enhanced translation and induced E7-specific antibody responses (Cid-Arregui et al. 2003). A DNA plasmid encoding HPV-16 L1 and codon-optimized E7 induced stronger cytotoxic and antibody responses than the wild type L1E7 vaccine (Cheung et al. 2004). Furthermore, a DNA vaccine encoding codon-optimized HPV-16 E6 also showed significantly enhanced E6-specific CD8+ T cell responses (Lin et al. 2006).

Another strategy to enhance antigen expression involves the use of demethylating agents. Methylation of CpG motifs has been shown to silence gene expression (Hirasawa et al. 2006). As a result, demethylation of genes encoding the antigen of interest may upregulate gene expression and thus antigen presentation. Use of 5-aza-2′-deoxycystidine (DAC), a demethylating agent, inhibits DNA methyltransferase and upregulates the expression of previously methylated genes (Suzuki et al. 2002). In mice, DAC treatment followed by a recombinant DNA vaccine of calreticulin and HPV-16 E7 (CRT/E7) showed enhanced E7-specific CD8+ T cell responses and antitumor effects than CRT/E7 alone (Lu et al. 2009).

Enhancing MHC Class I Presentation

MHC class I processing pathway presents endogenous antigen to naïve CD8+ T cells and induces a cellular immune response (Fig. 2.4). Intracellular antigen is degraded by the proteasome into short peptides and then sent to the endoplasmic reticulum (ER). Inside the ER, the peptide binds to a MHC class I molecule and forms a complex, which then travels to the cell surface to induce CD8+ T cell immune responses. Since CD8+ T cell immunity is important for antitumor effects, enhancing MHC class I presentation may increase vaccine immunogenicity.

Since endogenous antigens must be degraded by proteasomes before binding to MHC class I molecules, the rate of degradation by the ubiquitin-proteasome pathway influences MHC class I presentation (Grant et al. 1995). Therefore, linking antigens to molecules, such as ubiquitin, that target them to proteasomes stimulates a stronger immune response (Tobery and Siliciano 1997). One molecule, γ-tubulin, targets the molecule to the centrosome, a proteasome-rich organelle. Unlike wide type E7, HPV-16 E7 linked to γ-tubulin congregates at the centrosome instead of the cytoplasm and the nucleus. The linked vaccine generated a significantly stronger E7-specific CD8+ response than E7 alone (Hung et al. 2003). In addition, a DNA vaccine conjugating HPV-16 E7 with the coat protein of the potato virus X decreased antigen stability and increased degradation rate. The vaccine induced both E7-specific CD4+ and CD8+ T cell responses and inhibited tumor growth in mice (Massa et al. 2008).

MHC class I processing can also be enhanced by linking the antigen to a protein that targets to the ER. Calreticulin (CRT) is a binding protein in the ER that associates with peptides delivered into the ER by transporters for loading of MHC class I molecules. Vaccination of DNA encoding HPV-16 E7 linked with CRT generated stronger E7-specific CD8+ T cell responses than wild type E7 and demonstrated antitumor effects against existing tumors in mice (Cheng et al. 2001). A study of HPV-16 E6 linked with CRT demonstrated similarly enhanced cellular immunity

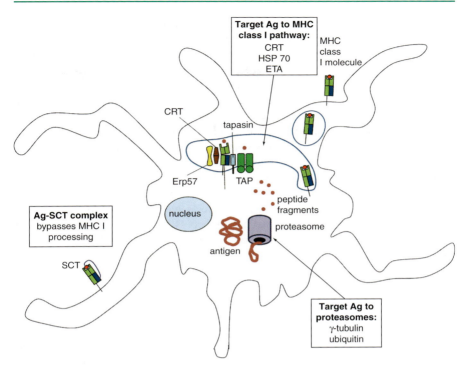

Fig. 2.4 Strategies to enhance MHC I processing and presentation. Endogenous antigens are presented by major histocompatibility class I (MHC I) molecules to prime CD8+ naïve T cells. In this pathway, proteasomes first degrade the antigenic protein into short peptides. Certain molecules, such as γ-tubulin and ubiquitin, target toward proteasomes and increase the rate of degradation of proteins. After degradation, the antigenic peptides (Ag) are transported into the endoplasmic reticulum (ER) by transporters associated with antigen processing (TAP) proteins. Certain proteins, such as calreticulin (CRT), heat shock protein (HSP) 70, and exotoxin A of *P. aeruginosa* (ETA), target linked molecules toward the ER. Inside the ER, the antigen binds with an empty MHC class I molecule through the help of chaperone proteins such as Erp57, CRT, and tapasin. After binding, peptide:MHC I complex travels to the cell surface for antigen presentation. DNA vaccines encoding a stable single chain trimer (SCT) of MHC I:peptide complex bypasses the MHC class I processing pathway completely in generating an immune response

and antitumor effects (Peng et al. 2004). A DNA vaccine encoding fusion of HPV-16 E6, E7, and L2 generated significant protective and therapeutic effects in mice, showing CRT's potential in enhancing both prophylactic and therapeutic vaccines (Kim et al. 2008a). Furthermore, DNA vaccine encoding antigen linked to ER insertion sequence (Ciernik et al. 1996) or translocation domain of bacteria *Pseudomonas aeruginosa* exotoxin A (Hung et al. 2001b) can also enhance MHC class I presentation of the antigen and improve DNA vaccine potency.

Several clinical trials have studied the effects of vaccines designed to improve MHC class I processing. A Phase I clinical trial involving 15 patients with high grade cervical intraepithelial neoplasia (CIN2/3) intramuscularly injected with

DNA encoding HPV-16 E7 and heat shock protein 70 (pNGVL4a-Sig/E7(detox)/HSP70) showed increased E7-specific T cell responses in eight patients. While the vaccine was well tolerated, subjects treated with the vaccine did not experience significantly enhanced therapeutic antitumor effects compared to unvaccinated subjects (Trimble et al. 2009). The same vaccine has also been used in patients with HPV-16+ head and neck cancer (Gillison and Wu, Personal communication). It is now clear that approximately 20% of head and neck cancers is associated with HPV, particularly HPV-16 [for review, see Chung and Gillison (2009)]. These early phase clinical trials demonstrate great safety without significant side effects. However, the immunogenicity of the HPV-16 E7-specific immune responses can be best appreciated in patients receiving the highest dose of DNA vaccine (Trimble et al. 2009). The results of the early phase clinical trials indicate that prime-boost with different expression vectors or delivery methods such as electroporation or intradermal administration via gene gun may be further necessary to increase DNA vaccine potency. An ongoing Phase I clinical trial involving women with grade 3 cervical intraepithelial neoplasia will investigate a prime-boost strategy combined with topical imiquimod to enhance immunogenicity. The subjects will be intramuscularly primed with pNGVL4a-Sig/E7(detox)/HSP70 and then boosted with a recombinant vaccinia virus encoding HPV-16 and 18 E6 and E7 (TA-HPV). Prime-boost strategies are discussed in depth in Chap. 9 of this book. Imiquimod, which may enhance DC activation, will also be applied topically to some patients to evaluate its ability to enhance immune responses (NCT00788164). As imiquimod is a TLR agonist and can enhance local inflammation to attract antigen-specific immune cells to the area of application, it represents a potentially promising adjuvant for DNA vaccines. Another ongoing clinical trial is a head-to-head comparison of the immunogenicity of three routes of administration (intradermal administration via gene gun, intramuscular administration, and intralesional delivery) of DNA vaccine encoding HPV-16 E7 and calreticulin (pNGVL4a-CRT/E7(detox)) in women with HPV-16+ high grade cervical intraepithelial neoplasia (NCT00988559). For safety reasons, the vaccines used in the above trials involve a mutated, non-oncogenic form of HPV-16 E7 (E7(detox)).

Bypassing MHC Class I Processing

The loading of antigen onto MHC class I molecules is a complex process with many steps of regulation (Fig. 2.4). These steps include degradation of antigen into antigenic peptides by the proteasome, entry of antigenic peptide into the ER by TAP proteins, formation of MHC class I complex by chaperone proteins, and sufficiently strong binding of antigen into MHC class I to be transported to the cell surface for antigen presentation. Any of these steps may affect the efficiency of the antigenic peptide to be presented by the MHC class I molecule on the surface of the APC. Therefore, a method to bypass MHC class I processing can allow for direct presentation of antigenic peptide through the MHC class I molecule on the surface of APCs will circumvent issues associated with antigen processing for significant enhancement of DNA vaccine potency to activate CD8+ T cell antitumor immunity.

One strategy to bypass MHC class I processing altogether is through the generation of a stable MHC class I molecule and peptide complex. A single chain trimer (SCT) comprised of an antigenic peptide linked to β_2 microglobulin and MHC class I heavy chain imitates the orientation of noncovalently-linked MHC complexes and increases the stability of the complex. A DNA vaccine encoding HPV-16 E6 peptide linked to β_2 microglobulin and H2-K^b-restricted MHC class I heavy chain SCT has been shown to stably express the molecules of transfected cells and was capable of activating E6-specific CD8+ T cell response compared to a wild type E6 vaccine (Huang et al. 2005). More importantly, vaccination with HPV-16 E6 peptide SCT intradermally via gene gun has been shown to result in potent E6-specific CD8+ T cell immune responses as well as antitumor effects against E6-expressing tumors in vaccinated mice. However, since DNA vaccine encoding SCT only effectively presents one antigenic peptide with a specific MHC class I molecule, it may not be applicable to a genetically outbred population with different MHC class I molecules. One potential solution is to combine multiple DNA vaccines encoding SCT comprised of highly immunogenic peptides linked to different MHC class I molecules that are highly prevalent in the general population.

Enhancing MHC Class II Antigen Presentation

The MHC class II processing pathway presents exogenous antigens to CD4+ T cells. In the ER, a MHC class II molecule binds to an invariant chain, whose class II-associated invariant-chain peptide (CLIP) region lies within the peptide-binding groove of the MHC molecule. The MHC class II then leaves the ER in an endosome where the Ii is clipped, leaving only CLIP. Meanwhile, exogenous antigens enter the cell via endosomes and are degraded into peptides. The two endosomes containing degraded peptides and MHC class II molecule respectively fuse into one vesicle. A chaperone protein, HLA-DM, then causes the MHC class II molecule to release CLIP and allows the antigenic peptide to bind to MHC class II. The peptide-MHC complex then travels to the cell surface and activates naïve CD4+ T cells to become activated T helper cells. These cells can then help activate macrophages or B cells to stimulate both cellular and humoral immunity.

Since activated CD4+ T cells help in the priming of CD8+ T cells, therapeutic DNA vaccines should also consider strategies to improve MHC class II antigen presentation to enhance vaccine immunogenicity (Fig. 2.5). It has been well established that the endosomal and lysosomal compartments are important sites for MHC class II presentation. The lysosomal-associated membrane protein (LAMP-1) is a transmembrane protein that is an important landmark molecule in the endosomal/lysosomal compartment. LAMP-1 contains a sorting signal located on its cytoplasmic domain that is responsible for the targeting of LAMP-1 to the endosomal and lysosomal compartments. A recombinant vaccinia-based vaccine encoding HPV-16 E7 linked to the sorting signal of LAMP-1 (Sig/E7/LAMP-1) rerouted the E7 protein from the original cytoplasmic/nuclear location into the endosomal/lysosomal compartment, resulting in MHC class II presentation of E7 to CD4+ T helper cells (Wu et al. 1995; Lin et al. 1996). Furthermore, vaccination with DNA encoding Sig/E7/LAMP-1 showed significantly improved E7-specific CD4+ and CD8+ T cell

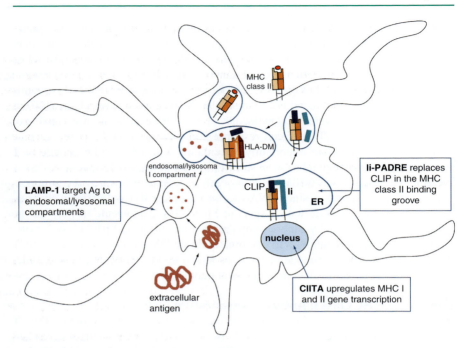

Fig. 2.5 Strategies to enhance MHC II processing and presentation. Exogenous antigens are presented by major histocompatibility class II (MHC II) molecules to prime CD4+ naïve T cells. The MHC class II transactivator (CIITA) gene regulates the creation of MHC I and II molecules. A newly synthesized MHC class II molecule in the ER contains an invariant chain (Ii), whose class II-associated invariant chain peptide (CLIP) region lies within the MHC binding groove. Replacement of CLIP with invariant Pan HLA-DR reactive epitope (Ii-PADRE) inside the ER generates strong PADRE-specific CD4+ responses once the MHC II:PADRE complex is exported. Otherwise, MHC II:CLIP leaves the ER in an endosome, where Ii is cleaved to leave only CLIP. Meanwhile, extracellular proteins enter the cell via endosomes and are degraded into peptides inside lysosomes. The sorting signal of the lysosomal-associated membrane protein (LAMP-1) targets to endosomal/lysosomal compartments and promotes the MHC II processing pathway. After degradation, the endosome containing the antigenic peptides (Ag) fuses with the endosome containing MHC II. A chaperone protein, HLA-DM, then causes CLIP to dissociate and allows the peptide to bind. The fully-assembled MHC II molecule is then transported to the cell surface to prime CD4+ naïve T cells

immune responses as well as potent antitumor effects in vaccinated mice (Ji et al. 1999). Thus, a strategy to enhance MHC class II antigen presentation can potentially be used to improve DNA vaccine potency.

Enhancing MHC Class I and II Transcription

Because the level of expression of MHC class I and II molecules on the surface of APCs is important for the activation of antigen-specific CD4+ and CD8+ T cells, a strategy to enhance MHC class I and II expression will potentially lead to improved vaccine potency. MHC class II transactivator (CIITA) is a well known master regulator of MHC class I and II expression and can increase MHC class I and II expression on transfected cells. It has been shown that HPV-16 E6 DNA vaccine coadministered with DNA encoding CIITA led to increased MHC I and MHC II expression on transfected cells, induced a stronger E6-specific CD8+ and CD4+ T cell immune responses, and prolonged survival of E6-expressing tumor-bearing mice compared to vaccination with DNA encoding E6 alone (Kim et al. 2008b).

Vaccine-Potentiating Strategies to Enhance DC and T cell Interaction

The maturation and activation of DCs is crucial for efficient priming of antigen-specific T cells. It is widely accepted that several Toll-like receptor (TLR) ligands, as well as cytokines, have been shown to be important for the activation of DCs and therefore represent a potential focus for improving DC and T cell interaction. Furthermore, strategies to prolong DC life or eliminate immunosuppressive factors in the microenvironment of DC and T cell interaction also serve as an important method to improve DNA vaccine potency. Likewise, approaches that lead to prolonged T cell survival and provide CD4+ T cell help have been used to enhance T cell priming to improve DNA vaccine potency. These strategies are discussed in the following.

Utilizing Adjuvants to Activate DCs

Since activated DCs are most effective in priming naïve T cells, promotion of DC activation and maturation may enhance vaccine efficacy. DCs contain TLRs that recognize different pathogenic characteristics, trigger innate immunity, and stimulate DC maturation in presence of TLR ligands [for review, see Iwasaki and Medzhitov (2004)]. Therefore, TLR ligands, such as lipopolysaccharide (LPS), double stranded RNA, or unmethylated DNA, may serve as adjuvants to activate DCs for the enhancement of vaccine potency. For example, imiquimod, a TLR7 ligand, has been shown to enhance DNA vaccination. Recently, Chuang et al. demonstrated that intradermal vaccination via gene gun of DNA vaccine encoding calreticulin (CRT) linked to HPV-16 E7 (CRT/E7) in combination with topical administration of imiquimod at the tumor site led to enhanced E7-specific CD8+ T cell immune responses, potent antitumor effects in E7-expressing tumor-bearing mice, and prolonged survival in treated mice (Chuang et al. 2010). Furthermore, treatment with imiquimod led to a decrease in the number of myeloid-derived suppressor cells and an increase in F4.80+ and NK1.1+ cells in the tumor microenvironment, implicating the role of macrophages and natural killer cells in antitumor effects mediated by treatment with imiquimod combined with therapeutic CRT/E7 DNA vaccine (Chuang et al. 2010). These preclinical results have translated to clinical studies. As mentioned above, a Phase I clinical trial is ongoing in CIN 3 patients primed with pNGVL4a-Sig/E7(detox)/HSP70 DNA vaccine, boosted with a recombinant vaccinia virus encoding HPV-16 and 18 E6 and E7

(TA-HPV) and topically administered with imiquimod on the CIN lesion (NCT00788164).

TLR-mediated cell activation proceeds through two distinct pathways. The first pathway depends on an adaptor molecule, myeloid differentiation factor 88 (MyD88) that transduces downstream events leading to nuclear factor κB (NF-κB) activation. MyD88-dependent pathway is triggered by TLR2, TLR4, TLR5, TLR7, TLR8, and TLR9. In contrast, the MyD88-independent pathway is mediated by Toll-IL-1 receptor domain-containing adaptor-inducing IFN-ß (TRIF) and the TRIF-related adaptor molecule (TRAM). Overexpression of these TLR adaptor molecules is proven to turn on downstream cellular signaling in the absence of TLRs or TLR ligands; thus, these TLR-adaptor molecules can also be used as genetic adjuvants. For example, a DNA vaccine encoding HPV-16 E7 linked to TRIF adaptor molecule has been shown to generate protective antitumor effects against E7-expressing tumors (Takeshita et al. 2006).

Another adjuvant to enhance DNA vaccine potency is the natural killer T cell ligand alpha-galactosylceramide (alpha-GalCer). It has been shown that priming with DNA encoding HPV-16 E7 combined with alpha-GalCer and boosting with E7-pulsed DC-1 dendritic cells led to a significant enhancement of E7-specific CD8+ effector and memory T-cells as well as significantly improved therapeutic and preventive effects against an E7-expressing tumor model in vaccinated mice (Kim et al. 2010). Additional adjuvants for activating DCs include growth factors such as Fms-like tyrosine kinase-3 (Flt3) ligand, which is a hematopoietic growth factor that can stimulate proliferation and differentiation of DC progenitors. A DNA vaccine encoding codon-optomized HPV-16 E6 and E7 linked to Flt3 ligand and a tissue plasminogen activator signal sequence generated significantly higher E6/E7-specific CD8+ T cell immune responses compared to DNA vaccine without Flt3 ligand (Seo et al. 2009). Flt3 ligand has also been shown to lead to accumulation of DCs in lymphoid tissues of vaccinated mice that can be cultivated with additional cytokines to result in large numbers of functionally active mature DCs (Shurin et al. 1997). Thus, adjuvants such as TLR ligands, TLR adaptor molecules, and immuno-stimulatory growth factors are potential methods to activate DCs to enhance therapeutic DNA vaccines.

Enhancing Cytokine/Chemokine Production for DC and T cell Activation

Antigen-presenting cells activate T cells through three main signals: recognition of MHC complex bound to peptide by the T cell receptor, costimulatory signal, and cytokines for proliferation and differentiation. Hence, research has focused on immunostimulatory cytokines for enhanced DC and T cell activation. DNA vaccines in conjunction with genetic adjuvants such as cytokines and chemokines can increase vaccine-elicited cellular immune responses. For example, DNA encoding HPV-16 E7 linked to IL-2 generated potent antitumor effects against E7-expressing tumors compared to HPV-16 E7 DNA alone (Lin et al. 2007). Other molecules that have been used as genetic adjuvants to enhance HPV-16 E7-specific CD8+ T cell immune responses

2 Strategies to Improve DNA Vaccine Potency: HPV-Associated Cervical Cancer

include IL-12, granulocyte-macrophage colony-stimulating factor (GM-CSF), macrophage inflammatory protein 1α (MIP-1α) and interferon-γ (IFN-γ) (Ohlschlager et al. 2009). In addition, it has been shown that DNA encoding HPV-16 E7 linked to Th1-polarizing chemokine IP-10 led to enhanced MHC class I presentation of E7 antigen and high chemotactic activity of the secreted IP-10/E7 protein, resulting in increased E7-specific CD4+ TH1 T cell and CD8+ T cell immune responses (Kang et al. 2010). Thus, the usage of cytokine genes to augment immune responses has been employed to improve DNA vaccine efficacy (also see Chap. 4 of this book).

Prolonging DC Survival

While DCs are crucial to triggering a strong adaptive immune response to treat tumors, they have limited life spans that may prevent long-term priming of naïve T cells into activated effector T cells. Hence, strategies to prolong survival of antigen-expressing DCs may increase the number of antigen-specific naïve T cells that a DC can activate in its lifetime, leading to the enhancement of DNA vaccine potency. Coadministration of DNA encoding HPV-16 E7 and various antiapoptotic proteins such as BCL-xL, BCL-2, X-linked inhibitor of apoptosis protein (XIAP), dominant negative capase-9, and negative capase-8, has been shown to prolong DC survival in vivo (Kim et al. 2003b). Furthermore, these antiapoptotic proteins, especially BCL-xL, were shown to significantly increase the number of E7-specific CD8+ T cells and lead to potent protective antitumor effects against E7-expressing tumors in vaccinated mice (Kim et al. 2003b). However, utilizing DNA encoding antiapoptotic proteins raises safety concerns on oncogenicity. Hence, research has focused on the employment of small interfering RNA (siRNA), which can transiently silence proapoptotic genes and thereby reduce the risk for oncogenicity. Delivery of DNA vaccine encoding HPV-16 E7 and siRNA targeting Bax and Bak, both proapoptotic proteins, significantly enhanced the E7-specific CD8+ T cell and E7-specific antitumor responses (Kim et al. 2005). Intradermal vaccination of DNA vaccines encoding IL-16 (Hsieh et al. 2007) and connective tissue growth factor (Cheng et al. 2008), cytokines inhibiting cell apoptosis and prolonging survival, also showed enhanced antigen-specific CD8+ immune responses and antitumor effects. These encouraging results have proven that prolonging transfected DC survival is a potential strategy to enhance DNA vaccine potency.

Modifying Immunosuppressive Microenvironment

One important category of immunosuppressive factors in the microenvironment of DC and T cell interaction are regulatory T cells (T_{reg}). After DC priming of naïve T cells to activated effector T cells, a subset of activated effector CD4+ T cells differentiates into T_{reg}. The CD4 + CD25+ T_{reg} release immunosuppressive cytokines such as IL-10 and TGF-β to inhibit T cell activation to prevent autoimmunity. However, T_{reg} that recognize tumor-associated-antigens can suppress antigen-specific immunity necessary to eradicate the antigen-expressing tumor cells. As a result, one strategy to enhance therapeutic vaccines focuses on elimination of T_{reg} for a stronger immune response. For example, the use of anti-CD25 monoclonal antibodies (PC61) followed by a DNA vaccine encoding HPV-16 E7 linked to heat shock protein 70 (E7/HSP70) successfully depleted CD4+CD25+ T_{reg} and generated increased levels of E7-specific CD8+ T cell responses compared to DNA vaccine delivery with a control antibody (Chuang et al. 2009a). Thus, elimination of immunosuppressive factors in the DC and T cell interaction microenvironment may enhance DNA vaccine potency.

Prolonging T Cell Survival

Strategies to prevent activated CD8+ T cell apoptosis may increase the number of activated T cells for mediating antitumor immunity, leading to enhanced DNA vaccine efficacy. The proapoptotic molecule Fas ligand (FasL) found on the surface of DCs interacts with its cognate receptor, Fas, located on T cells, to trigger apoptosis of the bound T cell. Therefore, DNA construct encoding short hairpin RNA (shRNA) targeting FasL can downregulate FasL expression on DCs, block binding of FasL on DCs to Fas on T cells, and subsequently prevent apoptosis of T cells. It has been shown that coadministration of HPV E7 DNA vaccine and DNA encoding shRNA targeting FasL led to significantly increased E7-specific CD8+ T cell activity and improved antitumor effects compared to HPV E7 DNA vaccine alone (Huang et al. 2008). These results show that targeting proapoptotic proteins in DCs to prolong activated T cell survival is an effective method to enhance DNA vaccine potency and warrants further exploration.

Utilizing CD4+ T Cell Help

While CD8+ T cells are well-known potent mediators of antitumor immunity, it has become clear that CD4+ T helper cells are also important for the induction of potent antitumor effects. It has been shown that in the absence of CD4+ T cell help, CD8+ T cells can be deleted or lose the capacity to develop into memory CD8+ T cells upon rechallenge (Janssen et al. 2003; Antony et al. 2005; Williams et al. 2006). Therefore, strategies to enhance CD4+ T cell activity may increase DNA vaccine potency.

One strategy to generate CD4+ T cell help is to use the molecules important for MHC class II presentation such as MHC class II-associated invariant chain (Ii). It has been shown that mice vaccinated with DNA encoding HPV-16 E7 linked to Ii led to increased number of E7-specific CD4+ T cells compared to DNA encoding unmodified HPV-16 E7, resulting in significantly better protective antitumor effects (Brulet et al. 2007). Another method to increase HPV antigen-specific CD4+ T cells is DNA encoding HPV antigen linked to sorting signal of LAMP-1 protein, as described above.

The enhancement of antigen-specific CD8+ T cell immune responses by CD4+ T cell help does not require antigen-specific CD4+ T cells. It has been shown that a DNA vaccine encoding Ii, in which the class II-associated Ii peptide (CLIP) region has been replaced by a high affinity CD4+ T-helper epitope called Pan HLA-DR epitope (PADRE) to form Ii-PADRE, can generate PADRE-specific CD4+ T cells in vaccinated mice (Hung et al. 2007). The coadministration of DNA encoding Ii-PADRE with DNA vaccines targeting HPV-16 E6 or E7 protein led to increased

2 Strategies to Improve DNA Vaccine Potency: HPV-Associated Cervical Cancer

HPV E6/E7-specific CD8+ T cell immune responses in vaccinated mice (Hung et al. 2007). An exploration of the mechanisms by which PADRE-specific CD4+ T cells enhance HPV E7-specific CD8+ T cell immune responses suggested the role of IL-2 secreted by PADRE-specific CD4+ T cells that led to the proliferation of E7-specific CD8+ T cells (Kim et al. 2008c).

The use of DNA encoding Ii-PADRE for providing PADRE-specific CD4+ T-helper cells to boost DNA vaccine potency can be further enhanced through combination with a strategy that employs Ii to increase antigen-specific CD8+ T cell immune responses. It has been shown that DNA vaccines encoding Ii linked to a model antigen on the carboxyl end of Ii can enhance antigen-specific CD8+ T-cell immune responses in vaccinated mice (Grujic et al. 2009). This raises the possibility that DNA vaccine encoding Ii-PADRE linked to target antigen may further enhance antigen-specific CD8+ T cell immune responses through PADRE-specific CD4+ T cell help. Wu et al. demonstrated that DNA vaccine encoding Ii-PADRE linked to HPV-16 E6 generated comparable levels of PADRE-specific CD4+ T-cell immune responses, as well as significantly stronger E6-specific CD8+ T-cell immune responses and antitumor effects against E6-expressing tumor compared with mice vaccinated with Ii-E6 DNA (Wu et al. 2010). In summary, DNA vaccine using strategy to provide CD4+ T cell help represents a potential approach to enhance DNA vaccine potency.

Conclusion

While the commercialization of prophylactic HPV vaccines, Gardasil® and Cervarix®, presents significant progress against cervical cancer, they do not have therapeutic effects against established HPV infections and HPV-associated lesions. Meanwhile, there is a significant number of established HPV dysplasias worldwide, which can progress to cancer. Thus, there remains an urgent need for safe, effective, and cost-efficient therapeutic vaccines. DNA vaccines have emerged as a promising approach to therapeutic vaccines. However, further advances are needed to improve the immunogenicity of most DNA vaccines. Strategies to increase vaccine potency by maximizing the ability of dendritic cells to trigger strong immune responses include optimizing the routes of administration, enhancing the intracellular processing of antigens by DCs, and improving the ability of DCs to uptake and present antigens. Increased understanding of the immunology involved in triggering a strong T-cell mediated response through DCs will lead to development of new strategies to enhance vaccine potency.

The diverse strategies to modify DCs through different mechanisms for enhanced DNA vaccine potency have created opportunities to combine them for optimal induction of HPV antigen-specific T cell-mediated immune responses for the control of HPV-associated disease.

For example, the strategy to prolong the life of DCs can be used in conjunction with an intracellular targeting strategy to further improve HPV DNA vaccine potency (Huang et al. 2007a; Kim et al. 2007; Kim et al. 2003a). Furthermore, the strategy to improve expression of MHC class I and MHC class II in the antigen-presenting cells can be used in combination with intracellular targeting strategy to further improve antigen-specific CD8+ and CD4+ T cell immune responses for therapeutic HPV DNA vaccine development (Kim et al. 2008b). It is foreseen that the best therapeutic HPV vaccine will most likely require the employment of various strategies that modify DCs through different mechanisms.

Conventional cancer therapies such as chemotherapy and radiation can also be used to improve therapeutic effects of DNA vaccination. Chemo/radiotherapy can lead to apoptosis of tumor cells, leading to the release of tumor antigens into the tumor microenvironment, which can facilitate cross priming of tumor antigen to DCs. This would result in tumor antigen-specific (i.e. HPV antigen-specific) CD8+ T cell precursors, which can be activated and increase upon vaccination with DNA targeting HPV antigen. Currently, cytotoxic drugs such as epigallocatechin-3-gallate (EGCG) (Kang et al. 2007), cisplatin (Tseng et al. 2008), and apigenin (Chuang et al. 2009b) have been used in conjunction with therapeutic HPV DNA vaccines to increase vaccine efficacy. Similarly, low dose radiation, which made tumor cells more susceptible to lysis, combined with the DNA vaccine CRT/E7(detox) has also showed enhanced CD8+ T cell responses and stronger antitumor effects (Tseng et al. 2009). For the control of advanced cancers, it is conceivable that combination of conventional cancer therapy with therapeutic HPV DNA vaccination will likely lead to better therapeutic effects.

It is clear that the tumor microenvironment plays a very important role to influence the therapeutic effect of cancer vaccines. There are a host of factors within the tumor microenvironment that may hinder the antigen-specific cell-mediated immunity generated by DNA vaccination. For example, T regulatory cells can release immune suppressive cytokines such as IL-10 (Yue et al. 1997) and TGF-β (Gorelik and Flavell 2001), which can paralyze T cell function. Other factors contributing to tumor immune suppression in tumor microenvironment include B7 homolog-1 (B7-H1) (Goldberg et al. 2007), signal transducer and activator of transcription 3 (STAT3) [for review, see Yu et al. (2007)] and MHC class I polypeptide-related sequence (MIC)-A and B (Groh et al. 2002), indoleamine 2,3-dioxygenase (IDO) enzyme (Munn and Mellor 2004), and galectin-1 (Rubinstein et al. 2004). These factors may serve as important potential targets for immune modulation to enhance therapeutic HPV vaccine potency [for review, see Kim et al. (2006)]. The combination of DNA vaccines with strategies to modulate the tumor microenvironment such that it is more favorable for tumor antigen-specific antitumor immunity warrants further exploration.

Currently, there are several therapeutic HPV DNA vaccines under different phases of clinical trials (Table 2.1). It is important to further advance through clinical trials for the eventual application of a therapeutic HPV vaccine to the general population. Continued advances in approaches to enhance DNA vaccine potency and the optimization of combinatorial approaches may lead to the control of HPV-associated lesions and malignancies.

Acknowledgements This review is not intended to be an encyclopedic one, and the authors apologize to those not cited. The work is supported by 5 R21 AI085380, 1 RO1 CA114425 01 and SPORE programs (P50 CA098252 and P50 CA96784-06) of the National Cancer Institute.

2 Strategies to Improve DNA Vaccine Potency: HPV-Associated Cervical Cancer

Table 2.1 Therapeutic HPV DNA vaccines in clinical trials

DNA vaccine	Disease	Antigen	Route of administration	Phase	Refereences
ZYC101	Anal dysplasia	HPV-16 E7	IM injection with microencapsulation of DNA vaccine	I	(Klencke et al. 2002)
	CIN 2/3			I	(Sheets et al. 2003)
ZYC101a (amolmigene bepiplasmid)	CIN 2/3	HPV-16/18 E6/E7	IM injection with microencapsulation of DNA vaccine	II	(Garcia et al. 2004)
pNGVL4a-Sig/E7(detox)•/HSP70	CIN 2/3	HPV-16 E7	IM injection	I	(Trimble et al. 2009)
	Advanced HNSCC			I	*
pNGVL4a-Sig/E7(detox)•/HSP70 prime and TA-HPV boost ± imiquimod	CIN 3	HPV-E7	IM injection (DNA vaccine and TA-HPV), Topical (imiquimod)	I	NCT00788 164
pNGVL4a-CRT/E7(detox)•	CIN 2/3	HPV-16 E7	Intradermal injection via gene gun	Ongoing, Phase I	NCT00988 559
VGX-3100	CIN 2/3	HPV-16/18 E6/E7	IM injection + electroporation	Ongoing Phase I	NCT00685 412

*M. Gillison, Personal communication
• Detox E7 mutated to abolish Rb binding site
CIN, cervical intraepithelial neoplasia; *CRT*, calreticulin; *HNSCC*, head and neck squamous cell carcinoma; *HPV*, human papillomavirus; *HSP*, heat shock protein; *IM*, intramuscular; *NCI*, National Cancer Institute; *NIH*, National Institutes of Health

References

Antony PA, Piccirillo CA, Akpinarli A, Finkelstein SE, Speiss PJ, Surman DR, Palmer DC, Chan CC, Klebanoff CA, Overwijk WW, Rosenberg SA, Restifo NP (2005) CD8+ T cell immunity against a tumor/self-antigen is augmented by CD4+ T helper cells and hindered by naturally occurring T regulatory cells. J Immunol 174(5):2591–2601

Babiuk S, Baca-Estrada ME, Foldvari M, Storms M, Rabussay D, Widera G, Babiuk LA (2002) Electroporation improves the efficacy of DNA vaccines in large animals. Vaccine 20(27–28):3399–3408

Best SR, Peng S, Juang CM, Hung CF, Hannaman D, Saunders JR, Wu TC, Pai SI (2009) Administration of HPV DNA vaccine via electroporation elicits the strongest CD8+ T cell immune responses compared to intramuscular injection and intradermal gene gun delivery. Vaccine 27:5450–5459

Brulet JM, Maudoux F, Thomas S, Thielemans K, Burny A, Leo O, Bex F, Hallez S (2007) DNA vaccine encoding endosome-targeted human papillomavirus type 16 E7 protein generates CD4+ T cell-dependent protection. Eur J Immunol 37(2):376–384

Buck CB, Pastrana DV, Lowy DR, Schiller JT (2004) Efficient intracellular assembly of papillomaviral vectors. J Virol 78(2):751–757

Buck CB, Pastrana DV, Lowy DR, Schiller JT (2005) Generation of HPV pseudovirions using transfection and their use in neutralization assays. Meth Mol Med 119:445–462

Cassaday RD, Sondel PM, King DM, Macklin MD, Gan J, Warner TF, Zuleger CL, Bridges AJ, Schalch HG, Kim KM, Hank JA, Mahvi DM, Albertini MR (2007) A phase I study of immunization using particle-mediated epidermal delivery of genes for gp100 and GM-CSF into uninvolved skin of melanoma patients. Clin Cancer Res 13(2 Pt 1):540–549

Chen CH, Wang TL, Hung CF, Yang Y, Young RA, Pardoll DM, Wu TC (2000) Enhancement of DNA vaccine potency by linkage of antigen gene to an HSP70 gene. Cancer Res 60(4):1035–1042

Chen CA, Chang MC, Sun WZ, Chen YL, Chiang YC, Hsieh CY, Chen SM, Hsiao PN, Cheng WF (2009) Noncarrier naked antigen-specific DNA vaccine generates potent antigen-specific immunologic responses and antitumor effects. Gene Ther 16(6):776–787

Cheng WF, Hung CF, Chai CY, Hsu KF, He L, Ling M, Wu TC (2001) Tumor-specific immunity and antiangiogenesis generated by a DNA vaccine encoding calreticulin linked to a tumor antigen. J Clin Invest 108(5):669–678

Cheng WF, Chang MC, Sun WZ, Lee CN, Lin HW, Su YN, Hsieh CY, Chen CA (2008) Connective tissue growth factor linked to the E7 tumor antigen generates potent antitumor immune responses mediated by an antiapoptotic mechanism. Gene Ther 15(13):1007–1016

Cheung YK, Cheng SC, Sin FW, Xie Y (2004) Plasmid encoding papillomavirus Type 16 (HPV16) DNA constructed with codon optimization improved the immunogenicity against HPV infection. Vaccine 23(5):629–638

Chuang CM, Hoory T, Monie A, Wu A, Wang MC, Hung CF (2009a) Enhancing therapeutic HPV DNA vaccine potency through depletion of CD4+CD25+ T regulatory cells. Vaccine 27(5):684–689

Chuang CM, Monie A, Wu A, Hung CF (2009b) Combination of apigenin treatment with therapeutic HPV DNA vaccination generates enhanced therapeutic antitumor effects. J Biomed Sci 16(1):49

Chuang CM, Monie A, Hung CF, Wu TC (2010) Treatment with imiquimod enhances antitumor immunity induced by therapeutic HPV DNA vaccination. J Biomed Sci 17:32

Chung CH, Gillison ML (2009) Human papillomavirus in head and neck cancer: its role in pathogenesis and clinical implications. Clin Cancer Res 15(22):6758–6762

Cid-Arregui A, Juarez V, zur Hausen H (2003) A synthetic E7 gene of human papillomavirus type 16 that yields enhanced expression of the protein in mammalian cells and is useful for DNA immunization studies. J Virol 77(8):4928–4937

Ciernik IF, Berzofsky JA, Carbone DP (1996) Induction of cytotoxic T lymphocytes and antitumor immunity with DNA vaccines expressing single T cell epitopes. J Immunol 156(7): 2369–2375

Dilber MS, Phelan A, Aints A, Mohamed AJ, Elliott G, Smith CI, O'Hare P (1999) Intercellular delivery of thymidine kinase prodrug activating enzyme by the herpes simplex virus protein, VP22. Gene Ther 6(1):12–21

Elliott G, O'Hare P (1997) Intercellular trafficking and protein delivery by a herpesvirus structural protein. Cell 88(2):223–233

Garcia F, Petry KU, Muderspach L, Gold MA, Braly P, Crum CP, Magill M, Silverman M, Urban RG, Hedley ML, Beach KJ (2004) ZYC101a for treatment of high-grade cervical intraepithelial neoplasia: a randomized controlled trial. Obstet Gynecol 103(2):317–326

Gnjatic S, Altorki NK, Tang DN, Tu SM, Kundra V, Ritter G, Old LJ, Logothetis CJ, Sharma P (2009) NY-ESO-1 DNA vaccine induces T-cell responses that are suppressed by regulatory T cells. Clin Cancer Res 15(6):2130–2139

Goldberg MV, Maris CH, Hipkiss EL, Flies AS, Zhen L, Tuder RM, Grosso JF, Harris TJ, Getnet D, Whartenby KA, Brockstedt DG, Dubensky TW Jr, Chen L, Pardoll DM, Drake CG (2007) Role of PD-1 and its ligand, B7-H1, in early fate decisions of CD8 T cells. Blood 110(1):186–192

Gorelik L, Flavell RA (2001) Immune-mediated eradication of tumors through the blockade of transforming growth factor-beta signaling in T cells. Nat Med 7(10):1118–1122

Graham BS, Kines RC, Corbett KS, Nicewonger J, Johnson TR, Chen M, LaVigne D, Roberts JN, Cuburu N, Schiller JT, Buck CB (2010) Mucosal delivery of human papillomavirus pseudovirus-encapsidated plasmids improves the potency of DNA vaccination. Mucosal Immunol 3(5):475–486

Grant EP, Michalek MT, Goldberg AL, Rock KL (1995) Rate of antigen degradation by the ubiquitin-proteasome pathway influences MHC class I presentation. J Immunol 155(8): 3750–3758

Groh V, Wu J, Yee C, Spies T (2002) Tumour-derived soluble MIC ligands impair expression of NKG2D and T-cell activation. Nature 419(6908):734–738

Grujic M, Holst PJ, Christensen JP, Thomsen AR (2009) Fusion of a viral antigen to invariant chain leads to augmented T-cell immunity and improved protection in gene-gun DNA-vaccinated mice. J Gen Virol 90(Pt 2):414–422

Harms JS, Ren X, Oliveira SC, Splitter GA (2000) Distinctions between bovine herpesvirus 1 and herpes simplex virus type 1 VP22 tegument protein subcellular associations. J Virol 74(7):3301–3312

Hauser H, Chen SY (2003) Augmentation of DNA vaccine potency through secretory heat shock protein-mediated antigen targeting. Methods 31(3):225–231

Hauser H, Shen L, Gu QL, Krueger S, Chen SY (2004) Secretory heat-shock protein as a dendritic cell-targeting molecule: a new strategy to enhance the potency of genetic vaccines. Gene Ther 11(11):924–932

Hirasawa Y, Arai M, Imazeki F, Tada M, Mikata R, Fukai K, Miyazaki M, Ochiai T, Saisho H, Yokosuka O (2006) Methylation status of genes upregulated by demethylating agent 5-aza-2′-deoxycytidine in hepatocellular carcinoma. Oncology 71(1–2):77–85

Hsieh CY, Chen CA, Huang CY, Chang MC, Lee CN, Su YN, Cheng WF (2007) IL-6-encoding tumor antigen generates potent cancer immunotherapy through antigen processing and anti-apoptotic pathways. Mol Ther 15(10):1890–1897

Huang CH, Peng S, He L, Tsai YC, Boyd DA, Hansen TH, Wu TC, Hung CF (2005) Cancer immunotherapy using a DNA vaccine encoding a single-chain trimer of MHC class I linked to an HPV-16 E6 immunodominant CTL epitope. Gene Ther 12(15):1180–1186

Huang B, Mao CP, Peng S, He L, Hung CF, Wu TC (2007a) Intradermal administration of DNA vaccines combining a strategy to bypass antigen processing with a strategy to prolong dendritic cell survival enhances DNA vaccine potency. Vaccine 25(45):7824–7831

Huang CY, Chen CA, Lee CN, Chang MC, Su YN, Lin YC, Hsieh CY, Cheng WF (2007b) DNA vaccine encoding heat shock protein 60 co-linked to HPV16 E6 and E7 tumor antigens generates more potent immunotherapeutic effects than respective E6 or E7 tumor antigens. Gynecol Oncol 107(3):404–412

Huang B, Mao CP, Peng S, Hung CF, Wu TC (2008) RNA interference-mediated in vivo silencing of fas ligand as a strategy for the enhancement of DNA vaccine potency. Hum Gene Ther 19(8):763–773

Hung CF, Cheng WF, Chai CY, Hsu KF, He L, Ling M, Wu TC (2001a) Improving vaccine potency through intercellular spreading and enhanced MHC class I presentation of antigen. J Immunol 166(9):5733–5740

Hung CF, Cheng WF, Hsu KF, Chai CY, He L, Ling M, Wu TC (2001b) Cancer immunotherapy using a DNA vaccine encoding the translocation domain of a bacterial toxin linked to a tumor antigen. Cancer Res 61(9):3698–3703

Hung CF, Hsu KF, Cheng WF, Chai CY, He L, Ling M, Wu TC (2001c) Enhancement of DNA vaccine potency by linkage of antigen gene to a gene encoding the extracellular domain of Fms-like tyrosine kinase 3-ligand. Cancer Res 61(3):1080–1088

Hung CF, He L, Juang J, Lin TJ, Ling M, Wu TC (2002) Improving DNA vaccine potency by linking Marek's disease virus type 1 VP22 to an antigen. J Virol 76(6):2676–2682

Hung CF, Cheng WF, He L, Ling M, Juang J, Lin CT, Wu TC (2003) Enhancing major histocompatibility complex class I antigen presentation by targeting antigen to centrosomes. Cancer Res 63(10):2393–2398

Hung CF, Tsai YC, He L, Wu TC (2007) DNA vaccines encoding Ii-PADRE generates potent PADRE-specific CD4+ T-cell immune responses and enhances vaccine potency. Mol Ther 15(6):1211–1219

Hung CF, Ma B, Monie A, Tsen SW, Wu TC (2008) Therapeutic human papillomavirus vaccines: current clinical trials and future directions. Expert Opin Biol Ther 8(4):421–439

Intra J, Salem AK (2009) Fabrication, characterization and in vitro evaluation of poly(D,L-lactide-co-glycolide) microparticles loaded with polyamidoamine-plasmid DNA dendriplexes for applications in nonviral gene delivery. J Pharm Sci 99:368

Iwasaki A, Medzhitov R (2004) Toll-like receptor control of the adaptive immune responses. Nat Immunol 5(10):987–995

Janssen EM, Lemmens EE, Wolfe T, Christen U, von Herrath MG, Schoenberger SP (2003) CD4+ T cells are required for secondary expansion and memory in CD8+ T lymphocytes. Nature 421(6925):852–856

Ji H, Wang TL, Chen CH, Pai SI, Hung CF, Lin KY, Kurman RJ, Pardoll DM, Wu TC (1999) Targeting human papillomavirus type 16 E7 to the endosomal/lysosomal compartment enhances the antitumor immunity of DNA vaccines against murine human papillomavirus type 16 E7-expressing tumors. Hum Gene Ther 10(17):2727–2740

Kang TH, Lee JH, Song CK, Han HD, Shin BC, Pai SI, Hung CF, Trimble C, Lim JS, Kim TW, Wu TC (2007) Epigallocatechin-3-gallate enhances CD8+ T cell-mediated antitumor immunity induced by DNA vaccination. Cancer Res 67(2):802–811

Kang TH, Chung JY, Monie A, Pai SI, Hung CF, Wu TC (2009) Enhancing DNA vaccine potency by co-administration of xenogenic MHC-class-I DNA. Gene Ther 17:531–540

Kang TH, Kim KW, Bae HC, Seong SY, Kim TW (2010) Enhancement of DNA vaccine potency by antigen linkage to IFN-gamma-inducible protein-10. Int J Cancer 128(3):702–714

Kim TW, Hung CF, Boyd D, Juang J, He L, Kim JW, Hardwick JM, Wu TC (2003a) Enhancing DNA vaccine potency by combining a strategy to prolong dendritic cell life with intracellular targeting strategies. J Immunol 171(6):2970–2976

Kim TW, Hung CF, Ling M, Juang J, He L, Hardwick JM, Kumar S, Wu TC (2003b) Enhancing DNA vaccine potency by coadministration of DNA encoding antiapoptotic proteins. J Clin Invest 112(1):109–117

Kim TW, Hung CF, Kim JW, Juang J, Chen PJ, He L, Boyd DA, Wu TC (2004) Vaccination with a DNA vaccine encoding herpes simplex virus type 1 VP22 linked to antigen generates long-term antigen-specific CD8-positive memory T cells and protective immunity. Hum Gene Ther 15(2):167–177

Kim TW, Lee JH, He L, Boyd DA, Hardwick JM, Hung CF, Wu TC (2005) Modification of professional antigen-presenting cells with small interfering RNA in vivo to enhance cancer vaccine potency. Cancer Res 65(1):309–316

Kim R, Emi M, Tanabe K, Arihiro K (2006) Tumor-driven evolution of immunosuppressive networks during malignant progression. Cancer Res 66(11):5527–5536

Kim D, Hoory T, Wu TC, Hung CF (2007) Enhancing DNA vaccine potency by combining a strategy to prolong dendritic cell life and intracellular targeting strategies with a strategy to boost CD4+ T cell. Hum Gene Ther 18(11):1129–1139

Kim D, Gambhira R, Karanam B, Monie A, Hung CF, Roden R, Wu TC (2008a) Generation and characterization of a preventive and therapeutic HPV DNA vaccine. Vaccine 26(3):351–360

Kim D, Hoory T, Monie A, Ting JP, Hung CF, Wu TC (2008b) Enhancement of DNA vaccine potency through coadministration of CIITA DNA with DNA vaccines via gene gun. J Immunol 180(10):7019–7027

Kim D, Monie A, He L, Tsai YC, Hung CF, Wu TC (2008c) Role of IL-2 secreted by PADRE-specific CD4+ T cells in enhancing E7-specific CD8+ T-cell immune responses. Gene Ther 15(9):677–687

Kim D, Hung CF, Wu TC, Park YM (2010) DNA vaccine with alpha-galactosylceramide at prime phase enhances anti-tumor immunity after boosting with antigen-expressing dendritic cells. Vaccine 28(45):7297–7305

Klencke B, Matijevic M, Urban RG, Lathey JL, Hedley ML, Berry M, Thatcher J, Weinberg V, Wilson J, Darragh T, Jay N, Da Costa M, Palefsky JM (2002) Encapsulated plasmid DNA treatment for human papillomavirus 16-associated anal dysplasia: a Phase I study of ZYC101. Clin Cancer Res 8(5):1028–1037

Le Borgne M, Etchart N, Goubier A, Lira SA, Sirard JC, van Rooijen N, Caux C, Ait-Yahia S, Vicari A, Kaiserlian D, Dubois B (2006) Dendritic cells rapidly recruited into epithelial tissues via CCR6/CCL20 are responsible for CD8+ T cell crosspriming in vivo. Immunity 24(2):191–201

Li Y, Subjeck J, Yang G, Repasky E, Wang XY (2006) Generation of anti-tumor immunity using mammalian heat shock protein 70 DNA vaccines for cancer immunotherapy. Vaccine 24(25):5360–5370

Lin KY, Guarnieri FG, Staveley-O'Carroll KF, Levitsky HI, August JT, Pardoll DM, Wu TC (1996) Treatment of established tumors with a novel vaccine that enhances major histocompatibility class II presentation of tumor antigen. Cancer Res 56(1):21–26

Lin CT, Tsai YC, He L, Calizo R, Chou HH, Chang TC, Soong YK, Hung CF, Lai CH (2006) A DNA vaccine encoding a codon-optimized human papillomavirus type 16 E6 gene enhances CTL response and anti-tumor activity. J Biomed Sci 13(4):481–488

Lin CT, Tsai YC, He L, Yeh CN, Chang TC, Soong YK, Monie A, Hung CF, Lai CH (2007) DNA vaccines encoding IL-2 linked to HPV-16 E7 antigen generate enhanced E7-specific CTL responses and antitumor activity. Immunol Lett 114(2):86–93

Liu R, Zhou C, Wang D, Ma W, Lin C, Wang Y, Liang X, Li J, Guo S, Zhang Y, Zhang S (2006) Enhancement of DNA vaccine potency by sandwiching antigen-coding gene between secondary lymphoid tissue chemokine (SLC) and IgG Fc fragment genes. Cancer Biol Ther 5(4):427–434

Lou PJ, Cheng WF, Chung YC, Cheng CY, Chiu LH, Young TH (2009) PMMA particle-mediated DNA vaccine for cervical cancer. J Biomed Mater Res A 88(4):849–857

Lu D, Hoory T, Monie A, Wu A, Wang MC, Hung CF (2009) Treatment with demethylating agent, 5-aza-2'-deoxycytidine enhances therapeutic HPV DNA vaccine potency. Vaccine 27(32):4363–4369

Lundberg M, Johansson M (2001) Is VP22 nuclear homing an artifact? Nat Biotechnol 19(8):713–714

Mao CP, Hung CF, Kang TH, He L, Tsai YC, Wu CY, Wu TC (2010) Combined administration with DNA encoding vesicular stomatitis virus G protein enhances DNA vaccine potency. J Virol 84(5):2331–2339

Massa S, Simeone P, Muller A, Benvenuto E, Venuti A, Franconi R (2008) Antitumor activity of DNA vaccines based on the human papillomavirus-16 E7 protein genetically fused to a plant virus coat protein. Hum Gene Ther 19(4):354–364

Munn DH, Mellor AL (2004) IDO and tolerance to tumors. Trends Mol Med 10(1):15–18

Munoz N, Bosch FX, de Sanjose S, Herrero R, Castellsague X, Shah KV, Snijders PJ, Meijer CJ (2003) Epidemiologic classification of human papillomavirus types associated with cervical cancer. N Engl J Med 348(6):518–527

Mwangi W, Brown WC, Splitter GA, Zhuang Y, Kegerreis K, Palmer GH (2005) Enhancement of antigen acquisition by dendritic cells and MHC class II-restricted epitope presentation to CD4+ T cells using VP22 DNA vaccine vectors that promote intercellular spreading following initial transfection. J Leukoc Biol 78(2):401–411

NCT00685412. Phase I of human papillomavirus (HPV) DNA plasmid (VGX-3100)+electroporation for CIN 2 or 3. http://clinicaltrials.gov/ct2/show/NCT00685412 Accessed 10 Oct 2010

NCT00788164. Vaccine therapy with or without imiquimod in treating patients with grade 3 cervical intraepithelial neoplasia. http://clinicaltrials.gov/ct2/show/NCT00788164 Accessed 11 Mar 2010.

NCT00859729. Dose finding study of a DNA vaccine delivered with intradermal electroporation in patients with prostate cancer. 3/10/09 edn

NCT00988559. Therapeutic vaccination for patients with HPV16+ cervical intraepithelial neoplasia (CIN2/3). http://clinicaltrials.gov/ct2/show/NCT00988559 Accessed 15 Aug 2010

NCT01064375. Safety study of DNA Vaccine delivered by intradermal electroporation to treat colorectal cancer (El-porCEA). http://clinicaltrials.gov/ct2/show/NCT01064375 Accessed 24 Mar 2010

Ohlschlager P, Quetting M, Alvarez G, Durst M, Gissmann L, Kaufmann AM (2009) Enhancement of immunogenicity of a therapeutic cervical cancer DNA-based vaccine by co-application of sequence-optimized genetic adjuvants. Int J Cancer 125(1):189–198

Otten G, Schaefer M, Doe B, Liu H, Srivastava I, zur Megede J, O'Hagan D, Donnelly J, Widera G, Rabussay D, Lewis MG, Barnett S, Ulmer JB (2004) Enhancement of DNA vaccine potency in rhesus macaques by electroporation. Vaccine 22(19):2489–2493

Peng S, Ji H, Trimble C, He L, Tsai YC, Yeatermeyer J, Boyd DA, Hung CF, Wu TC (2004) Development of a DNA vaccine targeting human papillomavirus type 16 oncoprotein E6. J Virol 78(16):8468–8476

Peng S, Monie A, Kang TH, Hung CF, Roden R, Wu TC (2010) Efficient delivery of DNA vaccines using human papillomavirus pseudovirions. Gene Ther 17:1453–1464

Phelan A, Elliott G, O'Hare P (1998) Intercellular delivery of functional p53 by the herpesvirus protein VP22. Nat Biotechnol 16(5):440–443

Qazi KR, Wikman M, Vasconcelos NM, Berzins K, Stahl S, Fernandez C (2005) Enhancement of DNA vaccine potency by linkage of *Plasmodium falciparum* malarial antigen gene fused with a fragment of HSP70 gene. Vaccine 23(9):1114–1125

Roos AK, Eriksson F, Timmons JA, Gerhardt J, Nyman U, Gudmundsdotter L, Brave A, Wahren B, Pisa P (2009) Skin electroporation: effects on transgene expression, DNA persistence and local tissue environment. PLoS ONE 4(9):e7226

Rubinstein N, Alvarez M, Zwirner NW, Toscano MA, Ilarregui JM, Bravo A, Mordoh J, Fainboim L, Podhajcer OL, Rabinovich GA (2004) Targeted inhibition of galectin-1 gene expression in tumor cells results in heightened T cell-mediated rejection; A potential mechanism of tumor-immune privilege. Cancer Cell 5(3):241–251

Safety and immunogenicity of a melanoma DNA vaccine delivered by electroporation. http://clinicaltrials.gov/ct2/show/NCT00471133. Accessed 25 Feb 2010

Scheerlinck JP, Karlis J, Tjelle TE, Presidente PJ, Mathiesen I, Newton SE (2004) In vivo electroporation improves immune responses to DNA vaccination in sheep. Vaccine 22(13–14):1820–1825

Seo SH, Jin HT, Park SH, Youn JI, Sung YC (2009) Optimal induction of HPV DNA vaccine-induced CD8(+) T cell responses and therapeutic antitumor effect by antigen engineering and electroporation. Vaccine 27(42):5906–5912

Sheets EE, Urban RG, Crum CP, Hedley ML, Politch JA, Gold MA, Muderspach LI, Cole GA, Crowley-Nowick PA (2003) Immunotherapy of human cervical high-grade cervical intraepithelial neoplasia with microparticle-delivered human papillomavirus 16 E7 plasmid DNA. Am J Obstet Gynecol 188(4):916–926

Shurin MR, Pandharipande PP, Zorina TD, Haluszczak C, Subbotin VM, Hunter O, Brumfield A, Storkus WJ, Maraskovsky E, Lotze MT (1997) FLT3 ligand induces the generation of functionally active dendritic cells in mice. Cell Immunol 179(2):174–184

Storrie H, Mooney DJ (2006) Sustained delivery of plasmid DNA from polymeric scaffolds for tissue engineering. Adv Drug Deliv Rev 58(4):500–514

Suzuki H, Gabrielson E, Chen W, Anbazhagan R, van Engeland M, Weijenberg MP, Herman JG, Baylin SB (2002) A genomic screen for genes upregulated by demethylation and histone deacetylase inhibition in human colorectal cancer. Nat Genet 31(2):141–149

Takeshita F, Tanaka T, Matsuda T, Tozuka M, Kobiyama K, Saha S, Matsui K, Ishii KJ, Coban C, Akira S, Ishii N, Suzuki K, Klinman DM, Okuda K, Sasaki S (2006) Toll-like receptor adaptor molecules enhance DNA-raised adaptive immune responses against influenza and tumors through activation of innate immunity. J Virol 80(13):6218–6224

Tobery TW, Siliciano RF (1997) Targeting of HIV-1 antigens for rapid intracellular degradation enhances cytotoxic T lymphocyte (CTL) recognition and the induction of de novo CTL responses in vivo after immunization. J Exp Med 185(5):909–920

Trimble C, Lin CT, Hung CF, Pai S, Juang J, He L, Gillison M, Pardoll D, Wu L, Wu TC (2003) Comparison of the CD8+ T cell responses and antitumor effects generated by DNA vaccine administered through gene gun, biojector, and syringe. Vaccine 21(25–26):4036–4042

Trimble CL, Peng S, Kos F, Gravitt P, Viscidi R, Sugar E, Pardoll D, Wu TC (2009) A phase I trial of a human papillomavirus DNA vaccine for HPV16+ cervical intraepithelial neoplasia 2/3. Clin Cancer Res 15(1):361–367

Tsen SW, Wu CY, Meneshian A, Pai SI, Hung CF, Wu TC (2009) Femtosecond laser treatment enhances DNA transfection efficiency in vivo. J Biomed Sci 16:36

Tseng CW, Hung CF, Alvarez RD, Trimble C, Huh WK, Kim D, Chuang CM, Lin CT, Tsai YC, He L, Monie A, Wu TC (2008) Pretreatment with cisplatin enhances E7-specific CD8+ T-Cell-mediated antitumor immunity induced by DNA vaccination. Clin Cancer Res 14(10):3185–3192

Tseng CW, Trimble C, Zeng Q, Monie A, Alvarez RD, Huh WK, Hoory T, Wang MC, Hung CF, Wu TC (2009) Low-dose radiation enhances therapeutic HPV DNA vaccination in tumor-bearing hosts. Cancer Immunol Immunother 58(5):737–748

Walboomers JM, Jacobs MV, Manos MM, Bosch FX, Kummer JA, Shah KV, Snijders PJ, Peto J, Meijer CJ, Munoz N (1999) Human papillomavirus is a necessary cause of invasive cervical cancer worldwide. J Pathol 189(1):12–19

Williams MA, Tyznik AJ, Bevan MJ (2006) Interleukin-2 signals during priming are required for secondary expansion of CD8+ memory T cells. Nature 441(7095):890–893

Wu TC, Guarnieri FG, Staveley-O'Carroll KF, Viscidi RP, Levitsky HI, Hedrick L, Cho KR, August JT, Pardoll DM (1995) Engineering an intracellular pathway for major histocompatibility complex class II presentation of antigens. Proc Natl Acad Sci USA 92(25):11671–11675

Wu A, Zeng Q, Kang TH, Peng S, Roosinovich E, Pai SI, Hung CF (2010) Innovative DNA vaccine for human papillomavirus (HPV)-associated head and neck cancer. Gene Ther 18:304–312

Wybranietz WA, Gross CD, Phelan A, O'Hare P, Spiegel M, Graepler F, Bitzer M, Stahler P, Gregor M, Lauer UM (2001) Enhanced suicide gene effect by adenoviral transduction of a VP22-cytosine deaminase (CD) fusion gene. Gene Ther 8(21):1654–1664

Ye J, Chen GS, Song HP, Li ZS, Huang YY, Qu P, Sun YJ, Zhang XM, Sui YF (2004) Heat shock protein 70/MAGE-1 tumor vaccine can enhance the potency of MAGE-1-specific cellular immune responses in vivo. Cancer Immunol Immunother 53(9):825–834

You Z, Huang X, Hester J, Toh HC, Chen SY (2001) Targeting dendritic cells to enhance DNA vaccine potency. Cancer Res 61(9):3704–3711

Yu H, Kortylewski M, Pardoll D (2007) Crosstalk between cancer and immune cells: role of STAT3 in the tumour microenvironment. Nat Rev Immunol 7(1):41–51

Yue FY, Dummer R, Geertsen R, Hofbauer G, Laine E, Manolio S, Burg G (1997) Interleukin-10 is a growth factor for human melanoma cells and down-regulates HLA class-I, HLA class-II and ICAM-1 molecules. Int J Cancer 71(4):630–637

Zeira E, Manevitch A, Manevitch Z, Kedar E, Gropp M, Daudi N, Barsuk R, Harati M, Yotvat H, Troilo PJ, Griffiths TG 2nd, Pacchione SJ, Roden DF, Niu Z, Nussbaum O, Zamir G, Papo O, Hemo I, Lewis A, Galun E (2007) Femtosecond laser: a new intradermal DNA delivery method for efficient, long-term gene expression and genetic immunization. FASEB J 21(13): 3522–3533

Zhang S, Zhang Y (2008) Novel chemotactic-antigen DNA vaccine against cancer. Future Oncol 4(2):299–303

Zheng C, Babiuk LA, van Drunen Littel-van den Hurk S (2005) Bovine herpesvirus 1 VP22 enhances the efficacy of a DNA vaccine in cattle. J Virol 79(3):1948–1953

Zheng CF, Brownlie R, Huang DY, Babiuk LA, van Drunen Littel-van den Hurk S (2006) Intercellular trafficking of the major tegument protein VP22 of bovine herpesvirus-1 and its application to improve a DNA vaccine. Arch Virol 151(5):985–993

Zhou C, Peng G, Jin X, Tang J, Chen Z (2010) Vaccination with a fusion DNA vaccine encoding hepatitis B surface antigen fused to the extracellular domain of CTLA4 enhances HBV-specific immune responses in mice: implication of its potential use as a therapeutic vaccine. Clin Immunol 137(2):190–198

zur Hausen H (2002) Papillomaviruses and cancer: from basic studies to clinical application. Nat Rev Cancer 2(5):342–350

Immune-Activating Mechanisms of Replicase-Based DNA and RNA Vaccines and Their Role in Immune-Apoptosis

3

Wolfgang W. Leitner

DNA vaccines have revolutionized the field of vaccinology and hold enormous promise due to their versatility, safety and simplicity. Although naked, non-adjuvanted DNA vaccines have proven their ability to prevent or treat a very broad range of diseases in animal models, their immunogenicity – not only in certain animal models but also when used in non-human primates or humans in general – has been unsatisfactory. Numerous strategies have been developed to improve the immunogenicity and efficacy of DNA vaccine. These range from modifications of the plasmid to improvements in the delivery method, the addition of immunostimulatory molecules (both conventional and molecular adjuvants) and the design of heterologous prime-boost regimens in which a DNA prime is followed by a booster immunization with another vaccine platform such as a recombinant virus. One of the more recent innovations is the incorporation of gene sequences for the alphaviral replicase complex into a naked DNA plasmid. The original objective was to significantly increased antigen production with the help of a viral enzyme which replicates (vaccine encoded-) mRNA in transfected cells. Although this mechanism continues to be cited in the literature as the reason for the higher immunogenicity and efficacy of replicase-based vaccines, antigen-levels induced by such vectors do not necessarily correlate with their immunogenicity. Instead, cells transfected with replicase-based vectors detect dsRNA generated by the RNA replicase through various RNA sensors and interpret the presence of those nucleic acid species as evidence of a viral infection. The role each of the currently known dsRNA sensors plays in this event is still not well known and the analysis is complicated by a high degree of redundancy in their functions. While the 2′,5′-oligoadenylate synthetase/RNase L pathway has been shown to be essential, the removal of another dsRNA sensing molecule that is triggered by replicase-based vaccines (toll like receptor (TLR) 3) did not affect the immunogenicity of these vaccines.

W.W. Leitner
National Institute of Allergy and Infectious Diseases, NIH,
Basic Immunology Branch,
Bethesda, MD, USA
e-mail: wleiter@niaid.nih.gov

J. Thalhamer et al. (eds.), *Gene Vaccines*,
DOI 10.1007/978-3-7091-0439-2_3, © Springer-Verlag/Wien, 2012

Signaling pathways induced by dsRNA-species results in innate immune activation and the induction of programmed cell death of the transfected host cell which in fact appears to curtail antigen production. Nevertheless, replicase-based nucleic acid vaccines induce superior immune responses due to the powerful immunostimulatory signals delivered by the dying transfected host cell which include the release of Type I interferon and most likely a variety of other stress signals such as heat shock proteins.

In addition to their much higher immunogenicity when compared to conventional counterparts, replicase-based DNA vaccines appear to be extremely safe and the "self-removal" of the injected vaccine through the apoptotic death of transfected host cells adds an additional attractive safety feature. The vaccine's safety profile is yet further improved by the fact that only minute amounts of plasmid are required to "optimally" transfect host cells due to the amplification of plasmid-encoded mRNA by the replicase enzyme complex. This allows even short-lived mRNA encoding alphaviral replicase and the antigen of interest (RNA replicon) to be used as vaccines. While conventional RNA is rapidly degraded by RNases which drastically limit their usefulness as vaccines, theoretically a single copy of replicase-based ("self-replicating") RNA in a transfected cell induces strong immune responses due to the amplification by the viral RNA-replicase.

Replicase-based nucleic vaccines hold the promise to move the DNA vaccine field significantly forward, but the lessons we have learned from studying the mechanism of action of these vaccines can also be used to improve the efficacy of other types of vaccines.

Introduction

DNA vaccines, consisting of "naked" DNA plasmids encoding the vaccine antigen under the control of either a strong viral promoter or a tissue-specific host-derived promoter, were introduced in the late 1980s (Dixon 1995). Due to their simplicity and effectiveness in rodent model systems, DNA vaccines rapidly became extremely popular and their potential usefulness was explored in virtually every disease model. Although their mechanism of action was poorly understood, DNA vaccines were rushed into non-human primates (NHP) and subsequently clinical trials, which initially yielded extremely disappointing results, leading many to believe that this novel technology was not suitable for human vaccines. Various factors have been proposed as reasons for inadequate immunogenicity in NHP or humans, including inadequate uptake of injected DNA plasmids by cells (Widera et al. 2000), the use of patients with advanced disease in early clinical trials of DNA vaccines (Leitner 2001), insufficient innate signaling of the plasmids in the primate host, the use of GLP or GMP-grade plasmids for primate or human trials which lack immunostimulatory contaminants (namely endotoxin) or technical issues such as the volume the vaccine was delivered in relation to the host's size and capacity of the target tissue (e.g., intramuscular injection leading to immunostimulatory mechanical damage to muscle fibers in mice).

Why Do DNA Vaccines Work?

The immunogenicity of pure, un-adjuvanted plasmid DNA was initially puzzling and seemed to contradict immunological principles. Unlike other vaccines, purified DNA did not provide any known signals to the innate immune system which could act as vaccine adjuvants, a prerequisite for the subsequent induction of adaptive immune responses. Publications going back several decades, which reported pro-inflammatory activities and adjuvant-like potential of nucleic acid derived from pathogens, were frequently dismissed as artifacts caused by trace amounts of contaminants (such as the above mentioned bacterial endotoxin). The discovery of specific DNA sequences with immunostimulatory properties, characterized by a central unmethylated CpG motif (Sato et al. 1996), represented not only a breakthrough in the understanding of the mechanism of action of this novel vaccine platform, but marked a milestone in the area of discovery of new Pathogen Associated Molecular Patterns (PAMPs) many of which are currently being explored as vaccine adjuvants.

The discovery of TLR9 provided the long-sought explanation for how DNA could induce innate immune responses and act as an adjuvant. Since then, additional innate immune receptors have been identified that recognize DNA (Deng 2008). TLR9 is expressed on a variety of cells of the immune system in a species-specific manner allowing those cells to selectively recognize different classes of immunostimulatory DNA sequences. While in vitro studies have clearly established the importance of sequences in activating TLR9-expressing cells, TLR9 knockout mice immunized with DNA vaccines, however, mount T and B cell responses comparable to those observed in their wildtype counterparts. This calls into question the relevance of this pathway for the immunogenicity of DNA vaccines. To further add to the confusion, some reports indicate that DNA-plasmid associated CpG recognition by TLR9 may, after all, be important for the adjuvanticity of DNA vaccines, but only during priming (Rottembourg et al. 2010). The seemingly contradictory results indicate that DNA recognition by the innate immune system is mediated by additional receptors, such as the recently identified cytoplasmid DNA receptor AIM2 (Hornung et al. 2009). Novel innate immune receptors continue to be discovered increasingly underscoring the highly redundant nature of innate immune responses. This assertion is supported by the finding in a large-scale mutagenesis program (Beutler 2009), which has failed to identify a single receptor or signaling pathway capable of significantly affecting innate immune responses to various pathogens. This is in stark contrast to numerous lymphocyte receptors and pathways, each of which is capable of completely disabling this arm of the immune system.

The rapidly expanding panel of PAMPs and the discovery of corresponding innate receptors represent an extremely valuable toolbox of novel adjuvants. Including additional CpG sequences into DNA plasmids or co-delivering such sequences in the form of DNA oligonucleotides was one of the first approaches to enhance the immunogenicity of DNA vaccines through a "molecular" adjuvant and countless other such approaches have been explored since.

Virus-Based Vaccine Platforms: Tapping into the Innate Immune Recognition of Viral PAMPs

Employing attenuated viruses as vaccines has a colorful history spanning several millennia and has evolved considerably since the use of scabs from smallpox patients in ancient China, and more recently, the injection of bovine tissue containing cowpox by Edward Jenner to cross-protect humans against smallpox. Current approaches include the much more sophisticated, rational design and modification of recombinant vaccine vectors to deliver non-viral target antigens.

Among the viruses used for vaccines as well as gene therapy vectors are several members of the alphavirus genus, which belong to the Togaviridae family of RNA viruses (small, lipid-enveloped, monopartite positive-stranded RNA viruses) such as Semliki forest virus, Sindbis virus and the Venezuelan equine encephalitis virus (Griffin 2007). Other members of the currently 27-member strong genus are the Chikungunya virus and the Ross River virus, all arthropod-transmitted viruses (arboviruses). By relying on a small RNA genome (encoding only seven multifunctional proteins (Ryman and Klimstra 2008)) these viruses, which unlike retroviruses do not go through a DNA stage, require replication of their RNA genome by an enzyme not supplied by their host and thus encoded in the viral genome. This alphaviral replicase is a polyprotein (called P1234), which is cleaved into multiple subunits. The cleavage intermediate P123 + nsp4 synthesizes approximately 200,000 copies of minus-strand copies of the viral RNA genome (Lundstrom 2005) (or entire self-replicating RNA construct) while the complex has to be processed into individual subunits for the synthesis of positive strand RNA species (Vasiljeva et al. 2003). Fully cleaved replicase subunits preferentially use the subgenomic mRNA binding site (Kim et al. 2004). In summary, the activity of the replicase results in the synthesis of genomic RNA copies, as well as the selective synthesis of sub-genomic segments of the viral genome, encoding viral capsid proteins (or target antigen, in case of recombinant self-replicating RNA constructs). Although RNA replicon vectors based on the genome of other RNA viruses have been generated, the discussion below focuses on alphavirus replicons. Replicon vaccines based on flaviviruses such as Kunjin virus (KUN) or Yellow Fever virus have also been shown to induce strong immune responses; a comparison of alphaviral and flaviviral replicon vectors indicates significant mechanistic differences (Tannis et al. 2005). The qualitative differences in the immune responses they induce may be due to the fact that alphaviral replicons are generally cytopathic (discussed below) while flaviviral replicons are generally not.

Recombinant virus-based vaccines in general, and alphavirus-based vaccines in particular (Karlsson and Liljestrom 2004), have been developed in different formats with three major categories being described below:

1. *Conventional recombinant viruses*: by replacing the gene sequences encoding the structural proteins of the virus with the RNA sequence of a pathogen-derived protein (i.e., the target antigen), recombinant vectors have been created which efficiently infect mammalian cells and deliver their payload in the form of the genetic information for the target protein. In contrast to the wildtype virus,

however, such vectors are only capable of one round of infection due to the lack of genetic information for structural genes. The strengths of these vectors include strong stimulation of innate immune responses (i.e., providing potent adjuvanticity) and efficient vaccine delivery. These strengths are counter-balanced by reduced efficacy in the face of pre-existing immunity to the parental vector (which also limits the repeated use of such vectors) the potential for immunological dominance of viral proteins over the target protein (particularly if the host had previously been exposed to related viruses) and, most importantly, safety concerns. Inadvertent recombination events between the replication-deficient vaccine vector, which lacks gene sequences for structural antigens, and helper viruses which provide those capsid proteins thus resulting in infectious viral particles.

2. *Recombinant viral particles as adjuvants*: Recombinant vectors require cloning of the nucleic acid sequence of the target antigen into the viral genome. Instead, recombinant proteins and other types of vaccines can simply be co-delivered with replication-incompetent viral particles in the same fashion as conventional vaccine adjuvants (Liljestrom and Garoff 1991). This approach bypasses a common shortcoming of viral vectors: the above-mentioned neutralizing anti-viral immunity. Pre-exposure to the parental virus (as in the case of adenovirus), related viruses, or repeated immunization with a particular viral vector results in (a) the induction of powerful neutralizing antibodies which interfere with the delivery of a recombinant virus' payload or (b) the induction of strong cytotoxic T cell responses which efficiently eliminate virus infected cells before a meaningful immune response is mounted against the encoded vaccine antigen. This problem can be circumvented by the use of "empty" viral particles not encoding the vaccine-target sequence. Replication-deficient particles represent off-the-shelf adjuvants which can be combined with potentially any vaccine, thus eliminating tedious custom production or formulation steps. The separation of antigen and viral adjuvant can overcome the problem of pre-existing anti-viral immune responses. Unlike in the case of recombinant viral vectors, the anti-viral immune responses accelerated due to the pre-exposure to this virus, will not affect the level of target antigen which is delivered with the viral particle as a final product (e.g., recombinant protein).

3. *Replicase-based nucleic acid vaccines* (Fig. 3.1): Recognizing the ability of the alphaviral genome to "self-replicate" led to the development of self-replicating RNA vaccines in which the sequence for structural (capsid) proteins was replaced by the sequence for the antigen of interest (Zhou et al. 1994; Ying et al. 1999). Using the alphaviral genome as a pure nucleic-acid vaccine eliminates the issue of pre-existing host immunity to viral capsid antigens. Furthermore, the absence of viral antigens also abolishes the potential immunodominance of viral antigens over the encoded target antigen which can focus the host's immune response to the viral antigens rather than the vaccine. The phenomenon of interference by an immunodominant antigen, used as a "helper-antigen," was recently reported for β-galactosidase, which was used in an attempt to provide a bystander response to a tumor antigen (Leitner et al. 2009). Any comparison of alphaviral with

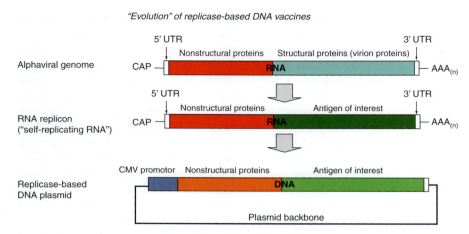

Fig. 3.1 The alphaviral genome (replicon) encodes nonstructural proteins (replicase enzyme complex) and structural proteins (viral capsid/virion proteins). In an RNA replicon vaccine, the genes for structural proteins are replaced with the RNA sequence of a target antigen ("antigen of interest"). DNA-based replicon vaccines contain the DNA sequence for the RNA replicon und the control of a promotor that is recognized by mammalian cells (most commonly one of viral origin such as the CMV promotor)

alphavirus-derived vectors (which lack capsid proteins) should take into account that the viral capsid not only protects the genomic RNA and mediates uptake of the viral particle by host cells, but also protects the active involvement of capsid proteins in the replication process. Binding of capsid to ribosomes may trigger uncoating of the genome which allows it to enter the cytoplasm from the lysosome and initiate its translational activity. Capsid proteins also appear to have a ribosome binding site at the same place where the protein interacts with viral RNA during encapsidation. The involvement of capsid proteins in the replication process may offer an explanation for the differences in replicon activity (and thus antigen levels) between attenuated alphaviral vaccines, (one-round infection only) alphaviral particles and replicon-based "naked" nucleic acid.

Replicon RNA: The First Generation of Replicase-Based Nucleic Acid Vaccines

Replicon-RNA (or "self-replicating" RNA) has previously successfully been used as an RNA vaccine (Ying et al. 1999; Zhou et al. 1994). In such constructs, the gene segments for structural proteins are replaced by mRNA encoding the vaccine antigen, keeping in place the gene sequence for the replicase enzyme complex as well as binding sites for the replicase on the modified viral genome (replicon) (Fig. 3.1). The difference in immunogenicity between such an RNA replicon vaccine and a conventional RNA vaccine (i.e., mRNA for the vaccine) are dramatic. Conventional RNA is largely inadequate as a vaccine when injected in the form of "naked" RNA due to several factors: (a) rapid degradation of extracellular RNA after injection,

3 Replicase-Based DNA and RNA Vaccines

(b) inefficient uptake of extracellular RNA into host cells and thus very low transfection efficiency, (c) limited half-life of cytoplasmic RNA and thus very limited antigen production, (d) insufficient or non-existent immunogenicity of mRNA and thus inadequate or missing adjuvanticity. Although RNA sensors, which assist in initiating inflammatory responses after viral infection have been identified, they are predominantly, if not exclusively, restricted to the cytoplasmic compartment and designed to recognize virus-specific RNA sequences. Nevertheless, "naked" replicon-RNA induces robust immune responses against the encoded antigen. Although subject to degradation by RNases, the amount of RNA available for antigen production is not limited by the inoculum. Instead, replicon-RNA molecules which successfully accessed the cytoplasm of host cells are amplified by the replicase enzyme. Therefore, in theory, a single copy of replicon-RNA per transfected host cell is sufficient for producing immunologically relevant amounts of vaccine antigen.

Replicon-DNA: The Second Generation of Replicase-Based Nucleic Acid Vaccines

Despite its immunogenicity, the usefulness of (self-replicating) RNA as a vaccine is limited by several factors, particularly because the production and handling of recombinant RNA is cumbersome. Plasmid DNA, in contrast, can easily and quickly be amplified in bacteria and is characterized by exceptional stability. In replicon-based DNA vaccines, a DNA-copy of the RNA-replicon is under the control of a viral promoter (generally, a CMV promoter), an approach initially used to generate alphaviral particles (DiCiommo and Bremner 1998). Unlike a conventional DNA vaccine, however, antigen-expression is not controlled by this promoter. Instead, the (viral) promoter only kick-starts the production of (self-replicating) mRNA in the transfected cells while antigen expression is under the control of the alphaviral replicase enzyme (DNA-launched RNA-replicon) resulting in antigen expression levels that are independent of the amount of plasmid delivered to each cell (Leitner et al. 2000). For most DNA vaccines, strong viral promoters such as the CMV promoter are used simply because of their ability to induce high-level antigen expression in a broad range of mammalian cells. Few studies – mostly in the area of gene therapy – have employed vectors with tissue-specific promoters which restrict antigen expression to specific cell types. The use of these promoters in nucleic acid vaccines was limited by often insufficient antigen expression levels although such promoters have provided important insights into the mechanism of action of DNA vaccines. Replacing the CMV promoter in a replicase-based DNA vaccine with a tissue-specific promoter offers exiting new opportunities for the development of novel vaccines: antigen expression will be restricted to specific cell types thus eliminating safety concerns related to antigen expression outside of the injection site. Antigen-expression will be under the control of the replicase enzyme and thus independent of the tissue-specific promoter. A brief, initial and low-level transcription from the plasmid is sufficient to initiate the production of self-replicating RNA transcripts (Figs. 3.1 and 3.2).

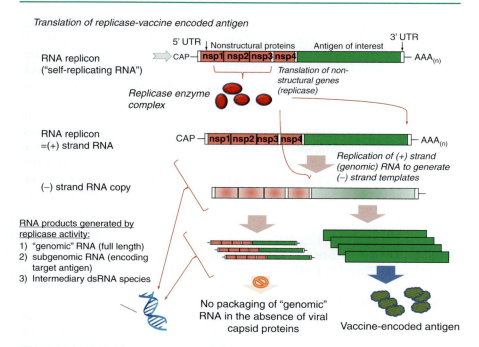

Fig. 3.2 The first product of the RNA replicon are the viral nonstructural proteins which form the replicase complex. The replicase binds to recognition sequences on the positive-strand ("genomic") RNA molecule resulting in negative-strand template and subsequently large numbers of positive-strand RNA copies. A subgenomic promotor (secondary replicase binding site) is used to generate shorter (subgenomic) RNA fragments which encode the antigen of interest. The entire replication process results in the production of several species of molecules which result in immune responses

Conventional vs. Replicase-Based Vectors: Comparing Apples to Oranges

The alphaviral replicase complex efficiently duplicates replicon RNA resulting in "massive production of the heterologous protein while competing out the host protein synthesis," as described for recombinant alphaviral particles (Liljestrom and Garoff 1991). The infection of a host cell with a single wildtype virus results in the release of a large number of offspring and the ability of alphavirus-derived vectors to produce large amounts of recombinant protein which has routinely been cited as the reason for why such vaccines tend to be much more immunogenic and efficacious. Interestingly, however, very few of those studies involving DNA vaccines include quantitative, side-by-side comparison analyses of replicase-based and conventional DNA vectors. Furthermore, antigen-expression experiments are almost exclusively done by transfecting cell lines in vitro with excessive amounts of plasmid. Such experiments, although useful for determining the functionality of

3 Replicase-Based DNA and RNA Vaccines

recombinant vectors, are not representative of what happens in vivo after DNA immunization for several reasons:

1. *Overall transfection efficiency*: The number of DNA plasmids per cell, regardless of the delivery method (injection by needle and syringe, electroporation, gene gun delivery) is unlikely to ever reach the levels seen in vitro when using highly efficient transfection reagents. This is exemplified by the observation that cell lines transfected in vitro (e.g., BHK-21 kidney cells) with a plasmid carrying antigens under the control of a tissue-specific promoter (e.g., a keratinocyte or dendritic cell-specific promoter) are still capable of producing the antigen due to the overwhelming copy number of plasmids per cell. The same plasmids, when injected in vivo, would only mediate antigen expression from the appropriate cell type (author's unpublished observation).

2. *Plasmid-dependent transfection efficiency*: When comparing different DNA vaccines, most studies do not take into account differences in the size of their DNA plasmids. This approach results in two common issues: (a) by basing the plasmid dose on weight only, fewer copies of the larger plasmid are injected; and (b) larger plasmids transfect cells less efficiently particularly when relying on uptake of injected, naked DNA in vivo.

3. *Immune response*: While studies conducted more than a decade ago have clearly shown that cells expressing a transgene after DNA immunization of animals are subject to lysis by antigen-specific T cells thus limiting the duration and extent of antigen production in vivo, it is less clear how innate immune responses affect antigen expression shortly after immunization. Different plasmids can be expected to provide different levels of innate immune activation depending on parameters such as the number of CpG motifs, the nature of the CpG sequence and various other, yet undefined signals. This is particularly evident in the case of replicase-based plasmids (as discussed below). Induction of any innate immune pathway (e.g., DNA sensors such as AIM2) has the potential to drastically affect the amount of plasmid-encoded antigen that the transfected cell will produce. In vitro studies with cell lines cannot predict the in vivo situation due to the differential expression of innate immune receptors in different types of cells as well as species-specific expression and recognition patterns.

In a side-by-side comparison of two replicase-based and two conventional (CMV-promoter driven) plasmids encoding the same antigen (β-galactosidase), we noticed that antigen expression levels after in vitro transfection of cell lines (and subsequently, after gene gun delivery of plasmids into mouse skin), induced by the plasmids did not correlate with their immunogenicity, with the most immunogenic replicase-driven plasmid inducing the lowest antigen production level (Leitner et al. 2000). The results from studies in which side-by-side comparison of conventional and replicase-based DNA plasmids indicate the expression of higher antigen levels in cells transfected with the alphaviral vector (such as the study by Ljungberg et al. (2007)) may be explained by the techniques used to evaluate the expression of reporter genes (such as green fluorescence protein): the replicase enzyme mediates the expression of distinct amounts of antigen regardless of the amount of DNA or RNA template. Thus, the level of antigen expression is maintained when transfected cells divide in vitro. In contrast, the transfection with a conventional plasmid results in antigen expression levels which depend on transfection efficiency and the amount of plasmid delivered to an individual cell. Therefore, varying plasmid doses used for transfection only drastically affects antigen expression from conventional, but not from replicase-based vectors (Leitner et al. 2000). Furthermore, each cell division of cultured cells carrying conventional plasmids cuts the amount of plasmid per cell (and thus antigen expression) in half resulting in a time-dependent "disappearance" of transfected cells not mediated by the death of transfected cells.

Although high antigen production continues to be cited in the literature as a distinguishing feature of replicase-based vectors, and antigen levels are frequently listed as a factor affecting DNA vaccine efficacy, antigen-levels alone do not explain the increased immunogenicity of plasmids in which antigen expression is under the control of an alphaviral replicase, prompting the search for other factors.

Innate Immune Responses and Replicase-Based Vaccines

Mammalian cells have acquired a broad range of receptors (such as TLR2, 3, 7, 8, 9, and RIG-I like receptors (RLRs)) and mechanisms to detect viruses and mount defensive responses. These include attempts to block RNA transcription, protein translation, production of anti-viral cytokines (and the initiation of innate immune responses), autophagy and apoptosis of the infected cell. Virus-derived structures recognized by mammalian pattern-recognition receptors include genomic DNA, single- or double-stranded RNA (ssRNA, dsRNA), RNA with 5'-triphosphate ends, and viral proteins (Takeuchi and Akira 2009). Different classes of viruses trigger overlapping sets of cellular receptors but determining the involvement of individual receptors and their signaling pathways is often complicated by the redundant nature of these sensors. Virus-based vaccines (attenuated or killed viruses, reassortant viruses, virosomes) owe their immunogenicity and efficacy to their ability to trigger these viral sensors, but the fact that viral RNA itself is recognized by specialized receptors has only been recognized recently.

After transfection of a cell with alphaviral ("pseudo-genomic") RNA vaccines, either directly (with "self-replicating" RNA replicon vaccines) or indirectly (self-replicating RNA is encoded on a DNA plasmid and generated by the transfected cell) the first product is the alphaviral replicase enzyme complex (encoded by the NS1-4 genes). This multi-subunit structure binds to recognition sequences on the alphavirus-derived RNA and is responsible for the synthesis of two RNA species: copies of the entire RNA molecule (which, in case of an alphaviral infection would be packaged as viral genome into the viral progeny) and short copies only encoding the structural (capsid) proteins (which, in the case of the vaccine, have been replaced by the sequences for the protein of interest) (Fig. 3.2). This process involves the creation of double-stranded RNA-intermediates. Although certain double-stranded RNA species can be found in mammalian cells, these tend to be restricted to short stretches of hairpin loops, for example, involving complementary RNA sequences within one RNA molecule but not long stretches of truly double-stranded RNA.

3 Replicase-Based DNA and RNA Vaccines

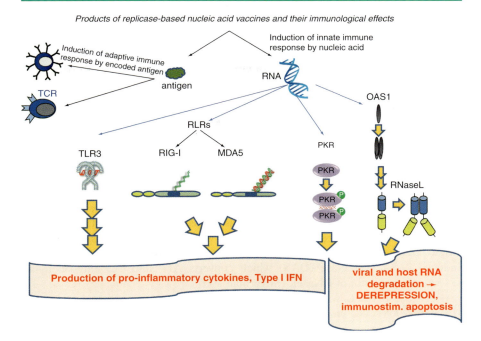

Fig. 3.3 Simplified summary of pathway and immune responses stimulated by replicase-based nucleic acid vaccines. Vaccine-encoded proteins, produced by transfected host cells, trigger both T and B cell responses. Innate immune stimulation is mediated by both DNA (in case of plasmid-based vaccines, not shown) and RNA (encoded by the DNA vector or in case of RNA replicon vaccines). DNA binds to TLR9 (CpG-mediated immune stimulation) and potentially to cytoplasmid DNA sensors such as MDA2. Double-stranded RNA binds to receptors such as TLR3, RIG-like receptors (RLRs, namely MDA5 while RIG-I recognizes ssRNA), PKR and 2′,5′-oligoadenylate synthetase 1 (OAS1). OAS-derived 2′–5′-oligoadenylate subsequently activates RNaseL which not simply degrades viral RNA, but (also) selectively eliminates host derived mRNA encoding inhibitors of innate immune responses thus inducing or enhancing inflammatory responses

The latter are recognized to be extremely efficient and lead to the rapid production of type I IFN designed to alert the immune system to the real or perceived viral infection of the dsRNA-carrying cell (Fig. 3.3). This phenomenon had been known for several decades and synthetic double-stranded RNA (poly-IC) is been used as an experimental adjuvant not only in animals but also with considerable success in clinical trials.

Receptors for double-stranded RNA molecules were only discovered relatively recently. Among the first pathways to be described were those involving RNA-dependent Protein Kinase (PKR) and Ribonuclease L (RNaseL), both shown to be important in the defense against viral infection. Transfection of mammalian cells with replicase-based DNA plasmids triggers a strong activation of PKR, as measured by the autophosphorylation of PKR-dimers which are generated when two molecules bind to the same dsRNA (Leitner et al. 2003). This finding indicated that the superior immunogenicity of nucleic acid vaccines appeared to be due to the activation of antiviral sensors and, thus, replicase-based vaccines, even in the absence of other viral proteins, mimic a viral infection. Interestingly, conventional DNA plasmids triggered some activation of PKR in transfected cells, albeit at much lower levels than replicase-based plasmids. It is still unclear how a DNA plasmid without a replicase or similar enzyme could produce RNA species that activate PRK, but this observation allows for the intriguing speculation that dsRNA-sensing pathways are also involved in the immunogenicity of conventional DNA vaccines.

A second dsRNA sensing pathway results in the activation of RNaseL (formerly 2–5A-dependent RNase) (an enzyme initially shown to be important for antiviral defense by degrading RNA, both viral and cellular) thus blocking viral infections. As many other anti-viral effector mechanisms, RNaseL is regulated by virus-induced interferons and recognizes various forms of viral dsRNA species which include replicative intermediates of single-stranded RNA (ssRNA) viruses, dsRNA genomes, annealed viral RNA of opposite polarities as well as stem structures of otherwise single-stranded viral RNAs. The recognition of these molecules is through the IFN-induced 2–5A synthetase (OAS) which converts ATP into $2',5'$-oligoadenylate (2–5A), the activator of RNaseL (Silverman 2007).

Recently, RNaseL was also implicated in immune responses against bacteria (Li et al. 2008). The enzyme does not simply degrade mRNA randomly, but upon activation appears to control innate immune pathways of infected cells by selectively degrading the mRNA of immune inhibitory molecules, namely anti-inflammatory cytokines. In vitro, Sindbis virus continuously triggers the synthesis of minus-strand templates in the absence of RNase-L, which is normally shut off by the enzyme within a few hours (Sawicki et al. 2003). Mice lacking this enzyme (RNaseL-KO mice) only mounted poor immune responses against B16 tumors after immunization with a replicase-based DNA vaccine which protects wildtype mice (Leitner et al. 2003). This protection was mediated by vaccine-induced CD8 T cells which drastically reduced tumor take in naïve mice after adoptive transfer from immunized mice. In hindsight, this finding is surprising and unexpected: several (viral) RNA sensing molecules and pathways have been identified since, namely TLR3 and the RLR-family (RIG-I and MDA5). Although RNAs from different viruses appear to be selectively recognized by different receptors, there appears to be a significant level of redundancy in the recognition of viral nucleic acid and thus, the elimination of a single pathway (i.e., RNaseL) would not be expected to have such a drastic effect. It may, however, indicate a central role that the RNaseL pathway plays in the intensity of an antiviral innate response through previously unappreciated mechanisms (Li et al. 2007).

As discussed above for TLR9, the discovery of TLR-molecules promised to provide the long-sought explanation for why and how pathogens are initially recognized by the innate immune system. Double-stranded RNA is the ligand of TLR3 (CD283), a strictly intracellular receptor expressed in the endosome of most cells (Ryman and Klimstra 2008) and thus, this receptor could be anticipated to play a role in the immunogenicity of a vaccine which generates dsRNA. Cells transfected with replicase-based DNA are readily phagocytized by dendritic cells in vitro and activated by the dsRNA inside the transfected cell. Surprisingly, however, the immunogenicity of a replicase-based DNA vaccine was unaffected in TLR3-knockout mice which generated the same number of antigen-specific CD8 T cells. Again, this underscores the highly redundant nature of innate sensing pathways and suggests that compensatory signaling pathways are at work (Diebold et al. 2009).

How Does a Perceived Viral Infection Enhance DNA Vaccine Efficacy?

Part 1: The Role of Type I IFNs

Mammalian cells respond to the infection with various viruses by producing interferon, a phenomenon known for almost half a century. Specifically, Type I interferons (IFN-α and β) are produced in direct response to a viral infection and, therefore, the IFN system represents one of the earliest, innate stages of an antiviral response (Palese 2005). In addition to their antiviral activity, Type I IFNs have important immunostimulatory functions such promoting dendritic cell-maturation or the stimulation of cross-presentation of antigens to CD8 T cells, making them attractive vaccine adjuvants (Tovey and Lallemand 2010). Viruses have evolved various immune escape mechanisms in an attempt to blunt or retard the host's anti-viral response. One of many such mechanisms is the recently described suppression of the Type I interferon response by one of the non-structural proteins in the alphaviral genome, nsp2 (Breakwell et al. 2007). This indicates that Type I IFNs are induced as a consequence of dsRNA recognition and alphaviral infection of cells (in vitro and in vivo) has been shown to trigger the release of IFN (Ryman and Klimstra 2008). Therefore, it was reasonable to postulate that the induction of Type I IFNs may be a contributing factor to the superior immunogenicity of replicase-based DNA vaccines. After in vitro transfection, replicase-based plasmids triggered the release of much higher levels of both IFN-α and β compared to conventional DNA vaccines (Leitner et al. 2006; Ljungberg et al. 2007). In vivo analysis of these cytokines is complicated by the large number of IFN-βs, however, since all Type I IFNs bind to the same receptor (IFNAR1/2), the question can be approached through the use of receptor knockout mice (Leitner et al. 2006). In these mice, which can produce Type I IFN but not respond to it, the efficacy of a replicase-based plasmid encoding a tumor antigen was drastically reduced. In this tumor model, protection is based predominantly on CD8 T cells and the Th1-promoting effects of type I IFNs have thoroughly been documented in the literature (Sinigaglia et al. 1999).

To confirm that the interferon does, indeed, act as an adjuvant for a DNA vaccine, a conventional DNA plasmid was "adjuvanted" through the co-delivery of a second plasmid encoding a Type I IFN (Leitner et al. 2006). Co-transfection to the same cells in vivo (in order to mimic the situation found in cells transfected with replicase-based plasmids) was insured by using gene gun delivery. This approach is extremely useful when analyzing any plasmid-based adjuvants since it permits the simple and efficient adjustment of the dose of the "adjuvant plasmid" (Leitner et al. 2009). The study clearly showed that Type I IFN, indeed, had adjuvant activity and significantly increased the efficacy of the conventional, poorly efficacious plasmid in a tumor model.

In the tumor model used for the studies described above, antibodies are induced by the vaccination with both conventional and replicase-based DNA vaccines, but they do not appear to contribute to tumor rejection. Interestingly, the IFN-αβR knockout mice produced significantly more antigen-specific antibodies after immunization with the replicase-based plasmid. This suggests that in the wildtype animal, the antiviral interferon response limits the amount of antigen produced by transfected cells. Suppression of gene expression by Type I interferons has previously been reported, for example after vaccination with conventional DNA (Sellins et al. 2005). A mechanistic explanation of these observations is complicated by the observation that in vitro, the Type I release of cells transfected with replicase-based vectors only affected host protein synthesis, but not the production of antigen encoded on the alphaviral vector (Liljestrom and Garoff 1991), suggesting that in vivo, Type I IFN does not affect the production of vaccine-encoded protein in an autocrine fashion (i.e., but preventing protein translation in general). Instead, the reduced antigen production is likely a result of the IFN-enhanced immune response targeted against the transfected cells.

Once again, the above described observations underscore the importance of developing and judging DNA vaccines not primarily based on the levels of (in vitro) antigen induction, but the intensity and quality of the innate (adjuvant-type) immune stimulatory signals they deliver. Surprisingly, in another study in which the authors investigated the involvement of Type I IFN in the immunogenicity of replicase-based DNA vectors, the alphaviral vector (which – as expected – triggered significant IFN-α/β secretion from transfected cells) provided superior humoral and cellular immunogenicity which did *not* appear to be different in the presence or absence of Type I IFN signaling (Ljungberg et al. 2007). Although this could indicate that the importance of Type I IFNs on vaccine-induced immunogenicity and efficacy may be dependent on the antigen or disease model, it may also reflect a technical artifact: The strength of the adaptive immune response induced by replicase-based vectors does not correlate with their dose (unlike conventional DNA plasmids), a phenomenon also observed in this study (Ljungberg et al. 2007). This is likely due to the induction of strong innate host responses when too much replicon RNA is present. Therefore, when investigating the role of a particular immune pathway on the immunogenicity or efficacy of a vaccine, it is important to use an optimized dose (or dose titration). The optimal dose for conventional and replicase-based DNA plasmids has repeatedly been shown to be very different and comparisons between the two should not be done using "comparable" (molar) amounts.

Part 2: The Role of Apoptosis

One downstream effect of interferon-signaling is the induction of genes involved in the elimination of viral components from the infected cells, the induction of an "anti-viral state" in non-infected bystander cells, as well as the induction of

3 Replicase-Based DNA and RNA Vaccines

programmed cell death (apoptosis) (Takeuchi and Akira 2009). Apoptosis is not only a constitutive mechanism by which unwanted (damaged or aged) cells are removed, but a common response to viral infections in an attempt to deprive the pathogen of its host. Thus, viral infections can be viewed as a race for time between the pathogen (attempting to successfully generate progeny before the host cell shuts down protein synthesis) and the host cell (trying to limit the spread of the virus to neighboring cells by interfering with viral replication, producing messengers, such as IFNs and heat shock proteins, and ultimately undergoing cell death). Numerous viral factors have been described which interfere with or divert the apoptotic process (reviewed in Tschopp et al. (1998)).

Host cells killed by many viruses are readily eliminated by phagocytic cells (dendritic cells, macrophages) after being tagged by apoptotic adaptor proteins, which bind to molecules exposed on the surface of the apoptotic cells such as phosphatidylserin. A number of apoptotic adaptor proteins have been identified (such as Annexin V or MFG-E8) and the redundancy in this system indicates how important the rapid removal of dying cells is. Deficiencies in this system result in the accumulation of immunogenic host-derived material and the ultimate induction of autoimmunity. Host cell death as a consequence of an infection fulfills distinct needs to the host. Massive apoptosis occurs after an infection has been cleared requiring large amounts of immune cells to be eliminated in order to re-establish immune cell homeostasis. In case of virus-infected cells, the desired outcome of host-cell death and its phagocytic removal by dendritic cells is

- Activation of the dendritic cell, and
- Presentation of virus-associated antigens to T cells in a pro-inflammatory context. In case of steady-state apoptosis (removal of aged and unwanted cells) such inflammatory processes need to be avoided or even suppressed.

After the initial discovery of at least two cell-death pathways, namely apoptosis and necrosis, it was initially suggested that apoptosis resulted in immune suppression (tolerance) while necrosis, the disintegration of cells which results in cytoplasmic content being released from dying cells, mediated the activation of dendritic cells and thus represents a pro-inflammatory stimulus. Recent studies have identified several cytoplasmic molecules, which when released from cells, can trigger vigorous inflammatory responses (Baccala et al. 2009). This provides a molecular mechanism for the immune stimulatory effect of necrosis by "misplaced" self-molecules. The immunological result of host cell apoptosis is much more complex and can be explained by the signals generated in the course of apoptosis and those depend on the signal which initiated apoptosis. Programmed cell death as part of a homeostatic mechanism would not be expected to produce signals leading to the activation of immune cells but only produce ligands for phagocyte receptors leading to their rapid, but immunologically "silent" removal. In contrast, in case of a viral infection, apoptosis of the infected cell is accompanied by the production of immunostimulatory signals such as heat shock proteins, Type I IFNs (see above) and others. Under those circumstances, phagocytosis of the apoptotic cell is accompanied by the activation of the dendritic cell followed by antigen presentation under stimulatory conditions.

The observation of caspase-dependent apoptosis of cells transfected with self-replicating RNA (RNA replicon) or replicase-based DNA raised an intriguing question: is this process simply a side effect of the perceived viral infection and the enhanced immunogenicity of the vectors driven by the signals the transfected cell produces (heat shock proteins, IFNs) or does apoptosis actively contribute to the superior immunogenicity of such vectors? The adjuvant effect of apoptosis has previously been shown and exploited in DNA vaccines which encoded pro-apoptotic molecules together with the antigen of interest. A major caveat of this approach is the need to "dial down" the efficacy of the pro-apoptotic protein to slow cell death and allow expression of the target antigen (Sasaki et al. 2001). This is a delicate balancing act which can be accomplished using different approaches: the two genes, i.e., pro-apoptotic antigen and vaccine antigen, need to be delivered to the same target cell for this approach to be efficacious. When delivering DNA vaccines by needle-and-syringe, co-delivery is accomplished by using either bi-cistronic plasmids or by separating the two genes by gene sequences, which mediate the production of two independent gene products (e.g., internal ribosomal entry sites (IRES)). When delivering DNA vaccines by gene gun, plasmids bound to gold particles are forced into cells of the epidermis mechanically as discrete aliquots of plasmid (i.e., the amount of plasmid bound to one gold particle). Co-delivery is achieved by the simple mixing of two or more types of plasmid to be coated onto the particle. Reducing the amount of one plasmid selectively decreases its expression level thus enabling the rapid, straight-forward testing of numerous pro- or anti- apoptotic genes at different "strengths" for their ability to modify the immune response to a DNA vaccine encoded protein (Bergmann-Leitner et al. 2009).

To determine the impact of apoptosis on the efficacy of replicase-based vectors, replicase-based DNA vaccines were co-delivered with an anti-apoptotic protein encoded on a separate plasmid using gene gun immunization as described above to ensure co-transfection of target cells. The efficacy of the replicase-based plasmid in a T cell dependent tumor model dropped significantly indicating that apoptosis, in fact does contribute to the immunogenicity of replicase-based vaccines. Interestingly, however, the inhibition of apoptosis resulted in enhanced antibody titers to the encoded antigen, consistent with prolonged survival of the transfected cells and increased antigen production (Leitner et al. 2004).

Less (Death) is More: How Lethal Hits Can Add Up

DNA-vaccine induced apoptosis is an important aspect not only from a safety and regulatory standpoint, as it ultimately leads to the removal of host cells carrying recombinant DNA, but mostly because of its adjuvant potential. Although this aspect has been acknowledged in the literature, the ability of transgenes themselves to induce host-cell apoptosis is still insufficiently appreciated. Depending on the source of the gene (virus, pathogen) and depending on its modifications (e.g., removal of certain sequences, re-coding of the entire gene), the pro-apoptotic effect of the antigen, such as the malaria parasite-derived CSP (Bergmann-Leitner et al. 2009), can affect its immunogenicity. When using vectors or vaccination approaches which already trigger significant apoptosis, host-cell death may be accelerated to a level where insufficient amounts of antigen are produced. Thus, not all antigens may be suitable for delivery in recombinant vectors which achieve high immunogenicity in part through the induction of apoptosis. Furthermore, modulating host cell apoptosis to enhance vaccine efficacy of DNA vaccines may have unexpected consequences as shown in the case of a DNA-based malaria vaccine, which modulated host cell apoptosis through the co-delivery of pro- or anti-apoptotic proteins and altered the Th-profiles of the vaccine-induced immune response and thus its efficacy (Bergmann-Leitner et al. 2009).

Lessons Learned from Replicase-Based Nucleic Acid Vaccines

The analysis of the mechanism of action of replicase-based DNA (and RNA) vaccines has provided important insights into how vaccines work and how their efficacy could be further improved. Some of these lessens had previously been learned in other systems but were not always thoroughly appreciated and applied in the design of novel vaccines.

Lesson 1: Less Is More

One criterion when evaluating recombinant vaccines routinely is the amount of antigen released from infected or transfected cells. In cells transfected with replicase-based vectors the amount of antigen is strictly controlled by the replicase and not the number of vaccine (RNA/DNA) molecules. Although this dose, both in vitro (as discussed above) and in vivo (unpublished observation) is lower than that induced by conventional vectors, superior T cell responses are induced. Both molecules discussed above which are involved in dsRNA-sensing, and likely additional anti-viral pathways, are responsible for limiting antigen production in cells transfected with replicase-based vectors (Terenzi et al. 1999). Therefore, providing adequate innate immune stimulation clearly appears to be more important than delivering more antigen. Moreover, immunization with high antigen doses promotes the expansion of T cells with low-avidity TCR (Alexander-Miller et al. 1996), which are undesirable when attempting to raise an effective T cell response against viruses or tumors. Although not formally shown yet, but based on this observation, replicase-based vectors can be expected to generate higher avidity T cells than conventional vectors.

Lesson 2: Follow the Pathogen's Lead

Viruses, bacteria and parasites present a large number of PAMPs to the host's immune system which trigger innate immune responses. These PAMPs have provided the adjuvant component of traditional vaccines such as attenuated or killed pathogens. In the case of recombinant protein vaccines, PAMPs which contaminate the preparation due to inadequate purification or their ability to bind to protein can provide potent adjuvant effects. A major challenge for modern vaccines is the development of efficacious but safe adjuvants that will be added back to vaccines which – by themselves – are non-immunogenic (purified recombinant proteins). Other vaccines could significantly benefit from an adjuvant to provide dose sparing or enhanced efficacy in special populations such as the elderly (e.g., seasonal flu vaccine). Many adjuvant candidates are based on pathogen-derived molecules which trigger inflammatory responses, but concerns over excessive inflammation and resulting side effects of adjuvants represent significant hurdles for the approval of such components as vaccine adjuvants. Understanding the immune escape mechanisms of pathogens (which include the production of immune-suppressive molecules such as soluble cytokine receptors) enables the design of recombinant vectors which only deliver adjuvant-type molecules and thus, immunostimulatory signals. Replicase-based vectors are a prototypic example of such vaccines albeit their actual mechanism of action was discovered in hindsight. The production of small amounts of immunostimulatory dsRNA molecules only in transfected cells provides a potent, but highly localized (thus highly contained) and safe adjuvant effect, resulting in "inflammatory apoptosis" (Restifo 2001). The subsequent elimination of vaccine-carrying host cells by vaccine-induced apoptosis and removal by dendritic cells represents an additional important safety feature of replicase-based nucleic acid vaccines.

Putting Replicase-Based Vaccines to the Test: Models, Formats and Regimens

The usefulness of replicase-based vectors as novel vaccine platforms has been explored in a wide variety of model systems. Only a limited number of studies, however, describe formal side-by-side comparisons of the different platforms, such as a comparison of conventional and replicase-based DNA vectors (e.g., for influenza (Miller et al. 2008) or a tumor model (Leitner et al. 2003; Leitner et al. 2000)). In general, these studies report higher immunogenicity and efficacy of replicase-based vectors.

Only selected studies involving replicase-based vectors can be discussed here. Among the replicase-based vaccines already being tested in humans are Sindbis-replicase encoding plasmids against measles (Ramirez et al. 2008) which are highly immunogenic in animal models. Importantly, unlike the conventional measles vaccine, a replicase-based plasmid (encoding the measles hemagglutinin) induces long lasting, high-avidity virus-neutralizing antibodies and T cell responses in neonates despite the presence of high levels of maternal antibodies (Capozzo et al. 2006). Although a measles vaccine is currently available, it is poorly efficacious in infants younger than 9 months. The virus, however, is responsible for significant morbidity and mortality in infants and young children in developing countries. In a side-by-side comparison of a replicon-particle vaccine encoding measles hemagglutinin with a non-protective formalin-inactivated, alum-precipitated measles vaccine, antibodies induced by the alphaviral particles exhibited higher avidity and had neutralizing activity (Bergen et al. 2010).

3 Replicase-Based DNA and RNA Vaccines

Numerous studies have described the usefulness of replicase-based vaccines (DNA or particles) in models of HIV, indicating that either DNA plasmids (Nordstrom et al. 2005), replicon particles or various heterologous prime-boost regimens involving either of the two platforms or both (Barnett et al. 2010; Ljungberg et al. 2007) are all promising approaches which may overcome the insufficient immunogenicity of previously tested HIV vaccines.

Outlook: Do Replicase-Based DNA Vaccines Have a Future?

A modern vaccine candidate which has shown efficacy in the laboratory needs to overcome yet additional hurdles before being considered for testing in humans and licensure: the legal acceptance by regulatory agencies as well as psychological acceptance by potential vaccine recipients. The main criterion for this acceptance is the actual and perceived safety of the vaccine. Preventive vaccines are expected to have few or no side effects, neither short term (such as local inflammation, fatigue, injection site pain) nor long term (risk of autoimmune disease, increased risk of other rare adverse effects). Based on the studies conducted so far, replicase-based nucleic acid vaccines appear to meet these requirements without exception. Replicase-based vectors are also very attractive due to their ability to induce potent immune responses even when minute amounts of vaccine are delivered. Up to 20,000-times less replicase-based than conventional plasmid was reported to be efficacious not only as a preventive, but also a therapeutic vaccine in experimental models of allergy (Scheiblhofer et al. 2006; Weiss et al. 2006). This phenomenon is a result of the alphaviral replicase controlling both the amount of antigen being produced in each transfected cells as well the production of a predictable amount of immunostimulatory material (mainly dsRNA) which is independent of the size of the inoculum.

Although the majority of nucleic acid vaccines that take advantage of a viral replicase are DNA (plasmid) based, self-replicating RNA vaccines (Ying et al. 1999) are still highly attractive if the (albeit short-term) persistence of foreign DNA in the host is a concern. Such RNA-replicon vaccines represent extremely safe but potentially very efficacious vaccines as shown in various models of Type I allergies (Roesler et al. 2009) thus keeping the door open for RNA-based vaccines.

References

Alexander-Miller MA, Leggatt GR, Berzofsky JA (1996) Selective expansion of high- or low-avidity cytotoxic T lymphocytes and efficacy for adoptive immunotherapy. Proc Natl Acad Sci USA 93(9):4102–4107

Baccala R, Gonzalez-Quintial R, Lawson BR, Stern ME, Kono DH, Beutler B, Theofilopoulos AN (2009) Sensors of the innate immune system: their mode of action. Nat Rev Rheumatol 5(8):448–456

Barnett SW, Burke B, Sun Y, Kan E, Legg H, Lian Y, Bost K, Zhou F, Goodsell A, Zur Megede J, Polo J, Donnelly J, Ulmer J, Otten GR, Miller CJ, Vajdy M, Srivastava IK (2010) Antibody-mediated protection against mucosal simian-human immunodeficiency virus challenge of macaques immunized with alphavirus replicon particles and boosted with trimeric envelope glycoprotein in MF59 adjuvant. J Virol 84(12):5975–5985

Bergen MJ, Pan CH, Greer CE, Legg HS, Polo JM, Griffin DE (2010) Comparison of the immune responses induced by chimeric alphavirus-vectored and formalin-inactivated alum-precipitated measles vaccines in mice. PLoS ONE 5(4):e10297

Bergmann-Leitner ES, Leitner WW, Duncan EH, Savranskaya T, Angov E (2009) Molecular adjuvants for malaria DNA vaccines based on the modulation of host-cell apoptosis. Vaccine 27(41):5700–5708

Beutler B (2009) Microbe sensing, positive feedback loops, and the pathogenesis of inflammatory diseases. Immunol Rev 227(1):248–263

Breakwell L, Dosenovic P, Karlsson Hedestam GB, D'Amato M, Liljestrom P, Fazakerley J, McInerney GM (2007) Semliki forest virus nonstructural protein 2 is involved in suppression of the type I interferon response. J Virol 81(16):8677–8684

Capozzo AV, Ramirez K, Polo JM, Ulmer J, Barry EM, Levine MM, Pasetti MF (2006) Neonatal immunization with a Sindbis virus-DNA measles vaccine induces adult-like neutralizing antibodies and cell-mediated immunity in the presence of maternal antibodies. J Immunol 176(9):5671–5681

Deng GM (2008) The role of bacterial DNA in inflammatory and allergic disease. Recent Pat Inflamm Allergy Drug Discov 2(2):117–122

DiCiommo DP, Bremner R (1998) Rapid, high level protein production using DNA-based Semliki forest virus vectors. J Biol Chem 273(29):18060–18066

Diebold SS, Schulz O, Alexopoulou L, Leitner WW, Flavell RA, Reis e Sousa C (2009) Role of TLR3 in the immunogenicity of replicon plasmid-based vaccines. Gene Ther 16(3):359–366

Dixon B (1995) The third vaccine revolution. Nat Biotechnol 13:420–442

Griffin DE (2007) Alphaviruses. In: Knipe DM, Howley PM, Griffin DE et al (eds) Fields Virology, 5th edn. Lippincott Williams & Wilkins, Philadelphia, PA, pp 1023–1067

Hornung V, Ablasser A, Charrel-Dennis M, Bauernfeind F, Horvath G, Caffrey DR, Latz E, Fitzgerald KA (2009) AIM2 recognizes cytosolic dsDNA and forms a caspase-1-activating inflammasome with ASC. Nature 458(7237):514–518

Karlsson GB, Liljestrom P (2004) Delivery and expression of heterologous genes in mammalian cells using self-replicating alphavirus vectors. Meth Mol Biol 246:543–557

Kim KH, Rumenapf T, Strauss EG, Strauss JH (2004) Regulation of Semliki forest virus RNA replication: a model for the control of alphavirus pathogenesis in invertebrate hosts. Virology 323(1):153–163

Leitner WW (2001) Myth, menace or medical blessing? The clinical potential and the problems of genetic vaccines. EMBO Rep 2(3):168–170

Leitner WW, Ying H, Driver DA, Dubensky TW, Restifo NP (2000) Enhancement of tumor-specific immune response with plasmid DNA replicon vectors. Cancer Res 60(1):51–55

Leitner WW, Hwang LN, deVeer MJ, Zhou A, Silverman RH, Williams BR, Dubensky TW, Ying H, Restifo NP (2003) Alphavirus-based DNA vaccine breaks immunological tolerance by activating innate antiviral pathways. Nat Med 9(1):33–39

Leitner WW, Hwang LN, Bergmann-Leitner ES, Finkelstein SE, Frank S, Restifo NP (2004) Apoptosis is essential for the increased efficacy of alphaviral replicase-based DNA vaccines. Vaccine 22(11–12):1537–1544

Leitner WW, Bergmann-Leitner ES, Hwang LN, Restifo NP (2006) Type I interferons are essential for the efficacy of replicase-based DNA vaccines. Vaccine 24(24):5110–5118

Leitner WW, Baker MC, Berenberg TL, Lu MC, Yannie PJ, Udey MC (2009) Enhancement of DNA tumor vaccine efficacy by gene gun-mediated codelivery of threshold amounts of plasmid-encoded helper antigen. Blood 113(1):37–45

Li XL, Andersen JB, Ezelle HJ, Wilson GM, Hassel BA (2007) Post-transcriptional regulation of RNase-L expression is mediated by the 3′-untranslated region of its mRNA. J Biol Chem 282(11):7950–7960

Li XL, Ezelle HJ, Kang TJ, Zhang L, Shirey KA, Harro J, Hasday JD, Mohapatra SK, Crasta OR, Vogel SN, Cross AS, Hassel BA (2008) An essential role for the antiviral endoribonuclease, RNase-L, in antibacterial immunity. Proc Natl Acad Sci USA 105(52):20816–20821

Liljestrom P, Garoff H (1991) A new generation of animal cell expression vectors based on the Semliki forest virus replicon. Biotechnology (NY) 9(12):1356–1361

Ljungberg K, Whitmore AC, Fluet ME, Moran TP, Shabman RS, Collier ML, Kraus AA, Thompson JM, Montefiori DC, Beard C, Johnston RE (2007) Increased immunogenicity of a DNA-launched Venezuelan equine encephalitis virus-based replicon DNA vaccine. J Virol 81(24): 13412–13423

Lundstrom K (2005) Biology and application of alphaviruses in gene therapy. Gene Ther 12(Suppl 1): S92–S97

Miller A, Center RJ, Stambas J, Deliyannis G, Doherty PC, Howard JL, Turner SJ, Purcell DF (2008) Sindbis virus vectors elicit hemagglutinin-specific humoral and cellular immune responses and offer a dose-sparing strategy for vaccination. Vaccine 26(44):5641–5648

Nordstrom EK, Forsell MN, Barnfield C, Bonin E, Hanke T, Sundstrom M, Karlsson GB, Liljestrom P (2005) Enhanced immunogenicity using an alphavirus replicon DNA vaccine against human immunodeficiency virus type 1. J Gen Virol 86(Pt 2):349–354

Palese P (ed) (2005) Modulation of host gene expression and innate immunity by viruses, 1st edn. Springer, Dordrecht, The Netherlands

Ramirez K, Barry EM, Ulmer J, Stout R, Szabo J, Manetz S, Levine MM, Pasetti MF (2008) Preclinical safety and biodistribution of Sindbis virus measles DNA vaccines administered as a single dose or followed by live attenuated measles vaccine in a heterologous prime-boost regimen. Hum Gene Ther 19(5):522–531

Restifo NP (2001) Vaccines to die for. Nat Biotechnol 19(6):527–528

Roesler E, Weiss R, Weinberger EE, Fruehwirth A, Stoecklinger A, Mostbock S, Ferreira F, Thalhamer J, Scheiblhofer S (2009) Immunize and disappear-safety-optimized mRNA vaccination with a panel of 29 allergens. J Allergy Clin Immunol 124(5):1070–1077, e1071-1011

Rottembourg D, Filippi CM, Bresson D, Ehrhardt K, Estes EA, Oldham JE, von Herrath MG (2010) Essential role for TLR9 in prime but not prime-boost plasmid DNA vaccination to activate dendritic cells and protect from lethal viral infection. J Immunol 184(12):7100–7107

Ryman KD, Klimstra WB (2008) Host responses to alphavirus infection. Immunol Rev 225:27–45

Sasaki S, Amara RR, Oran AE, Smith JM, Robinson HL (2001) Apoptosis-mediated enhancement of DNA-raised immune responses by mutant caspases. Nat Biotechnol 19(6):543–547

Sato Y, Roman M, Tighe H, Lee D, Corr M, Nguyen MD, Silverman GJ, Lotz M, Carson DA, Raz E (1996) Immunostimulatory DNA sequences necessary for effective intradermal gene immunization. Science 273(5273):352–354

Sawicki DL, Silverman RH, Williams BR, Sawicki SG (2003) Alphavirus minus-strand synthesis and persistence in mouse embryo fibroblasts derived from mice lacking RNase L and protein kinase R. J Virol 77(3):1801–1811

Scheiblhofer S, Gabler M, Leitner WW, Bauer R, Zoegg T, Ferreira F, Thalhamer J, Weiss R (2006) Inhibition of type I allergic responses with nanogram doses of replicon-based DNA vaccines. Allergy 61(7):828–835

Sellins K, Fradkin L, Liggitt D, Dow S (2005) Type I interferons potently suppress gene expression following gene delivery using liposome(-)DNA complexes. Mol Ther 12(3):451–459

Silverman RH (2007) Viral encounters with 2′,5′-oligoadenylate synthetase and RNase L during the interferon antiviral response. J Virol 81(23):12720–12729

Sinigaglia F, D'Ambrosio D, Rogge L (1999) Type I interferons and the Th1/Th2 paradigm. Dev Comp Immunol 23(7–8):657–663

Takeuchi O, Akira S (2009) Innate immunity to virus infection. Immunol Rev 227(1):75–86

Tannis LL, Gauthier A, Evelegh C, Parsons R, Nyholt D, Khromykh A, Bramson JL (2005) Semliki forest virus and Kunjin virus RNA replicons elicit comparable cellular immunity but distinct humoral immunity. Vaccine 23(33):4189–4194

Terenzi F, deVeer MJ, Ying H, Restifo NP, Williams BR, Silverman RH (1999) The antiviral enzymes PKR and RNase L suppress gene expression from viral and non-viral based vectors. Nucleic Acids Res 27(22):4369–4375

Tovey MG, Lallemand C (2010) Adjuvant activity of cytokines. Meth Mol Biol 626:287–309

Tschopp J, Thome M, Hofmann K, Meinl E (1998) The fight of viruses against apoptosis. Curr Opin Genet Dev 8(1):82–87

Vasiljeva L, Merits A, Golubtsov A, Sizemskaja V, Kaariainen L, Ahola T (2003) Regulation of the sequential processing of Semliki forest virus replicase polyprotein. J Biol Chem 278(43): 41636–41645

Weiss R, Scheiblhofer S, Gabler M, Ferreira F, Leitner WW, Thalhamer J (2006) Is genetic vaccination against allergy possible? Int Arch Allergy Immunol 139(4):332–345

Widera G, Austin M, Rabussay D, Goldbeck C, Barnett SW, Chen M, Leung L, Otten GR, Thudium K, Selby MJ, Ulmer JB (2000) Increased DNA vaccine delivery and immunogenicity by electroporation in vivo. J Immunol 164(9):4635–4640

Ying H, Zaks TZ, Wang RF, Irvine KR, Kammula US, Marincola FM, Leitner WW, Restifo NP (1999) Cancer therapy using a self-replicating RNA vaccine. Nat Med 5(7):823–827

Zhou X, Berglund P, Rhodes G, Parker SE, Jondal M, Liljestrom P (1994) Self-replicating Semliki forest virus RNA as recombinant vaccine. Vaccine 12(16):1510–1514

Cytokine Genes as Molecular Adjuvants for DNA Vaccines

4

Bin Wang, Youmin Kang, and Richard Ascione

DNA vaccines encoding a foreign antigen induce antigen-specific cellular and humoral immune responses to protect against viral and bacterial infections, parasites, cancers, and autoimmune diseases. However the relatively low efficacy of DNA vaccinations in large animal species and humans has hindered their practical use as therapeutics. Therefore, there is an urgent need to improve protective responses generated by DNA vaccines. Among various improvement strategies, the incorporation of cytokine expressing plasmids as molecular adjuvants have been widely studied in the past years, yet still without significant clinical application. Cytokines play critical roles in natural immune responses during the presentation of antigens, and in particular, in directing T-cell polarization. This chapter reviews recent progress in the co-application of cytokine-encoding genes used for enhancement and direction of immunogenicity, as well as discusses their therapeutic potential for future applications.

Introduction

DNA vaccines have been studied extensively in recent years since it is known to be a safe modality, simple to use and especially easy to store (Tang et al. 1992; Wang et al. 1993; Wolff et al. 1990). However, the relatively low efficacy of DNA vaccines in inducing immune responses, especially in large animal species and humans, has hampered their practical use (Sasaki et al. 1998). Thus many strategies have been employed to improve and modulate the immune response induced by DNA vaccines.

B. Wang (✉)
State Key Laboratory for Agro-Biotechnology, College of Biological Science,
China Agricultural University, Beijing, China
e-mail: bwang3@cau.edu.cn

J. Thalhamer et al. (eds.), *Gene Vaccines*,
DOI 10.1007/978-3-7091-0439-2_4, © Springer-Verlag/Wien, 2012

Cytokines are obvious choices for enhancing the immunogenicity of vaccines because of their recognized central role in modulating the hosts' immune responses.

The cytokine repertoire, with respect to DNA vaccines, currently extends to over 30 cytokines and all have the potential for significantly modulating immune responses. Cytokine expressing plasmids delivered simultaneously with DNA vaccines have proven useful for studying and understanding their particular roles in immune responses (Scheerlinck 2001). Different patterns of cytokine expression can influence the type of immune response that subsequently develops (Min et al. 2001). Co-administration of DNA vaccines with T-helper type 1 directing cytokine plasmids include: IL-2, IL-12, interferon γ (IFN-γ), IL-15, IL-18 and IL-23 (Lin et al. 1995). These cytokine-induced responses are associated with elevation of cellular and humoral immune responses manifested by increased CD8 cytotoxic T-lymphocyte activity, increased delayed type hypersensitivity responses, and preferential expression of complement fixing along with opsonizing IgG2a isotype antibodies. Th2 cytokine plasmids as adjuvants for DNA vaccines include: IL-4, IL-5, IL-6, IL-10 and IL-13 and induce augmented humoral immune responses along with a decrease in the IgG2a/IgG1 antibody isotype ratio, increased IgE expression, and a blunting of the cellular-type immune responses. Proinflammatory cytokine-expressing plasmids include granulocyte–macrophage colony stimulating factor (GM-CSF), IL-1α, IL-1β, and TNF-α, which, administered together with DNA vaccine constructs, enhance humoral and cellular immune responses while not substantially altering the Th1/Th2 cytokine balance (Egan and Israel 2002).

Th1 Plasmid Cytokines as DNA Vaccine Adjuvants

IL-2 Plasmid as DNA Vaccine Adjuvant

One of the first cytokines to be utilized with vaccines was the recombinant IL-2 protein, which was found to augment immune responses in mice; so IL-2 is a natural choice for use as an adjuvant. The use of IL-2 protein as a vaccine adjuvant is quite limited, due to its systemic toxicities and short in vivo half-life (West et al. 1989). The plasmid expressing IL-2 however, is the more practical strategy as a DNA vaccines adjuvant. Plasmid containing the IL-2 gene ("IL-2 plasmid" or "plasmid IL-2") was first shown to augment the immunogenicity of a transferring antigen in mice; IL-2 plasmids have subsequently been studied as vaccine adjuvants in a variety of small animal models of infectious diseases, autoimmunity, and cancer (Chow et al. 1998; Moore et al. 2002). The plasmid IL-2 has been reported to augment cellular and humoral immune responses elicited by DNA vaccines encoding hepatitis C virus core protein (Geissler et al. 1997), hepatitis B virus surface antigen (Chow et al. 1997), HIV-1 gp120 (Barouch et al. 1998), and herpes simplex virus (HSV) type 2gD in mice (Sin et al. 1999b). In rhesus monkeys, plasmid IL-2 has also been shown to increase humoral responses to HIV-1 gp120, although its adjuvant effects in monkeys appear substantially less notable than that in mice. Prior experimental results have shown that a plasmid expressing an IL-2/immunoglobulin (Ig) fusion protein was more effective than plasmid IL-2 in augmenting DNA vaccine-elicited immune responses in mice (Barouch et al. 1998), suggesting that increasing the half-life of the expressed cytokine can lead to improved potency. Moreover, delivering plasmid IL-2/Ig several days after the DNA vaccine led to optimal immune priming, perhaps reflecting the more natural kinetics of cytokine amplification of antigen-specific immune responses. It is also possible that the optimal time interval between vaccine and cytokine administration reflects the time required for increasing IL-2 receptor expression on antigen-primed T lymphocytes. In rhesus monkeys, plasmid IL-2/Ig was found to augment cellular immune responses to HIV/SIV DNA vaccines and to improve protective efficacy following a pathogenic SHIV challenge (Barouch et al. 2000). Moreover, plasmid IL-2/Ig has also been shown to augment cellular immune responses to a measles DNA vaccine in neonatal monkeys and to improve protective efficacy following a live measles virus challenge (Premenko-Lanier et al. 2003). A phase I human clinical trial to evaluate the safety and immunogenicity of multivalent HIV-1 DNA vaccines in conjunction with plasmid IL-2/Ig is currently in progress (NCT00069030 2009). Co-administration of murine IL-2 plasmid with a DNA vaccine expressing the HCV nucleocapsid protein increased the anti-HCV antibody seroconversion rate, elevated the CTL responses, and caused a dramatic increase in HCV-specific CD4 T-cell proliferative responses, along with a more Th1-like cytokine secretion profile (Geissler et al. 1997).

IL-12 Plasmid as DNA Vaccine Adjuvant

A considerable amount of attention has focused on IL-12, given its reported potency in driving Th1 responses and in stimulating effector T lymphocytes. Several studies have shown that plasmids containing the IL-12 gene ("plasmid IL-12") have the capacity to augment cellular responses to DNA vaccines encoding influenza (Iwasaki et al. 1997), FIV (Dunham et al. 2002) and HIV-1 (Tsuji et al. 1997). Plasmid IL-12 was also found to be a potent vaccine adjuvant necessary to afford long-term protection in a *Leishmania* model (Afonso et al. 1994).

Furthermore, plasmid IL-12 may exert synergistic effects when administered with plasmid GM-CSF in augmenting cellular immune responses to DNA vaccines (Ahlers et al. 1997).

Other studies, however, have underscored the complexities associated with cytokine augmentation of DNA vaccines. In contrast with its ability to augment cellular immune responses, plasmid IL-12 has been reported to suppress antibody responses to DNA vaccines in both mice (Kim et al. 1997b) and non-human primates (Kim et al. 2001a). In addition, although plasmid IL-12 administration was shown to afford major increases in primary CD8 T-lymphocyte responses elicited by an HIV-1 DNA vaccine, these apparent beneficial effects were lost following subsequent boost immunizations (Gherardi et al. 2000). It is therefore possible that plasmid IL-12 drives the selective expansion of effector memory cells rather than central memory cells, which may in fact limit its practical utility as a vaccine adjuvant.

It was thought that intramuscular co-administration of plasmid expressed IL-12 with HIV DNA vaccine could dramatically increase the HIV-1 *gag/pol*-specific CTL response; antigen-specific T-helper cell proliferation, but no effect on the antigen-specific serum antibody response was noted (Kim et al. 1999b). In mice, intramuscular co-injection of IL-12 plasmid with DNAs expressing SIV *gag/pol*, HIV-1 *env*, *vif*, and *nef* increased the CTL responses, enhanced antigen-specific proliferative responses and augmented *env*-specific CTL activity, but failed to augment serum anti-HIV-1 *env* antibody titers (Kim et al. 1997b). Thus, co-injection of IL-12 plasmid with HIV-1 DNA vaccines in the rhesus macaque model could shift the DNA vaccine-elicited immune response in a more Th1-like direction (Kim et al. 1999a).

Gene gun co-delivery of feline IL-12 plasmid with a DNA vaccine expressing the FIV *env* protein protected cats from homologous FIV challenge, whereas FIV *env* *plasmid* alone delayed seroconversion, and failed to protect the animals from viral infection (Boretti et al. 2000). Co-administration feline IL-12 plasmid with FeLV *gag/pol* and *env* DNA vaccines failed to protect cats from homologous virus challenge, however, a significant level of protection against FeLV challenge was achieved by immunization with FeLV DNA in combination with IL-12 and IL-18 plasmids (Hanlon et al. 2001).

Co-administration of IL-12 cDNA with HSV-2 gD DNA vaccine inhibited gD-specific humoral immune responses, enhanced cell-mediated immune responses, and significantly decreased morbidity and mortality following a lethal virus challenge (Sin et al. 1999a). Co-delivery of IL-12 plasmid with HBV surface antigen (HBVsAg) DNA vaccine augmented both humoral and cellular immune responses and enhanced protection against the growth and establishment of syngeneic HBVsAg expressing tumors, when compared to mice vaccinated with the HBVsAg DNA vaccine alone (Chow et al. 1998).

IFN-γ Plasmid as DNA Vaccine Adjuvant

INF-γ produced mainly by CD8 T cells and NK cells, has been proven to have antiviral effects that include activating CTLs, enhancing macrophage function, and upregulating MHC Class I and II expression on APCs and myoblasts. The ability of plasmid expressed INF-γ to modulate the immune response elicited by DNA vaccination has been extensively studied. The first report evaluating the effect of INF-γ co-expression with rabies virus gene was tested in the mouse model of a rabies virus infection. In this study, it was found that INF-γ co-expression had a slightly negative effect on vaccine immunogenicity by inhibiting T-helper cell proliferative responses and decreasing the induction of rabies virus-specific neutralizing antibodies (Xiang et al. 1997). By contrast, INF-γ co-expression with a DNA vaccine expressing the surface antigen of HBVsAg in mice resulted in increased antigen-specific humoral and cellular immune responses and a more Th1-like cytokine expression profile (Chow et al. 1998). The ability of plasmid expressed INF-γ to modulate immune responses elicited by HIV-1 DNA vaccine has been evaluated in the mouse, rat, and

4 Cytokine Genes as Molecular Adjuvants for DNA Vaccines

rhesus macaque. In the mouse model, INF-γ co-administration generally results in increased antigen-specific proliferative responses, enhanced antigen-specific humoral immune responses, and a more Th1-like cytokine expression profile. The positive immunomodulatory effects mediated by INF-γ in the mouse model were either significantly reduced or absent in the rhesus macaque studies (Kim et al. 1999a, 2001b). Therefore, additional studies in non-human primates will be required to completely evaluate the potential clinical utility of INF-γ as a genetic adjuvant.

Other Th1 Cytokine Plasmids as DNA Vaccine Adjuvants

IL-7 promotes lymphocyte growth and differentiation as well as affects CTL activity and maintenance of CD8 T cell memory (Wolowczuk et al. 1999), giving it excellent potential as a vaccine adjuvant for HIV therapy. In vitro, IL-7 has been shown to enhance the proliferative response to HIV antigens in lymphocytes derived from HIV vaccine recipients (Kim et al. 1997a). Immunization studies in mice have further revealed that co-injection of IL-7 DNA with HIV-1 gp120 DNA resulted in enhanced Th1-type immune responses (Kim et al. 1997a).

IL-9, a cytokine produced by T cells, mast cells, eosinophils, and neutrophils, stimulates cell proliferation and prevents apoptosis. IL-9 plasmid used as molecular adjuvant for foot and mouth virus DNA vaccine could enhance the immunogenicity of DNA vaccination, in augmenting humoral and cellular responses and particularly promoting Tc1 activation (Zou et al. 2010). Thus, IL-9 may be utilized as a potent Tc1 adjuvant for DNA vaccines.

IL-15 plays a critical role in establishing and especially maintaining memory CD8 T lymphocytes (Giri et al. 1995). Intramuscular injection of an IL-15 expression plasmid with an HIV-1 DNA vaccine enhanced antigen-specific CTL activity compared to HIV-1 DNA vaccination alone (Xin et al. 1999). In mice, the intramuscular administration of plasmid expressed IL-15 with a DNA vaccine expressing HSV-2 gD resulted in enhanced gD-specific T-helper cell proliferative responses and decreased morbidity and mortality following HSV-2 challenge (Sin et al. 1999b). The intranasal co-delivery of plasmid expressed IL-15 with a DNA vaccine expressing HIV-1 *gp160* elicited enhanced levels of antigen-specific CTL activity and increased DTH responses when compared to mice just receiving the DNA vaccine alone. The simultaneous administration of plasmid DNAs expressing IL-2 and IL-15 with an HIV-1 *gp160* expressing plasmid in mice did not significantly alter the pattern of immune responses when compared to responses of individually co-administered cytokine genes (Xin et al. 1999). Intranasal delivery of IL-15 plasmid as a mucosal adjuvant of FMDV DNA vaccine induced not only humoral immune responses but also higher levels of mucosal sIgA, serum IgG, and higher level of FMDV neutralizing antibodies as well as cellular immune responses including higher levels of antigen-specific T-cell proliferation and CTL responses (Wang et al. 2008).

Co-vaccination of IL-15 expressing plasmid with *Brucella abortus* DNA vaccine yielded a robust humoral response displaying a high ratio of IgG2a/IgG1 and significantly higher levels of IFN-γ and CD8$^+$ T cell responses, suggesting induction of a T-helper-1-dominated immune response (Hu et al. 2010).

IL-18 plasmid as a genetic adjuvant of mouse herpes simplex virus 1 (HSV-1) DNA vaccine increased the serum IgG2a/IgG1 ratio and the expression of Th1 cytokines, as well as antigen-specific lymphocyte proliferation and DTH, while inhibiting the production of IL-10. When mice were challenged with HSV-1 administered into the cornea, co-injection of IL-18 plasmid with gD DNA vaccine showed significantly better protection, which was manifested as fewer corneal lesion scores and faster recovery times suggesting that co-injection of an IL-18 plasmid with gD DNA vaccine efficiently induces Th1-dominant immune responses and substantially improves the protective effect against HSV-1 infection (Zhu et al. 2003). The plasmid encoding feline IL-18 co-immunized with DNA vaccination expressing the gag/pol and env genes of feline leukaemia virus (FeLV) completely protected cats from viraemia following challenge. Feline leukaemia virus DNA vaccine efficacy is enhanced by co-administration with IL-18 plasmid as the adjuvant suggesting further that the adjuvant effect on the FeLV DNA vaccine appears to reside in the expression of IL-18 (O'Donovan et al. 2005):

IL-23, a cytokine described in the last decade, can stimulate CD4$^+$ and CD8$^+$ T cell proliferation and induce the production of IFN-γ. Because IL-23 is primarily produced by APCs and exerts its effects on T cells, this cytokine is a good candidate for modulating vaccine-induced antigen-specific T-cell expansion. One preclinical study showed that IL-23 plasmid co-administered with hepatitis C virus (HCV) antigen resulted in enhanced induction and increased numbers of HCV-specific IFN-γ secreting CTL. Interestingly, if IL-23 was pre-administered prior to HCV antigen, then the HCV-specific responses were of a greater magnitude and persisted longer than when co-administered which indicates IL-23 is also having a potential adjuvant effect (Ha et al. 2004). The genes encoding p19 and p40 chains of IL-23 were cloned on either side of a self-cleaving peptide from the FMDV2A protein (p2AIL-23). The p2AIL-23-transfected cells induced the release of IL-17 from activated lymphocytes, suggesting the presence of a bioactive IL-23 (Wozniak et al. 2006a). Co-immunization of C57BL/6 mice with a DNA vaccine expressing M. tuberculosis antigen 85B and IL-23 plasmid stimulated stronger Ag85B-specific T-cell proliferative and IFN-gamma responses (Wozniak et al. 2006b).

Th2 Cytokine Plasmids as DNA Vaccine Adjuvants

DNA vaccines co-injected with plasmids encoding Th2 inducing cytokines have a tendency to induce immune responses characterized by higher levels of IgG1 antibodies resulting in both a higher level of total antibodies and a higher ratio of IgG1:IgG2a. Most of these cytokines induced either similar or lower CTL responses or DTH reactions in vivo. IL-10 however has been reported to augment DTH responses when measured as a reaction to the contact allergen oxazalone, whereas decreased responses were observed with Ag-specific DTH induction (Kim et al. 1998a).

IL-4 Plasmid as DNA Vaccine Adjuvant

IL-4 functions as a co-stimulant to B-cell growth, increasing cell surface expression of MHC II, and also serves to regulate immunoglobulin class switching. A large body of work has been done to evaluate the effect of plasmid expressed IL-4 on the immunogenicity of HIV-1 DNA vaccines in both the mouse model and in nonhuman primates (Kim et al. 1999b, 2000b). The effect of plasmid encoded IL-4 co-administration on vaccine antigen specific antibody responses is somewhat varied, with some studies demonstrating a decrease in antigen-specific antibody titers, while others have demonstrated an increase in antibody titers (Kim et al. 2001b). The effect of IL-4 co-administration on HIV-1 antigen-specific T-helper cell proliferation is even less clear.

Numerous studies have been conducted in mice to evaluate the ability of plasmid encoded IL-4 to augment HCV-specific cellular and humoral immune responses. It was found that IL-4 co-administration in conjunction with a plasmid DNA vaccine expressing the HCV nucleocapsid protein resulted in an increased anti-HCV antibody seroconversion rate, but this treatment did not significantly increase anti-HCV antibody titers. Also, IL-4 appeared to drive the resulting immune response in a more Th0-like direction by augmenting HCV-specific T-helper cell proliferative responses, and by increasing the antigen-specific secretion of both IL-2 and IL-4, while suppressing the induction of functional CTL responses (Geissler et al. 1997). In contrast, studies conducted in the HBV mouse tumor-challenge model showed that co-administration of an IL-4 plasmid with an HBVsAg plasmid resulted in a Th1 to Th2 shift in the vaccine elicited immune response. IL-4 co-expression resulted in a slight increase in HBVsAg-specific T-helper cell proliferation with a clear shift towards a Th2 cytokine expression profile. This Th2-like cytokine expression profile, moreover, was associated with an increase in IgG1 antibody isotype titers, a decrease in IgG2a antibody isotype and CTL activity, and a complete loss of vaccine-mediated protection against syngeneic HBVs antigen transfected tumor cells (Chow et al. 1998).

Plasmid IL-4 co-administration with an HSV-2 gD DNA immunogen in mice, directed the resulting immune response towards a more Th2-like profile. Mice co-administered the DNA vaccine along with an IL-4 expression plasmid showed similar levels of elevated gD-specific T-helper cell proliferation and total gD-specific IgG antibody responses compared to animals that received the gD-expressing DNA vaccine alone, but increased the rate of mortality and morbidity of the challenged mice (Sin et al. 1999b).

All in all, the co-administration of IL-4 DNA generally results in a more Th2-like immune response characterized by a decrease in the IgG2a/IgG1 isotype antibody ratio; by a failure to augment cellular immune response, and by decreased vaccine efficacy following viral or tumor challenge.

IL-6 Plasmid as DNA Vaccine Adjuvant

IL-6 is a Th2 type cytokine involved in end-stage differentiation of B-cells into antibody secreting plasma cells and is vital for the maintenance of mucosal IgA responses. In contrast to most other Th2 type cytokines, IL-6 has been shown to augment the activity of antigen-specific CTLs, natural killer cells, lymphokine-activated killer cells, and tumor-infiltrating lymphocytes.

The first evidence that IL-6 could substantially augment the immunomodulatory effect of DNA immunization comes from studies done in a mouse tumor model. It had been reported that vaccination of mice bearing established pulmonary metastases with a DNA vaccine expressing the model tumor-associated antigen β-gal, while capable of eliciting antigen-specific antibody and cell-mediated immune responses, failed to demonstrate any active therapeutic effect. However, co-administration of mouse rIL-6 significantly reduce the number of established metastases indicating a potent adjuvant effect of this cytokine (Irvine et al. 1996). On the other hand, mice vaccinated with plasmids expressing HA and IL-6 were completely protected from challenge with influenza virus. Virus titers in the lungs of mice that received the IL-6 expressing DNA without HA DNA were comparable to control-vaccinated mice, confirming that the protection could not be attributed to the effect of plasmid expressed IL-6 alone. Pre-challenge virus-specific humoral immune responses in serum were similar in the mice immunized with the HA-expressing DNA alone, compared to the mice that received HA plus IL-6 DNA. However, there was a substantial difference in the levels of virus-specific IgG in nasal secretions at the time of challenge (Larsen et al. 1998). Co-inoculation of IL-6 plasmid with FMDV DNA vaccine induced higher ratios of IgG2a/IgG1, higher levels of expression of IFN-γ in CD4$^+$ and CD8$^+$ T cells, expression of IL-4 in CD4$^+$ T cells, and a CTL response, as well as maturation of DCs, all of which demonstrates that IL-6 used as a molecular adjuvant can enhance the antigen-specific cell-mediated responses elicited by VP1 DNA vaccine (Su et al. 2008). When IL-6 plasmid was co-inoculated with a HIV-1 DNA vaccine, immunized BALB/c mice displayed enhanced specific humoral and cellular immunity including specific killing activities of spleen CTLs (Jiang et al. 2006).

IL-10 Plasmid as DNA Vaccine Adjuvant

Several studies have been conducted in the mouse model to evaluate the ability of plasmid expressed IL-10 to modulate the immune response to DNA vaccination (Daheshia et al. 1997). Plasmid IL-10 co-administration with DNA vaccines expressing HIV-1 antigens resulted in increased serum antigen-specific IgG antibody titers, and increased antigen-specific T-helper cell proliferative responses, but had no significant effect on CTL activity (Kim et al. 1999b). In contrast to the results achieved with the HIV-1 DNA vaccines, IL-10 co-administration with a DNA vaccine expressing HSV gD failed to augment serum IgG responses or gD-specific proliferation, and IL-10 co-administration had a distinct Th2-like effect by decreasing

4 Cytokine Genes as Molecular Adjuvants for DNA Vaccines

the secretion of the Th1 cytokines, here after IL-2 and INF-γ. Consistent with a Th2-like effect, IL-10 administration like IL-4, showed a significantly reduced survival following subsequent HSV-2 challenge (Sin et al. 1999b). When IL-10 plasmid was used as an adjuvant of sheep DNA vaccine encoding an antigen of *Haemonchus contortus* (pNPA), antibody responses of the sheep were decreased significantly suggesting IL-10 plasmid suppressed the humoral immune response (Yen and Scheerlinck 2007).

Other Th2 Cytokine Plasmids as DNA Vaccine Adjuvants

IL-5 has been shown to be critically involved in the differentiation of B-cells into antibody secreting plasma cells; able to induce antigen-specific IgA antibody responses and to promote eosinophilia. However the ability of plasmid expressed IL-5 to modulate the immune response elicited by DNA vaccination has only been evaluated in the mouse model thus far. Intramuscular injection of a plasmid expressing IL-5, with either HIV-1 *gag/pol* or *env* expressing DNA vaccines resulted in enhanced antigen-specific serum IgG responses similar to what was seen with IL-4 co-administration. However, co-inoculation with IL-5 DNA did not significantly alter the DNA vaccine elicited cellular immune response (Kim et al. 1998b).

IL-13 is a Th2 type cytokine produced by T-cells and mast cells that has many biological properties in common with IL-4. Unlike IL-4, co-administration of a plasmid expressing IL-13 with DNA vaccines expressing HIV-1 *env* or *gag/pol* failed to augment antigen-specific serum antibody or T-helper cell proliferative responses in vaccinated mice. However, like IL-4, IL-13 co-expression resulted in decreased IFN-γ expression following antigen stimulation and failed to augment cell-mediated immune response (Kim et al. 2000b).

Proinflammatory Cytokine Plasmids as DNA Vaccine Adjuvants

GM-CSF Plasmid as DNA Vaccine Adjuvant

The GM-CSF gene has been one of the most studied genetic adjuvants and has a good track record for enhancing humoral responses. GM-CSF has only moderate effects on the antibody isotype induced when injected simultaneously with the DNA vaccine, suggesting little influence on the balance between Th1 and Th2 type responses.

Plasmid GM-CSF was first shown to enhance antibody and helper T-lymphocyte responses when used with a rabies virus DNA vaccine. Co-administration of a GM-CSF expressing plasmid together with a DNA vaccine expressing the rabies virus G protein increased G protein-specific antibody responses as well as the expression of Th1-type cytokines, augmenting virus-specific neutralizing antibody responses. Most importantly, this regimen completely protects the animal from a lethal rabies virus challenge (Xiang and Ertl 1995). In addition, plasmid GM-CSF has been shown to augment antibody and/or CD4 Th responses to DNA vaccines encoding HSV and HIV-1 antigens (Kim et al. 1999b; Sin et al. 1998). Co-administration of DNA vaccine encoding the idiotype (Id) of a murine B-cell lymphoma fused to GM-CSF resulted in a more rapid antibody response to the tumor Id; it also increased the frequency of responding mice, and enhanced survival after lethal tumor challenge when compared to mice vaccinated with the Id DNA alone. However, GM-CSF plasmid failed to significantly alter the cytokine expression profile or augment antigen-specific CTL responses (Syrengelas et al. 1996). In other studies, it was consistently found that the co-administration of plasmid encoded GM-CSF with the plasmid DNA vaccine against hepatitis C virus antigen could augment antigen-specific antibody responses and T-helper cell proliferative response (Geissler et al. 1997; Cho et al. 1999). In the majority of such studies, GM-CSF co-administration was shown to effectively augment antigen-specific antibody responses and T-helper cell proliferative responses. However, the effect of GM-CSF on functional CTL activity was less clear.

Although plasmid GM-CSF consistently augments DNA vaccine-elicited CD4 T-lymphocyte responses in mice, the effects of plasmid GM-CSF in monkeys and humans have been considerably less impressive. Plasmid GM-CSF was found to provide minimal adjuvant effects when administered with a malaria DNA vaccine in rhesus monkeys (Kumar et al. 2002) and it had no detectable adjuvant effects in a phase I human clinical study (Barbaro et al. 1997). Other studies have reported that plasmid GM-CSF modestly improved antibody responses to an SIV DNA vaccine in rhesus monkeys. Furthermore, plasmid GM-CSF in conjunction with plasmid IL-12 may be more effective than plasmid GM-CSF alone in augmenting SIV-specific T-lymphocyte responses in rhesus monkeys (Kim et al. 1999b). The reasons that plasmid GM-CSF appears less effective in primates than in mice are not entirely clear but may reflect lower levels of expression, or perhaps a different GM-CSF receptor distribution in primates as compared with mice. Similarly with plasmid IL-2 and plasmid IL-12, the timing of plasmid GM-CSF administration in relation to DNA vaccination also appears to be important in determining the magnitude of responses, and nature of these adjuvant effects.

IL-1α and IL-1β Plasmids as DNA Vaccine Adjuvants

IL-1 is a multifunctional cytokine expressed in two biologically indistinguishable forms, IL-1α and IL-1β. IL-1 has been shown to influence the differentiation, growth, and antibody production by B-cells (Lipsky et al. 1983) and to activate T-cells by up-regulating IL-2 receptor expression through the indirect production of IL-2 (Kaye et al. 1984). A functionally active peptide fragment derived from IL-1β, expressed as a fusion protein of a DNA vaccine expressing a tumor specific antigen (TSA), was first investigated in a mouse model of B-cell lymphoma immunotherapy. The IL-1β derived peptide was selected based on its ability to augment T-cell dependent and T-cell independent immune responses. The plasmid expressed TSA/ IL-1β fusion protein elicited an increased antigen-specific IgG response and increased survival after a lethal tumor challenge (Hakim et al. 1996). By contrast, co-administration of a plasmid expressing the full length IL-1β protein with a DNA vaccine expressing a soluble form of the bovine herpes virus-1 gD protein failed to augment gD-specific serum IgG titers (Lewis et al. 1997). Co-immunization of an IL-1α plasmid with HIV-1 DNA vaccines induced a moderate increase in antigen-specific IgG antibody titers with little effect on immune responses (Kim et al. 1998b).

IFN-α Plasmid as DNA Vaccine Adjuvant

IFN-α, a type I interferon produced by dendritic cells, augments the generation and cytotoxicity of natural killer cells and CD8 CTL, and upregulates the expression of MHCII and the co-stimulatory molecules B7.1 and B7.2 on DCs. Only a single study has been published evaluating the ability of IFN-α to modulate immune responses elicited by DNA vaccination. Co-transfection of a plasmid expressing IFN-α with plasmid DNA as an immunogen, demonstrated that the primary CTL responses against several melanoma antigens could be elicited in vitro and augmented the resulting antigen-specific T-cell response (Tuting et al. 1999). The adjuvant effect of IFN-α with HIV-1 DNA vaccine was studied in a mouse model. After BALB/c mice were immunized by three intramuscular inoculations of the HIV-1 DNA vaccine plasmid alone or in combination with IFN-α expression plasmid, the different levels of anti-HIV-1 humoral and cellular responses were measured. The percentage of CD3$^+$CD4$^+$ and CD3$^+$CD8$^+$ subgroups of spleen T lymphocytes and the specific CTLs were all significantly enhanced and were also noted for antibody response (Jiang et al. 2007). These findings suggest IFN-α can be an effective immunological adjuvant in DNA vaccination against HIV-1.

Other Proinflammatory Cytokines

TNF-α and TNF-β play key roles in the initiation of an inflammatory response and bind to the same cell-surface receptors. TNF- α is produced by a wide variety of cell types including activated macrophages, monocytes, neutrophils, and natural killer cells; whereas TNF-β is produced mainly by lymphocytes. During the development of an immune response, TNF-α acts as a primary mediator of the inflammatory response, so TNF-α may exhibit important immunomodulatory effects following co-injection with DNA vaccines. The ability of plasmid expressed TNF-α was initially tested to modulate the immune response elicited by a suboptimal dose of DNA-encoding bovine herpes virus-1 (BHV-1)gD. In mice, TNF-α co-administration failed to increase the gD-specific humoral immune response, but did increase the seroconversion rate and effect a Th1-like serum antibody isotype switch from IgG1 to IgG2a (Lewis et al. 1997). Intramuscular injection of plasmid expressed TNF-α with HIV-1 *gag/pol* or *env* DNA vaccines resulted in a dramatic enhancement of humoral and cellular immune responses in immunized mice.

In contrast to the encouraging results observed after co-injection of TNF-α DNA, co-administration of TNF-β DNA only moderately augmented the immune responses to HIV-1 antigens in the mouse model (Kim et al. 1998b). Co-inoculation of TNF-α plasmid with FMDV DNA vaccine can increase cellular immune responses; including higher ratios of IgG2a/IgG1, higher levels of IFN-γ in T cells, and stimulation of DC maturation (Su et al. 2008), collectively suggesting a correlation between the initiating innate immune response and subsequent activating adaptive immune responses.

Granulocyte-colony stimulating factor (G-CSF) is a growth factor produced by macrophages, fibroblasts, endothelial cells, and bone marrow stromal cells. G-CSF can activate neutrophils and endothelial cells but has been shown to have little effect on professional APCs. Macrophage-colony stimulating factor (M-CSF) is a potent activator of macrophages and regulator of mononuclear phagocytes. The ability of plasmid encoded G-CSF and M-CSF to modulate the immune responses elicited by DNA vaccines expressing HIV-1 *env* and *gag/pol* in mice was tested. In contrast to results achieved with GM-CSF, the co-administration of plasmid expressed G-CSF and M-CSF had no effect, or only a moderate enhancing effect on serum antibody responses respectively. G-CSF and M-CSF co-delivery resulted in a moderate increase in T-helper cell proliferative responses. However, only M-CSF had a beneficial effect on CTL activity. Both G-CSF and M-CSF elicited a more Th1-like immune response by upregulating INF-γ production in antigen-stimulated splenocytes and increased the serum IgG2a/IgG1 antibody isotype ratio. Additionally, histological analysis revealed that M-CSF resulted in a dramatic infiltration of lymphocytes and dendritic cells at the site of vaccine administration (Kim et al. 2000a). These preliminary results suggest M-CSF may be useful as a genetic adjuvant based on its ability to modulate the function of APCs and to upregulate humoral and cellular immune responses.

Combinations of Cytokine Plasmids as DNA Vaccine Adjuvants

The co-delivery of several genetic adjuvants has been attempted to further modulate the immune response to DNA vaccines. When co-delivering two cytokines, the immune response is enhanced compared to each of the cytokine genes individually. Co-delivery of proinflammatory cytokines, Th1 cytokines and Th2 cytokines were tested for induction and regulation of immune responses. Co-delivery of Th2 cytokines IL-4, IL-5, and IL-10 as well as that of IL-2 and IL-18 enhanced antigen-specific humoral responses, whereas a dramatic increase in antigen-specific T helper cell proliferation was induced by IL-2 and TNF-α co-injections. Co-administration of TNF-α and IL-15 genes with HIV-1 DNA immunogens increased both MHC class I-restricted and CD8+ T cell-dependent CTL responses (Kim et al. 1998b). The adjuvant effect of Th1-type and Th2-type cytokines plasmids were tested by vaccination with DNA expression constructs encoding HSV-2gD proteins. Results showed Th1 cytokine gene co-administration not only enhanced survival rate, but also reduced the frequency and severity of herpetic lesions following intravaginal HSV challenge; whereas co-injection with Th2 cytokine genes increased the rate of mortality and morbidity of the challenged mice (Sin et al. 1999b).

The addition of IL-4 or IL-2 to GM-CSF is of particular interest, because it demonstrates that two quite separate functions of genetic adjuvants can be combined. Indeed, while GM-CSF enhances the immune response with minimal effect on the Th1:Th2 balance, the addition of IL-4 biases this response towards Th2, and IL-2 biases the response to Th1. When IL-12 and GM-CSF were combined with CD80 but not CD86, a further enhancement of the CTL response occurred (Iwasaki et al. 1997). GM-CSF plasmid in combination with other genetic adjuvants such as IL-2, IL-4, IL-12, and CD40 ligand (CD40L) have been tested to augment DNA vaccine-elicited immune responses. In mice, the co-delivery of GM-CSF with IL-2 or IL-4 in combination with a DNA vaccine expressing HIV-1 *gp160* was found to augment the *gp160*-specific serum and mucosal antibody response compared to mice immunized with GM-CSF and HIV-1 DNA alone. In the same study, the co-administration of IL-2 or IL-12 with GM-CSF and HIV-1 DNA resulted in an increased antigen-specific DTH reaction compared to GM-CSF and HIV-1 DNA alone. The intranasal co-administration of plasmid expressed IL-12 along with a DNA vaccine expressing HIV-1 *gp160* resulted in an enhanced CTL response. Interestingly, the co-administration of HIV-1 DNA plus IL-12 and GM-CSF further increased the antigen-specific CTL response, whereas HIV-1 DNA plus GM-CSF alone fails to alter the CTL response (Okada et al. 1997). In the SIV/Rhesus macaque rectal challenge model, the co-administration of GM-CSF and IL-12 in combination with an SIV DNA prime followed by a virus-like particle boost was shown to improve vaccine efficacy following SIV challenge (O'Neill et al. 2002). It was shown that the co-administration of plasmids expressing GM-CSF and CD40L further increased β-gal specific antibody and CTL responses above that seen with either GM-CSF or CD40L alone (Burger et al. 2001). GM-CSF and IL-12 co-delivery with DNA immunogen encoding influenza NP resulted in enhanced cellular immune responses (Iwasaki et al. 1997). The plasmid encoding IL-4 and GM-CSF used as adjuvant with the sheep DNA vaccine encoding an antigen of *H. contortus* (pNPA), significantly enhanced both antibody responses and T cell proliferation responses. This study suggested co-delivery of plasmid-encoded IL-4 and GM-CSF genes has the ability to effectively modulate DNA vaccine immune responses in a large animal (Yen and Scheerlinck 2007).

A fusion gene of porcine IL-4 and IL-6 (PIL4/IL6) packaged with chitosan nanoparticles (CNPs) was utilized to orally inoculate 21-day-old female Kunming mice that simultaneously received an intramuscular injection of inactivated *Escherichia coli* vaccine. 35 days later, the mice were challenged by oral feeding with virulent O139: K88 strain EPEC *E. coli* bacteria. The immunoglobulins and specific antibodies to *E. coli* were seen to increase significantly as also the levels of IL-2, IL-4 and IL-6 cytokines. The immunized mice all survived the challenge and did not show any symptoms or lesions, whereas the control mice manifested obvious clinical symptoms and hemorrhagic lesions in the digestive tracts (Zhang et al. 2007).

Summary

A large number of plasmid cytokine adjuvants have proven remarkably effective in augmenting DNA vaccine-elicited immune responses in small animal models. Several approaches have also proven successful in non-human primates; however, few plasmid cytokines have been assessed to date in humans. Plasmid cytokines can be organized into two major categories based on their presumed mechanism of action. The first category involves cytokines that enhance the stimulation, proliferation, and/or function of T lymphocytes. The second category involves cytokines that recruit or activate APCs and enhance their ability to prime adaptive immune responses. Scientific challenges for advancing plasmid cytokines into clinical trials include our current inability to predict which preclinical models, immunization parameters, and specific cytokines will translate successfully to humans. Regulatory challenges for advancing plasmid cytokines into clinical trials include the theoretical possibilities of persistent cytokine expression, chronic immune stimulation, autoimmune anti-cytokine antibodies, and cytokine-specific toxicities. Fortunately, these possibilities have not been observed in preclinical toxicology studies (Barouch et al. 2004; Parker et al. 2001) or in any clinical studies to date. Several phase I trials are currently in progress or planned using plasmid cytokines (NCT00069030 2009; NCT00111605 2010; NCT00137865 2011; NCT00455221 2011; NCT00528489 2010; NCT00991354 2010; NCT01070797 2011; NCT01300858 2011). Over the next several years, these studies should yield valuable information regarding the safety and potential utility of these approaches in humans. Meanwhile, growing numbers of preclinical studies will continue to support recent advances of molecular immunology, in attempts designed to improve immune responses to both traditional and DNA vaccines. It is hoped that these basic research advances can be translated effectively and harnessed to accelerate vaccine development.

References

Afonso LC, Scharton TM, Vieira LQ, Wysocka M, Trinchieri G, Scott P (1994) The adjuvant effect of interleukin-12 in a vaccine against *L. major*. Science 263(5144):235–237

Ahlers JD, Dunlop N, Alling DW, Nara PL, Berzofsky JA (1997) Cytokine-in-adjuvant steering of the immune response phenotype to HIV-1 vaccine constructs: granulocyte-macrophage colony-stimulating factor and TNF-alpha synergize with IL-12 to enhance induction of cytotoxic T lymphocytes. J Immunol 158(8):3947–3958

Barbaro G, Di Lorenzo G, Grisorio B, Soldini M, Barbarini G (1997) Effect of recombinant human granulocyte-macrophage colony-stimulating factor on HIV-related leukopenia: a randomized, controlled clinical study. AIDS 11(12):1453–1461

Barouch DH, Santra S, Steenbeke TD, Zheng XX, Perry HC, Davies ME, Freed DC, Craiu A, Strom TB, Shiver JW, Letvin NL (1998) Augmentation and suppression of immune responses to an HIV-1 DNA vaccine by plasmid cytokine/Ig administration. J Immunol 161(4): 1875–1882

Barouch DH, Santra S, Schmitz JE, Kuroda MJ, Fu TM, Wagner W, Bilska M, Craiu A, Zheng XX, Krivulka GR, Beaudry K, Lifton MA, Nickerson CE, Trigona WL, Punt K, Freed DC, Guan L, Dubey S, Casimiro D, Simon A, Davies ME, Chastain M, Strom TB, Gelman RS, Montefiori DC, Lewis MG, Emini EA, Shiver JW, Letvin NL (2000) Control of viremia and prevention of

4 Cytokine Genes as Molecular Adjuvants for DNA Vaccines

clinical AIDS in rhesus monkeys by cytokine-augmented DNA vaccination. Science 290(5491):486–492

Barouch DH, Truitt DM, Letvin NL (2004) Expression kinetics of the interleukin-2/immunoglobulin (IL-2/Ig) plasmid cytokine adjuvant. Vaccine 22(23–24):3092–3097

Boretti FS, Leutenegger CM, Mislin C, Hofmann-Lehmann R, Konig S, Schroff M, Junghans C, Fehr D, Huettner SW, Habel A, Flynn JN, Aubert A, Pedersen NC, Wittig B, Lutz H (2000) Protection against FIV challenge infection by genetic vaccination using minimalistic DNA constructs for FIV env gene and feline IL-12 expression. AIDS 14(12):1749–1757

Burger JA, Mendoza RB, Kipps TJ (2001) Plasmids encoding granulocyte-macrophage colony-stimulating factor and CD154 enhance the immune response to genetic vaccines. Vaccine 19(15–16):2181–2189

Cho JH, Lee SW, Sung YC (1999) Enhanced cellular immunity to hepatitis C virus nonstructural proteins by codelivery of granulocyte macrophage-colony stimulating factor gene in intramuscular DNA immunization. Vaccine 17(9–10):1136–1144

Chow YH, Huang WL, Chi WK, Chu YD, Tao MH (1997) Improvement of hepatitis B virus DNA vaccines by plasmids coexpressing hepatitis B surface antigen and interleukin-2. J Virol 71(1):169–178

Chow YH, Chiang BL, Lee YL, Chi WK, Lin WC, Chen YT, Tao MH (1998) Development of Th1 and Th2 populations and the nature of immune responses to hepatitis B virus DNA vaccines can be modulated by codelivery of various cytokine genes. J Immunol 160(3):1320–1329

Daheshia M, Kuklin N, Kanangat S, Manickan E, Rouse BT (1997) Suppression of ongoing ocular inflammatory disease by topical administration of plasmid DNA encoding IL-10. J Immunol 159(4):1945–1952

Dunham SP, Flynn JN, Rigby MA, Macdonald J, Bruce J, Cannon C, Golder MC, Hanlon L, Harbour DA, Mackay NA, Spibey N, Jarrett O, Neil JC (2002) Protection against feline immunodeficiency virus using replication defective proviral DNA vaccines with feline interleukin-12 and -18. Vaccine 20(11–12):1483–1496

Egan MA, Israel ZR (2002) The use of cytokines and chemokines as genetic adjuvants for plasmid DNA vaccines. Clin Appl Immunol Rev 2(4–5):255–287

Geissler M, Gesien A, Tokushige K, Wands JR (1997) Enhancement of cellular and humoral immune responses to hepatitis C virus core protein using DNA-based vaccines augmented with cytokine-expressing plasmids. J Immunol 158(3):1231–1237

Gherardi MM, Ramirez JC, Esteban M (2000) Interleukin-12 (IL-12) enhancement of the cellular immune response against human immunodeficiency virus type 1 env antigen in a DNA prime/vaccinia virus boost vaccine regimen is time and dose dependent: suppressive effects of IL-12 boost are mediated by nitric oxide. J Virol 74(14):6278–6286

Giri JG, Anderson DM, Kumaki S, Park LS, Grabstein KH, Cosman D (1995) IL-15, a novel T cell growth factor that shares activities and receptor components with IL-2. J Leukoc Biol 57(5):763–766

Ha SJ, Kim DJ, Baek KH, Yun YD, Sung YC (2004) IL-23 induces stronger sustained CTL and Th1 immune responses than IL-12 in hepatitis C virus envelope protein 2 DNA immunization. J Immunol 172(1):525–531

Hakim I, Levy S, Levy R (1996) A nine-amino acid peptide from IL-1beta augments antitumor immune responses induced by protein and DNA vaccines. J Immunol 157(12):5503–5511

Hanlon L, Argyle D, Bain D, Nicolson L, Dunham S, Golder MC, McDonald M, McGillivray C, Jarrett O, Neil JC, Onions DE (2001) Feline leukemia virus DNA vaccine efficacy is enhanced by coadministration with interleukin-12 (IL-12) and IL-18 expression vectors. J Virol 75(18):8424–8433

Hu XD, Chen ST, Li JY, Yu DH, Yi Z, Cai H (2010) An IL-15 adjuvant enhances the efficacy of a combined DNA vaccine against Brucella by increasing the CD8+ cytotoxic T cell response. Vaccine 28(12):2408–2415

Irvine KR, Rao JB, Rosenberg SA, Restifo NP (1996) Cytokine enhancement of DNA immunization leads to effective treatment of established pulmonary metastases. J Immunol 156(1):238–245

Iwasaki A, Stiernholm BJ, Chan AK, Berinstein NL, Barber BH (1997) Enhanced CTL responses mediated by plasmid DNA immunogens encoding costimulatory molecules and cytokines. J Immunol 158(10):4591–4601

Jiang W, Jin N, Cui S, Li Z, Zhang L, Wang H, Han W (2006) Enhancing immune responses against HIV-1 DNA vaccine by coinoculating IL-6 expression vector. J Virol Methods 136(1–2):1–7

Jiang W, Ren L, Jin N (2007) HIV-1 DNA vaccine efficacy is enhanced by coadministration with plasmid encoding IFN-alpha. J Virol Methods 146(1–2):266–273

Kaye J, Gillis S, Mizel SB, Shevach EM, Malek TR, Dinarello CA, Lachman LB, Janeway CA Jr (1984) Growth of a cloned helper T cell line induced by a monoclonal antibody specific for the antigen receptor: interleukin 1 is required for the expression of receptors for interleukin 2. J Immunol 133(3):1339–1345

Kim JH, Loveland JE, Sitz KV, Ratto Kim S, McLinden RJ, Tencer K, Davis K, Burke DS, Boswell RN, Redfield RR, Birx DL (1997a) Expansion of restricted cellular immune responses to HIV-1 envelope by vaccination: IL-7 and IL-12 differentially augment cellular proliferative responses to HIV-1. Clin Exp Immunol 108(2):243–250

Kim JJ, Ayyavoo V, Bagarazzi ML, Chattergoon MA, Dang K, Wang B, Boyer JD, Weiner DB (1997b) In vivo engineering of a cellular immune response by coadministration of IL-12 expression vector with a DNA immunogen. J Immunol 158(2):816–826

Kim JJ, Maguire HC Jr, Nottingham LK, Morrison LD, Tsai A, Sin JI, Chalian AA, Weiner DB (1998a) Coadministration of IL-12 or IL-10 expression cassettes drives immune responses toward a Th1 phenotype. J Interferon Cytokine Res 18(7):537–547

Kim JJ, Trivedi NN, Nottingham LK, Morrison L, Tsai A, Hu Y, Mahalingam S, Dang K, Ahn L, Doyle NK, Wilson DM, Chattergoon MA, Chalian AA, Boyer JD, Agadjanyan MG, Weiner DB (1998b) Modulation of amplitude and direction of in vivo immune responses by co-administration of cytokine gene expression cassettes with DNA immunogens. Eur J Immunol 28(3):1089–1103

Kim JJ, Nottingham LK, Tsai A, Lee DJ, Maguire HC, Oh J, Dentchev T, Manson KH, Wyand MS, Agadjanyan MG, Ugen KE, Weiner DB (1999a) Antigen-specific humoral and cellular immune responses can be modulated in rhesus macaques through the use of IFN-gamma, IL-12, or IL-18 gene adjuvants. J Med Primatol 28(4–5):214–223

Kim JJ, Simbiri KA, Sin JI, Dang K, Oh J, Dentchev T, Lee D, Nottingham LK, Chalian AA, McCallus D, Ciccarelli R, Agadjanyan MG, Weiner DB (1999b) Cytokine molecular adjuvants modulate immune responses induced by DNA vaccine constructs for HIV-1 and SIV. J Interferon Cytokine Res 19(1):77–84

Kim JJ, Yang JS, Lee DJ, Wilson DM, Nottingham LK, Morrison L, Tsai A, Oh J, Dang K, Dentchev T, Agadjanyan MG, Sin JI, Chalian AA, Weiner DB (2000a) Macrophage colony-stimulating factor can modulate immune responses and attract dendritic cells in vivo. Hum Gene Ther 11(2):305–321

Kim JJ, Yang JS, Montaner L, Lee DJ, Chalian AA, Weiner DB (2000b) Coimmunization with IFN-gamma or IL-2, but not IL-13 or IL-4 cDNA can enhance Th1-type DNA vaccine-induced immune responses in vivo. J Interferon Cytokine Res 20(3):311–319

Kim JJ, Yang JS, Dang K, Manson KH, Weiner DB (2001a) Engineering enhancement of immune responses to DNA-based vaccines in a prostate cancer model in rhesus macaques through the use of cytokine gene adjuvants. Clin Cancer Res 7(3 Suppl):882s–889s

Kim JJ, Yang JS, Manson KH, Weiner DB (2001b) Modulation of antigen-specific cellular immune responses to DNA vaccination in rhesus macaques through the use of IL-2, IFN-gamma, or IL-4 gene adjuvants. Vaccine 19(17–19):2496–2505

Kumar S, Villinger F, Oakley M, Aguiar JC, Jones TR, Hedstrom RC, Gowda K, Chute J, Stowers A, Kaslow DC, Thomas EK, Tine J, Klinman D, Hoffman SL, Weiss WW (2002) A DNA vaccine encoding the 42 kDa C-terminus of merozoite surface protein 1 of *Plasmodium falciparum* induces antibody, interferon-gamma and cytotoxic T cell responses in rhesus monkeys: immuno-stimulatory effects of granulocyte macrophage-colony stimulating factor. Immunol Lett 81(1):13–24

4 Cytokine Genes as Molecular Adjuvants for DNA Vaccines

Larsen DL, Dybdahl-Sissoko N, McGregor MW, Drape R, Neumann V, Swain WF, Lunn DP, Olsen CW (1998) Coadministration of DNA encoding interleukin-6 and hemagglutinin confers protection from influenza virus challenge in mice. J Virol 72(2):1704–1708

Lewis PJ, Cox GJ, van Drunen Littel-van den Hurk S, Babiuk LA (1997) Polynucleotide vaccines in animals: enhancing and modulating responses. Vaccine 15(8):861–864

Lin R, Tarr PE, Jones TC (1995) Present status of the use of cytokines as adjuvants with vaccines to protect against infectious diseases. Clin Infect Dis 21(6):1439–1449

Lipsky PE, Thompson PA, Rosenwasser LJ, Dinarello CA (1983) The role of interleukin 1 in human B cell activation: inhibition of B cell proliferation and the generation of immunoglobulin-secreting cells by an antibody against human leukocytic pyrogen. J Immunol 130(6):2708–2714

Min W, Lillehoj HS, Burnside J, Weining KC, Staeheli P, Zhu JJ (2001) Adjuvant effects of IL-1beta, IL-2, IL-8, IL-15, IFN-alpha, IFN-gamma TGF-beta4 and lymphotactin on DNA vaccination against *Eimeria acervulina*. Vaccine 20(1–2):267–274

Moore AC, Kong WP, Chakrabarti BK, Nabel GJ (2002) Effects of antigen and genetic adjuvants on immune responses to human immunodeficiency virus DNA vaccines in mice. J Virol 76(1):243–250

NCT00069030 (2009) Safety of and immune response to an HIV vaccine (VRC-HIVDNA009-00-VP) administered with interleukin-2/immunoglobulin (IL-2/Ig) DNA adjuvant in uninfected adults. http://clinicaltrials.gov/ct2/show/NCT00069030. Accessed on 13th jul 2011

NCT00111605 (2010) Study of an HIV preventive vaccine given with or without an adjuvant in HIV uninfected adults. http://www.clinicaltrials.gov/ct2/show/NCT00111605. Accessed on 13th jul 2011

NCT00137865 (2011) Safety study of phIL-12-005/PPC to treat recurrent ovarian cancer. http://www.clinicaltrials.gov/ct2/show/NCT00137865. Accessed on 13th jul 2011

NCT00455221 (2011) Safety assessment of a multipeptide-gene vaccine in CML. http://www.clinicaltrials.gov/ct2/show/NCT00455221. Accessed on 13th jul 2011

NCT00528489 (2010) Safety and effectiveness of PENNVAX-B vaccine alone, with IL-12, or IL-15 in healthy adults. http://www.clinicaltrials.gov/ct2/show/NCT00528489. Accessed on 13th jul 2011

NCT00991354 (2010) Safety of and immune response to the PENNVAX-B DNA vaccine with and without IL-12 in HIV-uninfected adults. http://www.clinicaltrials.gov/ct2/show/NCT00991354. Accessed on 13th jul 2011

NCT01070797 (2011) Administration of rapidly generated multivirus-specific cytotoxic T-lymphocytes (VIRAGE). http://www.clinicaltrials.gov/ct2/show/NCT01070797. Accessed on 13th jul 2011

NCT01300858 (2011) A study of the safety and biological activity of intraperitoneal (IP) EGEN-001 administered alone and in combination with standard chemotherapy in colorectal peritoneal carcinomatosis patients. http://www.clinicaltrials.gov/ct2/show/NCT01300858. Accessed on 13th jul 2011

O'Donovan LH, McMonagle EL, Taylor S, Bain D, Pacitti AM, Golder MC, McDonald M, Hanlon L, Onions DE, Argyle DJ, Jarrett O, Nicolson L (2005) A vector expressing feline mature IL-18 fused to IL-1beta antagonist protein signal sequence is an effective adjuvant to a DNA vaccine for feline leukaemia virus. Vaccine 23(29):3814–3823

O'Neill E, Martinez I, Villinger F, Rivera M, Gascot S, Colon C, Arana T, Sidhu M, Stout R, Montefiori DC, Martinez M, Ansari AA, Israel ZR, Kraiselburd E (2002) Protection by SIV VLP DNA prime/protein boost following mucosal SIV challenge is markedly enhanced by IL-12/GM-CSF co-administration. J Med Primatol 31(4–5):217–227

Okada E, Sasaki S, Ishii N, Aoki I, Yasuda T, Nishioka K, Fukushima J, Miyazaki J, Wahren B, Okuda K (1997) Intranasal immunization of a DNA vaccine with IL-12- and granulocyte-macrophage colony-stimulating factor (GM-CSF)-expressing plasmids in liposomes induces strong mucosal and cell-mediated immune responses against HIV-1 antigens. J Immunol 159(7):3638–3647

Parker SE, Monteith D, Horton H, Hof R, Hernandez P, Vilalta A, Hartikka J, Hobart P, Bentley CE, Chang A, Hedstrom R, Rogers WO, Kumar S, Hoffman SL, Norman JA (2001) Safety of a GM-CSF adjuvant-plasmid DNA malaria vaccine. Gene Ther 8(13):1011–1023

Premenko-Lanier M, Rota PA, Rhodes G, Verhoeven D, Barouch DH, Lerche NW, Letvin NL, Bellini WJ, McChesney MB (2003) DNA vaccination of infants in the presence of maternal antibody: a measles model in the primate. Virology 307(1):67–75

Sasaki S, Tsuji T, Asakura Y, Fukushima J, Okuda K (1998) The search for a potent DNA vaccine against AIDS: the enhancement of immunogenicity by chemical and genetic adjuvants. Anticancer Res 18(5D):3907–3915

Scheerlinck JY (2001) Genetic adjuvants for DNA vaccines. Vaccine 19(17–19):2647–2656

Sin JI, Kim JJ, Ugen KE, Ciccarelli RB, Higgins TJ, Weiner DB (1998) Enhancement of protective humoral (Th2) and cell-mediated (Th1) immune responses against herpes simplex virus-2 through co-delivery of granulocyte-macrophage colony-stimulating factor expression cassettes. Eur J Immunol 28(11):3530–3540

Sin JI, Kim JJ, Arnold RL, Shroff KE, McCallus D, Pachuk C, McElhiney SP, Wolf MW, Pompa-de Bruin SJ, Higgins TJ, Ciccarelli RB, Weiner DB (1999a) IL-12 gene as a DNA vaccine adjuvant in a herpes mouse model: IL-12 enhances Th1-type CD4+ T cell-mediated protective immunity against herpes simplex virus-2 challenge. J Immunol 162(5):2912–2921

Sin JI, Kim JJ, Boyer JD, Ciccarelli RB, Higgins TJ, Weiner DB (1999b) In vivo modulation of vaccine-induced immune responses toward a Th1 phenotype increases potency and vaccine effectiveness in a herpes simplex virus type 2 mouse model. J Virol 73(1):501–509

Su B, Wang J, Wang X, Jin H, Zhao G, Ding Z, Kang Y, Wang B (2008) The effects of IL-6 and TNF-alpha as molecular adjuvants on immune responses to FMDV and maturation of dendritic cells by DNA vaccination. Vaccine 26(40):5111–5122

Syrengelas AD, Chen TT, Levy R (1996) DNA immunization induces protective immunity against B-cell lymphoma. Nat Med 2(9):1038–1041

Tang DC, DeVit M, Johnston SA (1992) Genetic immunization is a simple method for eliciting an immune response. Nature 356(6365):152–154

Tsuji T, Hamajima K, Fukushima J, Xin KQ, Ishii N, Aoki I, Ishigatsubo Y, Tani K, Kawamoto S, Nitta Y, Miyazaki J, Koff WC, Okubo T, Okuda K (1997) Enhancement of cell-mediated immunity against HIV-1 induced by coinoculation of plasmid-encoded HIV-1 antigen with plasmid expressing IL-12. J Immunol 158(8):4008–4013

Tuting T, Gambotto A, Robbins PD, Storkus WJ, DeLeo AB (1999) Co-delivery of T helper 1-biasing cytokine genes enhances the efficacy of gene gun immunization of mice: studies with the model tumor antigen beta-galactosidase and the BALB/c Meth A p53 tumor-specific antigen. Gene Ther 6(4):629–636

Wang B, Ugen KE, Srikantan V, Agadjanyan MG, Dang K, Refaeli Y, Sato AI, Boyer J, Williams WV, Weiner DB (1993) Gene inoculation generates immune responses against human immunodeficiency virus type 1. Proc Natl Acad Sci USA 90(9):4156–4160

Wang X, Zhang X, Kang Y, Jin H, Du X, Zhao G, Yu Y, Li J, Su B, Huang C, Wang B (2008) Interleukin-15 enhance DNA vaccine elicited mucosal and systemic immunity against foot and mouth disease virus. Vaccine 26(40):5135–5144

West WH, Tauer KW, Yannelli JR, Marshall GD, Orr D, Lewis M, Birch R, Oldham RK (1989) Multiple cycles of constant infusion recombinant interleukin-2 in adoptive cellular therapy of metastatic renal carcinoma. Mol Biother 1(5):268–274

Wolff JA, Malone RW, Williams P, Chong W, Acsadi G, Jani A, Felgner PL (1990) Direct gene transfer into mouse muscle in vivo. Science (New York) 247(4949 Pt 1):1465–1468

Wolowczuk I, Roye O, Nutten S, Delacre M, Trottein F, Auriault C (1999) Role of interleukin-7 in the relation between *Schistosoma mansoni* and its definitive vertebrate host. Microbes Infect 1(7):545–551

Wozniak TM, Ryan AA, Britton WJ (2006a) Interleukin-23 restores immunity to *Mycobacterium tuberculosis* infection in IL-12p40-deficient mice and is not required for the development of IL-17-secreting T cell responses. J Immunol 177(12):8684–8692

Wozniak TM, Ryan AA, Triccas JA, Britton WJ (2006b) Plasmid interleukin-23 (IL-23), but not plasmid IL-27, enhances the protective efficacy of a DNA vaccine against *Mycobacterium tuberculosis* infection. Infect Immun 74(1):557–565

Xiang Z, Ertl HC (1995) Manipulation of the immune response to a plasmid-encoded viral antigen by coinoculation with plasmids expressing cytokines. Immunity 2(2):129–135

4 Cytokine Genes as Molecular Adjuvants for DNA Vaccines

Xiang ZQ, He Z, Wang Y, Ertl HC (1997) The effect of interferon-gamma on genetic immunization. Vaccine 15(8):896–898

Xin KQ, Hamajima K, Sasaki S, Tsuji T, Watabe S, Okada E, Okuda K (1999) IL-15 expression plasmid enhances cell-mediated immunity induced by an HIV-1 DNA vaccine. Vaccine 17(7–8):858–866

Yen HH, Scheerlinck JP (2007) Co-delivery of plasmid-encoded cytokines modulates the immune response to a DNA vaccine delivered by in vivo electroporation. Vaccine 25(14):2575–2582

Zhang H, Cheng C, Zheng M, Chen JL, Meng MJ, Zhao ZZ, Chen Q, Xie Z, Li JL, Yang Y, Shen Y, Wang HN, Wang ZZ, Gao R (2007) Enhancement of immunity to an Escherichia coli vaccine in mice orally inoculated with a fusion gene encoding porcine interleukin 4 and 6. Vaccine 25(41):7094–7101

Zhu M, Xu X, Liu H, Liu X, Wang S, Dong F, Yang B, Song G (2003) Enhancement of DNA vaccine potency against herpes simplex virus 1 by co-administration of an interleukin-18 expression plasmid as a genetic adjuvant. J Med Microbiol 52(Pt 3):223–228

Zou Q, Wu B, He X, Zhang Y, Kang Y, Jin J, Xu H, Liu H, Wang B (2010) Increasing a robust antigen-specific cytotoxic T lymphocyte response by FMDV DNA vaccination with IL-9 expressing construct. J Biomed Biotechnol 2010:562356

Pharmaceutical Non-Viral Formulations for Gene Vaccines

5

Glen Perera and Andreas Bernkop-Schnürch

Ever since the ground-breaking findings that immune responses can be provoked by biolistic application of pDNA and subsequent protein expression, no effort has been spared in order to make genetic vaccination feasible. Unfortunately, most approaches failed to convert the promising results from rodents to larger animals and human beings. To make such systems available for a global community, simple, safe and highly effective delivery systems are highly on demand. Since physical methods like the "gene gun" are neither cost-effective nor applicable in an everyday use and viral systems are still subject to heavy safety concerns, chemo-pharmaceutical approaches have become a major area of interest within the field of genetic vaccination. This chapter will shine a light on the barriers that need to be overcome by genetic vaccination systems and on the major approaches to achieve this aim. In particular, approaches based on (cationic) polymers, cationic lipids, combinations of these two major strategies and their in vivo performance will be discussed in detail. Besides, immunostimulatory agents and targeting ligands will be discussed as options to improve the in vivo efficiency of a genetic vaccination system. Finally, alternative routes to intradermal and intramuscular injections will be highlighted as part of future developments in this field.

Introduction

Genetic vaccines represent one of the most modern and most valuable contributions to the vaccination area in the past two decades because of their numerous advantageous features like comparably simple customization of the DNA sequence, low

G. Perera (✉)
Department of Pharmaceutical Technology, Institute of Pharmacy,
University of Innsbruck,
Innsbruck, Austria
e-mail: glen.perera@uibk.at

J. Thalhamer et al. (eds.), *Gene Vaccines*,
DOI 10.1007/978-3-7091-0439-2_5, © Springer-Verlag/Wien, 2012

production costs, high storage stability and their potential to induce robust cellular and humoral immune responses.

Ever since Wolff et al. achieved protein expression after intramuscular plasmid DNA (pDNA) application in mice (Wolff et al. 1990) and Tang et al. could demonstrate that an immune response can be induced by proteins which are expressed after biolistic application of pDNA in mice (Tang et al. 1992), it is the aim to make genetic vaccination feasible in humans. Unfortunately, the very promising results from pre-clinical studies in small laboratory animals could not be reproduced in man with naked DNA formulations.

Limited efficacy of DNA vaccines may be attributed to extracellular barriers such as nucleolytic degradation or adhesion to non-target tissues. Upon arrival at the target, further barriers like the cell membrane, entrapment in endosomal vesicles and lysosomal degradation as well as the nuclear membrane need to be overcome.

A variety of strategies have been developed in order to tackle these problems. Recombinant viruses have been proven to be effective as vectors for genetic vaccination but due to justified safety concerns like immune response, insertional mutagenesis, carcinogenesis and germ-cell-line alterations they could never be established as genetic vaccination system. Hence, numerous non-viral delivery methods have been developed in order to increase the efficiency of pDNA vaccines.

Aside from physical methods like biolistics, electroporation, sonoporation, magnetofection or intracellular microinjection and biological methods like optimization of the expression cassette, various chemo-pharmaceutical approaches have been pursued. This section will mainly focus on the latter including addition of immunostimulatory adjuvants, formulation of polymeric micro- and nanoparticles including dendrimer-based formulations as well as lipid-based particulate formulations.

Delivery of DNA Vaccines

Studies with naked pDNA showed that translation of the results obtained in mice to larger animals and humans is often problematic due to impractical dosing. As an example, if a mouse shows an immunogenic effect after receiving 50 µg of pDNA, an average adult human being would probably need a dose of more than 100 mg of pDNA.

Hence, development of more effective delivery systems is highly on demand in order to make genetic vaccination in human beings feasible. For this purpose, Cui and Mumper have defined numerous requirements for an efficient DNA vaccine delivery system (Cui and Mumper 2003). Accordingly, an ideal delivery system should be (i) easy to synthesize and characterize, (ii) inexpensive, (iii) non-toxic and generally regarded as safe, (iv) non-immunogenic, (v) biodegradable, (vi) easy to scale up, (vii) stable upon storage, (viii) able to provide protection towards nucleases, (ix) stable in biological fluids, (x) able to be taken up by specific cells, (xi) capable of releasing pDNA from endosomal/lysosomal compartments and (xii) able to improve pDNA trafficking to the nucleus. Such delivery systems will be most helpful in order to overcome the obstacles set by almost omnipresent nucleases and cellular membranes.

Most strategies for efficient genetic vaccine delivery are currently based on DNA complexation either with cationic lipids or cationic polymers. Moreover, DNA gets incorporated into various polymer micro- and nanoparticles. Hence, a lot of research has been done in order to find the ideal conditions in order to achieve high transfection rates and finally high immune responses. A major focus has been set on physicochemical properties of such particulate systems like particle size and surface charge. Currently, there is broad consensus that particles below 200 nm allow more efficient transfection than larger particles even though the latter are likely to be taken up exclusively by professional antigen-presenting cells (APC) (van den Berg et al. 2010; Foged et al. 2005). Moreover, it is beyond dispute that a positive surface charge supports the internalization of such a delivery system due to ionic interactions with heparan sulfate proteoglycans which are present on cell surfaces (Mislick and Baldeschwieler 1996; Mounkes et al. 1998). Unfortunately, cationic particles also interact with serum proteins, extracellular matrix components and blood cells which may significantly limit their in vivo performance due to aggregation and immobilization effects. In particular, extracellular polyanions like glycosaminogylcans (GAGs) appear to limit in vivo transfection (Ruponen et al. 1999). Moreover, cytotoxic side effects need to be evaluated carefully considering cationic gene vaccine delivery systems (Lv et al. 2006). Interestingly, there are also indications that a dendritic cell targeting can be achieved with anionic particles (Foged et al. 2005) or particles with a particle size between 0.5 and 5 μm (van den Berg et al. 2010).

Aside from formulation issues, the route of vaccine application highly influences its efficacy. Currently, most delivery systems for genetic vaccines are designed either for intramuscular or intradermal application due to the highest vaccine efficiency achieved on these routes. Besides, the skin contains numerous antigen-presenting cells like Langerhans cells that contribute to an immune response. Nevertheless, other routes are subject to intensive research. Among these, oral, nasal, pulmonary and vaginal administration are of certain interest since mucosal immunity might be generated which, in turn, would guarantee an immune response prior to systemic entry of a potential pathogen.

Adjuvants for Genetic Vaccination

Since antigen-encoding pDNA proved to be inefficient as a vaccine in man, many studies have been conducted with different chemical and biological immunostimulatory adjuvants. These adjuvants aim to enhance activation of antigen-presenting cells (APC), attract APC to the vaccination site or co-stimulate T-cells in order to induce immune responses.

Biological adjuvants are mainly cytokines like several interleukins, tumor necrosis factor (TNF)-α, interferon (IFN)-γ or granulocyte-macrophage colony stimulating factor (GM-CSF). These cytokines may stimulate the immune response by recruiting and stimulating APC. Moreover, they can directly act on infected cells.

IL-2, in particular, has been shown to induce proliferation and activation of T-cells (Smith 1980). Due to their short half-life in vivo, they are usually expressed from pDNA just as the actual antigen (Barouch et al. 2004).

Chemical adjuvants are mostly Toll-like receptor (TLR) ligands. Major representatives of this class are monophosphoryl lipid A (MPLA, TLR-4) (Lodmell et al. 2000), imiquimod (TLR-7) (Thomsen et al. 2004) and CpG motifs (TLR-9) (Zhang et al. 2005). These adjuvants may be directly added to the DNA vaccine formulation, preferably in a sustained release system in order to improve their efficiency. Besides TLR-ligands, emulsion-based adjuvants like MF59 were investigated in order to provide a better DNA uptake (Ott et al. 2002). QS-21, a saponin-fraction from *Quillaja saponaria*, was shown to be a potential adjuvant for DNA vaccine formulations due to induction of IL-2 and IFN-γ (Sasaki et al. 1998). It has also been investigated in clinical trials with DNA prime/protein boost regimen since it is believed to enhance cell-mediated and humoral immune response (Wang et al. 2008).

Polymer-Based Delivery Systems for Genetic Vaccines

Polyplexes with Cationic Polymers

Most current polymer-related approaches are based on formation of micro- and nanoparticles, usually in the range between 50 nm and a few micrometers.

The lion's share of polymeric formulations is based on the principle of electrostatic interactions between the anionic phosphate groups of DNA and a cationic polymer. A summary of the cationic polymers described herein is provided in Fig. 5.1. In general, DNA gets condensed into positively charged, nano-sized particles (so called polyplexes) by an excess of a cationic polymer. This is generally done by simple complexation-coacervation methods. Since this complexation is usually based on interactions between a positively charged nitrogen and the mentioned phosphate group, the term N/P ratio was established in order to define the charge ratio between polymer and DNA. This N/P ratio is crucial for the success of a genetic vaccine delivery system as it influences size and charge of such polyplexes and by these means the transfection efficiency of a formulation. On the one hand, a positive surface charge supports the cellular uptake of such particles but on the other hand cytotoxic effects need to be carefully investigated when positively charged delivery systems are utilized. The ideal surface charge depends on the cell type and the nature of the application environment and may be correlated to the characteristics of GAGs present on the cell surface and in the extracellular matrix (Mislick and Baldeschwieler 1996; Ruponen et al. 1999).

One of the first cationic polymers, investigated for gene delivery, was poly(L-lysine) (PLL). Hence, this polypeptide was also investigated as a carrier material for genetic vaccine delivery. PLL-polyplexes containing DNA encoding herpes simplex virus type-1 glycoprotein D were shown to target hepatocytes after intravenous administration when an asialooromucoid ligand was coupled (Rogers et al. 2000).

5 Pharmaceutical Non-Viral Formulations for Gene Vaccines 113

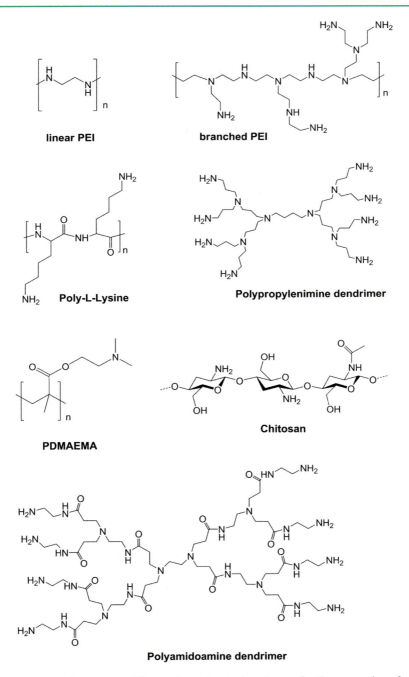

Fig. 5.1 Chemical structures of frequently used cationic polymers for the preparation of gene vaccine containing polyplex formulations

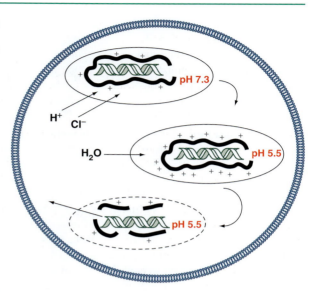

Fig. 5.2 Schematic depiction of the endosomal escape via proton sponge effect based on the buffering capacities of certain cationic polymers

Unfortunately, PLL polyplexes are rapidly bound to plasma proteins and cleared from systemic circulation which limits their in vivo efficacy. Moreover, PLL suffers from its poor endosomolytic activity. Hence, release of complexed pDNA into the cytoplasma is usually insufficient without co-administration of lytic agents. An endosomolytic effect can, for example, be generated by incorporation of histidine moieties (Pichon et al. 2001) or by coupling PLL with lytic agents such as mellitin (Meyer et al. 2007). Histidine moieties will cause a so-called proton sponge effect. Vesicular ATPase accumulates high proton concentrations within the endosome due to the buffering capacity of histidine which causes passive chloride diffusion into the endosome and subsequent osmotic swelling and subsequent rupture (Fig. 5.2). More recently, PLL was also used as a linker in order to adsorb pDNA to the surface of inert polystyrene nanoparticles (Minigo et al. 2007). It was observed that this formulation induced high levels of CD8[+] T cells as well as antigen-specific antibodies. The cellular response appeared to be slightly higher than with protein-controls while a superior humoral response was observed with protein-control.

Polyethylenimine (PEI) is probably the most investigated polymer for gene delivery systems. PEI polyplexes show several beneficial properties for gene delivery such as a membrane destabilization potential, high charge density (necessary for effective DNA condensation) and protective effects towards nucleolytic enzymes. Moreover, PEIs are capable of inducing endosomal disruption by acting as a proton sponge. These different properties are influenced by the chemical properties of different PEIs like molecular mass and its arborization. On the one hand, the toxicity of PEIs is positively correlated to their molecular mass (MM) while, on the other hand, linear PEIs are less toxic than branched ones due to their negligible amount of primary amines. However, primary amines in branched PEIs render them more suitable for chemical modifications. Secondary and tertiary amines provide a high buffering capacity which is necessary for the mentioned proton sponge effect. Hence, PEIs are mainly used for their DNA condensing and their endosomolytic properties. Nevertheless, PEI polyplexes could not be established as a genetic vaccine delivery system due to significant cytotoxic effects. Combinations with other strategies like polyplex-encapsulation into non-toxic shells are therefore subject to extensive investigations.

Similar to PEI, poly[(2-N,N-dimethylamino) ethyl methacrylate] (PDMAEMA) displays strong DNA condensing and thus protecting properties (Verbaan et al. 2005). PDMAEMA has shown great promise as a transfection agent but suffers from a high cytotoxicity just like PEI. Hence, its usage has been limited to preliminary studies thus far and combinatory strategies will be needed in the future.

Chitosan takes an exceptional position among cationic polymers, consisting of randomly distributed β-(1–4)-linked D-glucosamine and N-acetyl-D-glucosamine, which displays notable beneficial properties within the field of gene vaccine delivery. Chitosan has shown great promise for gene delivery due to its unique properties such as biocompatibility, biodegradability and its outstandingly low cytotoxicity for a cationic polymer (Guliyeva et al. 2006). Moreover, chitosan polyplexes guarantee protection towards nuclease degradation. However, its modest solubility marks a major drawback. Moreover, transfection efficiency and buffering capacity of chitosan polyplexes are quite low in comparison to PEI. Yang et al. postulate that chitosans with lower MM may be more effective as transfection agent than those with higher MM. Improved solubility and facilitated dissociation of such polyplexes might be the cause for this effect. On the contrary, chitosans with higher MM appear to provide superior protection towards nucleases (Yang et al. 2009). Moreover, several chitosan modifications have been synthesized in order to improve its transfection efficiency. Conjugates of chitosan with enzyme inhibitors like aurintricarboxylic acid were shown to enhance the transfection properties of chitosan which was attributed to the enhanced protection towards degradation by nucleases (Martien et al. 2006). A further promising approach which has been investigated in order to enhance the properties of chitosan consists of covalent attachment of thiol-bearing small molecules to its backbone. Thiol groups may play an important role for the stabilization of polyplexes and consequently their gene release features as well as nuclease inhibition which could make an important contribution to the area of oral gene delivery (Martien et al. 2007). The solubility issues of chitosan might be addressed by quaternization. In particular, trimethylated chitosan was investigated as a material for gene delivery within this context. This modification was demonstrated to be superior to unmodified chitosan but did not reach the potential of commonly used liposome formulations (Thanou et al. 2002). Like other polymers, chitosan has also been used in combination with several other strategies.

Dendrimers are special polymeric structures of polymers, such as PEI, poly(propylene imine) or poly(amidoamines), with highly branched, three-dimensional chains originating from one core. These dendrimers are highly reactive owing to their big amount of primary amino groups on their surface. This structure allows various chemical modifications, encapsulation of guest molecules in the internal cavity and formulation of stable complexes with DNA through electrostatic interactions. Complexes with

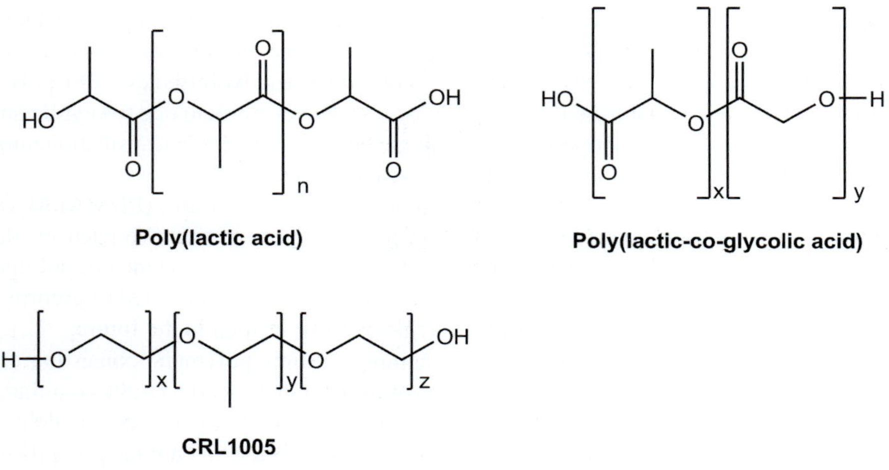

Poly(lactic acid)

Poly(lactic-co-glycolic acid)

CRL1005

Fig. 5.3 Chemical structures of commonly used uncharged polymers for the delivery of gene vaccines

dendrimers are sometimes referred to as dendriplexes. However, despite their very promising properties, dendrimers share the problem of high cytotoxicity with other cationic polymers (Jain et al. 2010). A more recent strategy combines poly(propylene imine) dendrimers with a shell of phosphatidylcholine (PC) and cholesterol which is supposed to mask primary amino groups. These so-called dendrosomes have a comparatively lower cytotoxicity while displaying improved transfection efficiency and immune response in mice (Dutta et al. 2008).

Miscellaneous Polymeric Micro- and Nanoparticles

Numerous other polymers than cationic ones have become interesting as potential materials for particulate delivery systems of genetic material over the years. Popular examples are synthetic polymers like poly(ε-caprolacton) (PCL), poly(vinylpyridine) (PVP), poly(lactic acid) (PLA), poly(lactic-co-glycolic acid) (PLGA) or polyoxypropylene/polyoxyethylene co-polymers such as CRL1005. The most prominent of these polymers are depicted in Fig. 5.3.

Among these polymers, PLGA is one of the most commonly used polymers for the delivery of gene material as it is highly biocompatible and biodegradable Therefore, it is already approved by the FDA. PLGA particles are usually prepared by solvent evaporation methods. Like other uncharged polymers, PLGA lacks the ability to condense DNA. Therefore, PLGA often gets combined with a cationic agent. A well established approach that has successfully been investigated in mice consists of DNA adsorption to the surface of PLGA micro- or nanoparticles which contain the positively charged surfactant cetyltrimethylammonium bromide (CTAB). These particles showed superior immune responses after intramuscular administration in mice compared to particles without CTAB and naked DNA control formulations (He et al. 2005). A similar approach was pursued with PEI. In this study, mixing PEI and PLGA led to increased transfection efficiencies which were in the range of DNA/PEI mixtures while membrane toxicity was significantly reduced in comparison to PEI/DNA polyplexes. PLGA/PEI was also shown to be superior to PLGA/CTAB mixtures within this study (Oster et al. 2005). Similar to this approach, Ribeiro et al. encapsulated dendriplexes based on two different PLL-dendrons in PLGA nanoparticles and showed significantly pronounced antibody formation after immunization of BALB/c mice (Ribeiro et al. 2007).

Besides PLGA, CRL1005 is a another non-ionic polymer, consisting of a 12 kDA polyoxypropylene core and 5% polyoxyethylene, which is frequently used for vaccine delivery systems, either peptide-based or DNA-based. CRL1005 microparticles can be generated by heating CRL1005 solutions above their phase-transition temperature. In this context, one major approach has been intensively investigated. Microparticles of CRL1005 including benzalkonium chloride (BAK), as a DNA-complexing agent, could be identified as potential delivery systems for pDNA vaccination which elicited robust cellular and humoral immune responses in rhesus macaques and BALB/c mice (Evans et al. 2004; Hartikka et al. 2008).

LIPID-Based Delivery Systems for Genetic Vaccines

Cationic lipids are probably the oldest non-viral carrier system for genetic vaccinations. In principle, cationic liposomes are usually formulated with cationic lipids and neutral helper lipids. Structures of lipids described in this section are depicted in Fig. 5.4. Different techniques like the dehydration-rehydration technique, lipid film hydration, ethanol injection, detergent dialysis and reversed-phase evaporation can be utilized in order to formulate cationic liposomes. These liposomes can in turn form electrostatic complexes with anionic DNA which is often incorporated during the formulation process. These so-called lipoplexes are usually in the submicron range. Moreover, various liposomal formulations are already commercially available. Hence, these formulations can be diluted and mixed with DNA. By these means very simple lipoplex formulations can be obtained.

Like polyplex formulations, lipoplex formulations provide a valuable protection from nuclease attack in biological milieu. The cationic charge supports cell uptake similar to polyplex uptake by interactions via heparan sulfate proteoglycans. Besides, the lipophilic chains can also interact with the phospholipid bilayer of the cell membrane. Furthermore, there are indications that liposomes are appropriate vehicles for APC and lymph node targeting.

In order to transfer the knowledge that has been gained regarding general gene delivery to genetic vaccination, various different lipids have been investigated for these applications. 1,2-Dimyristyoxypropyl-3-dimethyl-hydroxyethylammonium bromide (DMRIE) is one of the key lipids, which has been widely investigated in laboratory animals as well as in patients. DMRIE is usually combined either with cholesterol (DMRIE-C) or with dioleoylphosphatidylethanolamine (DOPE) as helper lipids in order to form liposomes. Moreover, DOPE is widely used within such applications since it supports the endosomal escape within the cell. DMRIE-DOPE

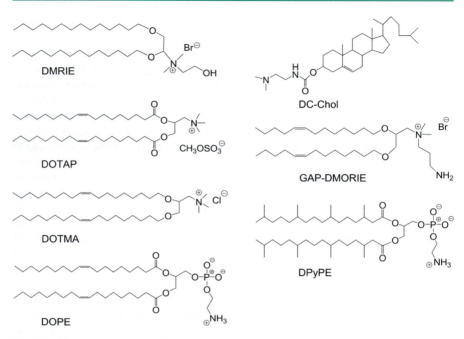

Fig. 5.4 Chemical structures of the most frequently used lipids for the preparation of cationic liposomal gene vaccine (lipoplex) formulations

liposomes have been prepared by a lipid film hydration method according to Felgner et al. (1994) and pDNA encoding different antigens have been incorporated into this system. It was shown that this system provides notable rabies antibody titres in animals as large as horses after intramuscular administration of a comparatively low single dose of 200 μg of pDNA. A further increase in the antibody titre was observed after a second injection (Fischer et al. 2003). Vaxfectin® is a commercially available and widely investigated liposome formulation for DNA vaccines. It consists of (±)-*N*-(3-aminopropyl)-*N,N*-dimethyl-2,3-bis(cis-9-tetradecenyloxy)-1-propanaminium bromide (GAP-DMORIE), structurally similar to DMRIE, and the helper lipid 1,2-diphytanoyl-sn-glycero-3-phosphoethanolamine (DPyPE) in a 1:1 ratio. Usually, Vaxfectin® gets diluted with sterile water for injection and finally mixed with pDNA in an appropriate ratio. It could be demonstrated that such formulations are capable of inducing humoral as well as cellular immune responses towards *Plasmodium falciparum*, influenza, rabies and further genetically encoded antigens (Sedegah et al. 2010; Smith et al. 2010; Margalith and Vilalta 2006). Margalith et al. compared DMRIE-DOPE and Vaxfectin® formulations regarding neutralizing antibody titres towards rabies antigens and concluded that Vaxfectin® formulations are more effective in this case (Margalith and Vilalta 2006).

The research group of Gregoriadis and co-workers has intensively studied multilamellar vesicles, prepared by the dehydration-rehydration method, as vehicles for

5 Pharmaceutical Non-Viral Formulations for Gene Vaccines

genetic vaccine delivery. Within this context, two further lipids have been investigated in particular: 1,2-dioleoyl-3-(trimethylammonium) propane (DOTAP) and cholesteryl 3-*N*-(dimethyl amino ethyl) carbamate (DC-Chol). Two different approaches were investigated. Plasmid DNA was either incorporated during the formation of small unilamellar vesicles (SUV) by sonication of lipids, helper lipids and phosphatidylcholin (PC) or during formation of multilamellar vesicles by rehydration of the freeze-dried SUV. Incorporation was similarly efficient in both cases but the smallest particles with the highest zeta potential were obtained when pDNA was incorporated during formation of SUV (Perrie et al. 2003). Within in vivo studies DOTAP formulations appeared to show longer lasting antibody titres than DC-Chol formulations while both lipids showed clearly superior results in comparison to naked DNA controls.

Further Modifications of Delivery Systems

The mentioned delivery systems have been further modified in order to pass the physiological barriers.

Cationic dosage forms tend to interact with serum proteins, extracellular matrix components or blood cells. Immobilization of poly(ethylene glycol) to the surface of cationic particles can shield ionic charges and thus limits interactions with the mentioned components (Lee and Kim 2005). Since cationic charges, on the other hand, help to increase transfection of cells PEGylation needs to be balanced carefully.

Other agents that have been attached to particulate delivery systems in order to improve their in vivo performance are cell-penetrating peptides (CPP) and nuclear localization signals (NLS). While CPP facilitate the cellular uptake across the cell membrane, NLS may increase the transport to the nucleus within the cell.

APC-targeting and targeting of dendritic cells in particular is regarded as an effective strategy for eliciting robust immune responses with DNA vaccines. For this purpose, targeting ligands can be attached to one of the mentioned delivery systems. Most commonly, C-type lectin receptors, which are sensitive to mannose-rich glycoproteins, like DC-SIGN are targeted. Hence, attachment of mannose or mannose-type carbohydrates to the surface of particulates has become a major strategy in order to achieve APC-targeting (Jain et al. 2005).

Route of Vaccine Administration

Up to now, formulations for intradermal and intramuscular administration of genetic vaccines dominate contemporary research due to the most reliable antigen expression. Nevertheless, interest in formulations for mucosal vaccination is persistently growing as mucosal tissues are the most likely portal of entry for pathogens and local immune responses at mucosal surfaces after parenteral administration are negligible.

Furthermore, investigations regarding needle-free transcutaneous delivery systems based on liposomes may be a potential alternative to intradermal injections.

Mucosal Vaccination

Regarding mucosal vaccination systems, three routes of administration are of particular interest: the oral, the nasal and the pulmonary route.

Exploitation of the oral route can serve several purposes. Besides improved mucosal immunity, convenient administration, improved patient compliance and administration without trained personnel are the most important advantages of oral delivery systems. Nevertheless, development of an oral delivery system for gene vaccines must be regarded as one of the biggest challenges within this evolving field due to mechanical, chemical and enzymatic barriers present in the gastrointestinal tract. Thus, breakdown of poly- or lipoplexes must be regarded as a major threat to the above mentioned formulations (Howard et al. 2004).

Earliest approaches for the mentioned purpose focused on simple encapsulation of the vaccine into PLGA microparticles by solvent evaporation methods (Kaneko et al. 2000) or chitosan nanoparticles by the complexation-coacervation method (Bivas-Benita et al. 2003). Kaneko et al. could demonstrate the expression of mRNA specific to the HIV envelope glycoprotein (env) in the gastrointestinal tract of BALB/c mice after oral administration of PLGA-encapsulated pDNA encoding env. More importantly, mucosal env-specific IgA could be detected in fecal samples (Kaneko et al. 2000). Unfortunately, similar studies with different plasmids did not deliver comparably promising results. Bivas-Benita and associates prepared chitosan-nanoparticles for oral delivery of pDNA encoding a granule protein of *Toxoplasma gondii*. These displayed promising physico-chemical properties and shielded pDNA from DNase I degradation. However, an intramuscular boost injection with the utilized plasmid was necessary in order to achieve a significant difference from empty control particles (Bivas-Benita et al. 2003). More advanced studies combine different strategies in order to make oral vaccination with genetic material feasible. Usually, an electrostatic complex, either lipoplex or polyplex, gets coated with a polymer-shell which is supposed to prevent complex breakdown. Somavarapu et al. prepared liposomes including PC, cholesterol, stearylamine and pDNA encoding hepatitis B surface antigen (HBsAg) and coated them with poly(DL-lactic acid) (PLA). They investigated transgene specific cytokine production (IFN-γ and IL-6) which was significantly pronounced after oral administration of the polymer-modified liposomes (Somavarapu et al. 2003). In a similar approach, polyplexes of PEI and pDNA were pre-formed and subsequently PEGylated. These polyplexes were finally incorporated into PLGA microparticles by a solvent evaporation method. Within in vivo studies, it could be demonstrated with a β-galactosidase-encoding plasmid that this delivery system is capable of inducing in vivo gene expression (Howard et al. 2004). Unfortunately, these last two studies did not investigate the production of secretory IgA that can be achieved with these systems. Jain et al. prepared niosomes of Span 60, cholesterol and stearylamine by reversed phase evaporation and

5 Pharmaceutical Non-Viral Formulations for Gene Vaccines

subsequently coated them with o-palmitoyl mannan (OPM) (Jain et al. 2005). OPM-coating serves two different purposes. On the one hand, this coating is supposed to prevent bile salt caused dissolution as well as enzymatic degradation and thus stabilizes the niosomes. On the other hand mannan can also act as a ligand for mannose receptors of APC that can be found in the vicinity of Peyer's patches of the intestine. Within immunization studies antibody titers, sufficient for seroprotection, were found. Regarding secretory IgA, OPM-coated niosomes showed the highest levels of salivary and intestinal IgA of all investigated formulations. Unfortunately, all mentioned studies suffer from a giant drawback, namely huge doses of plasmid that will probably turn out to be impractical in larger animals than small laboratory rodents.

Since many diseases enter the human body via the airways nasal and pulmonary vaccine delivery appear to be useful strategies in order to face these threats. Moreover, convenient administrations systems are available for these routes and a dose reduction compared to oral systems might be feasible due to reduced dilution in the nasal cavity or within the lungs. Hence, chitosan nanoparticles containing a HBsAg-encoding plasmid were prepared by complexation-coacervation by Khatri et al. These microparticles elicited a systemic humoral immune response after nasal administration comparable to that of naked DNA after intramuscular administration. It is believed that these nanoparticles are capable of passing the nasal membranes in order to finally reach the underlying lymphoid tissue where the systemic immune response can be generated. Another option might be uptake by M-cells of the nasal-associated lymphoid tissue (NALT). Interestingly, chitosan-nanoparticles caused secretion of mucosal IgA in nasal, salivary and vaginal samples after nasal administration. IgA levels of chitosan-nanoparticles were significantly superior to those of naked DNA, after intranasal as well as intramuscular administration (Khatri et al. 2008b). Similar observations were made by the same authors when they investigated liposomes consisting of PC, DOPE and cholesterol coated with glycol chitosan for nasal gene vaccine delivery (Khatri et al. 2008a). A PLGA-based formulation with pDNA encoding HIV-1 gag absorbed to its surface by means of CTAB was investigated by Singh et al. The authors demonstrated cell- and antibody-mediated responses in local as well as systemic lymphoid tissues. Secretory IgA were found in nasal washes (Singh et al. 2001).

Pulmonary delivery systems for genetic vaccines have been studied extensively by Bivas-Benita and different co-workers. Beside other systems, they investigated chitosan-nanoparticles, PEI-polyplexes and PLGA-PEI nanoparticles (Bivas-Benita et al. 2004, 2009, 2010). Unfortunately, IgA production in mucosal tissue was not investigated within these studies. Nevertheless, cytokine production was investigated as part of cellular immune responses. It could be demonstrated for all three systems that pulmonary administration leads to an increased cytokine production that was even superior to intramuscular administration of naked DNA. Most recently, Bivas-Benita et al. reported that PEI-DNA complexes induce robust local and systemic CD8[+] T-cell responses after pulmonary administration. The magnitude of the systemic response was similar to that after intramuscular administration. Interestingly, there was no significant difference between complexed and naked DNA after i.m. administration. On the contrary, CD8[+] T-cell responses in pulmonary tissue and in mediastinal lymph nodes were approximately 10-fold higher after pulmonary administration. CD8+ T-cell responses were also detected in the reproductive and the GI tract. However, no significant difference to i.m. administration could be demonstrated in these mucosal tissues.

Many of the mentioned studies managed to demonstrate the production of systemic as well as mucosal antibodies. Moreover, cellular immune responses were observed in most studies. Unfortunately, most of these studies still rely on very high pDNA doses. On the one hand, this would make a potential commercialized product highly expensive. On the other hand, a transfer of these delivery systems to humans would be rather difficult due to the high amounts of pDNA and adjuvants.

Needle-Free Transcutaneous Delivery Systems

Liposomes have been reported to be able to overcome the stratum corneum of the skin. Hence, liposomes appear to be an interesting alternative to intradermal application of genetic vaccines.

Based on this knowledge, Mahor et al. developed a cationic formulation which they call transferosomes (Mahor et al. 2007). It consists of sodium deoxycholate and N-[(1-(2,3)-dioleyloxy)-propyl]-N,N,N-trimethylammonium chloride (DOTMA). Plasmid DNA was adsorbed to their surface by electrostatic interactions between DOTMA and pDNA. Antibody-mediated response of this transcutaneous formulation was comparable to an intramuscular injection of a control protein but inferior to intramuscular naked DNA. Cytokine production was found to be at a similar level after intramuscular administration of naked DNA and transcutaneous application of transferosomes, respectively. Promising results were also obtained with a lipoplex-patch system consisting of DC-Chol, DOPE and DOTAP (Cheng et al. 2009). However, as promising as these results may appear, the development of such transcutaneous systems is still in its infancy. One major issue in these studies is surely the limited comparability of human skin and murine skin. Moreover, the problem of high dosings could not be solved on these routes, either.

However, a formulation of plasmid DNA encapsulated within a mannobiosylated PEI delivered via the skin is under clinical evaluation for treatment of HIV patients. Chapter 6 in this book provides detailed information about this technology.

Concluding Remarks

The methods described herein were shown to be valuable tools in order to improve the low transfection efficiency and immunogenicity of naked DNA vaccines. However, their in vivo performances suggest that a more precise knowledge about cellular trafficking and mode of action of such vaccines will be needed in order to develop efficient delivery systems. Major steps in the development of such a system will be the optimization of physico-chemical properties in the first place and finally investigations regarding suitable targeting ligands for the different stages of action.

5 Pharmaceutical Non-Viral Formulations for Gene Vaccines

Moreover, reliable evaluation models need to be chosen in order to allow an appropriate dose estimation prior to potential clinical trials.

References

Barouch DH, Letvin NL, Seder RA (2004) The role of cytokine DNAs as vaccine adjuvants for optimizing cellular immune responses. Immunol Rev 202:266–274

Bivas-Benita M, Laloup M, Versteyhe S, Dewit J, De Braekeleer J, Jongert E, Borchard G (2003) Generation of *Toxoplasma gondii* GRA1 protein and DNA vaccine loaded chitosan particles: preparation, characterization, and preliminary in vivo studies. Int J Pharm 266(1–2):17–27

Bivas-Benita M, van Meijgaarden KE, Franken KL, Junginger HE, Borchard G, Ottenhoff TH, Geluk A (2004) Pulmonary delivery of chitosan-DNA nanoparticles enhances the immunogenicity of a DNA vaccine encoding HLA-A*0201-restricted T-cell epitopes of *Mycobacterium tuberculosis*. Vaccine 22(13–14):1609–1615

Bivas-Benita M, Lin MY, Bal SM, van Meijgaarden KE, Franken KL, Friggen AH, Junginger HE, Borchard G, Klein MR, Ottenhoff TH (2009) Pulmonary delivery of DNA encoding *Mycobacterium tuberculosis* latency antigen Rv1733c associated to PLGA-PEI nanoparticles enhances T cell responses in a DNA prime/protein boost vaccination regimen in mice. Vaccine 27(30):4010–4017

Bivas-Benita M, Bar L, Gillard GO, Kaufman DR, Simmons NL, Hovav AH, Letvin NL (2010) Efficient generation of mucosal and systemic antigen-specific CD8+ T-cell responses following pulmonary DNA immunization. J Virol 84(11):5764–5774

Cheng JY, Huang HN, Tseng WC, Li TL, Chan YL, Cheng KC, Wu CJ (2009) Transcutaneous immunization by lipoplex-patch based DNA vaccines is effective vaccination against Japanese encephalitis virus infection. J Control Release 135(3):242–249

Cui Z, Mumper RJ (2003) Microparticles and nanoparticles as delivery systems for DNA vaccines. Crit Rev Ther Drug Carrier Syst 20(2–3):103–137

Dutta T, Garg M, Jain NK (2008) Poly(propyleneimine) dendrimer and dendrosome mediated genetic immunization against hepatitis B. Vaccine 26(27–28):3389–3394

Evans RK, Zhu DM, Casimiro DR, Nawrocki DK, Mach H, Troutman RD, Tang A, Wu S, Chin S, Ahn C, Isopi LA, Williams DM, Xu Z, Shiver JW, Volkin DB (2004) Characterization and biological evaluation of a microparticle adjuvant formulation for plasmid DNA vaccines. J Pharm Sci 93(7):1924–1939

Felgner JH, Kumar R, Sridhar CN, Wheeler CJ, Tsai YJ, Border R, Ramsey P, Martin M, Felgner PL (1994) Enhanced gene delivery and mechanism studies with a novel series of cationic lipid formulations. J Biol Chem 269(4):2550–2561

Fischer L, Minke J, Dufay N, Baudu P, Audonnet JC (2003) Rabies DNA vaccine in the horse: strategies to improve serological responses. Vaccine 21(31):4593–4596

Foged C, Brodin B, Frokjaer S, Sundblad A (2005) Particle size and surface charge affect particle uptake by human dendritic cells in an in vitro model. Int J Pharm 298(2):315–322

Guliyeva U, Oner F, Ozsoy S, Haziroglu R (2006) Chitosan microparticles containing plasmid DNA as potential oral gene delivery system. Eur J Pharm Biopharm 62(1):17–25

Hartikka J, Geall A, Bozoukova V, Kurniadi D, Rusalov D, Enas J, Yi JH, Nanci A, Rolland A (2008) Physical characterization and in vivo evaluation of poloxamer-based DNA vaccine formulations. J Gene Med 10(7):770–782

He X, Jiang L, Wang F, Xiao Z, Li J, Liu LS, Li D, Ren D, Jin X, Li K, He Y, Shi K, Guo Y, Zhang Y, Sun S (2005) Augmented humoral and cellular immune responses to hepatitis B DNA vaccine adsorbed onto cationic microparticles. J Control Release 107(2):357–372

Howard KA, Li XW, Somavarapu S, Singh J, Green N, Atuah KN, Ozsoy Y, Seymour LW, Alpar HO (2004) Formulation of a microparticle carrier for oral polyplex-based DNA vaccines. Biochim Biophys Acta 1674(2):149–157

Jain S, Singh P, Mishra V, Vyas SP (2005) Mannosylated niosomes as adjuvant-carrier system for oral genetic immunization against hepatitis B. Immunol Lett 101(1):41–49

Jain K, Kesharwani P, Gupta U, Jain NK (2010) Dendrimer toxicity: let's meet the challenge. Int J Pharm 394(1–2):122–142

Kaneko H, Bednarek I, Wierzbicki A, Kiszka I, Dmochowski M, Wasik TJ, Kaneko Y, Kozbor D (2000) Oral DNA vaccination promotes mucosal and systemic immune responses to HIV envelope glycoprotein. Virology 267(1):8–16

Khatri K, Goyal AK, Gupta PN, Mishra N, Mehta A, Vyas SP (2008a) Surface modified liposomes for nasal delivery of DNA vaccine. Vaccine 26(18):2225–2233

Khatri K, Goyal AK, Gupta PN, Mishra N, Vyas SP (2008b) Plasmid DNA loaded chitosan nanoparticles for nasal mucosal immunization against hepatitis B. Int J Pharm 354(1–2):235–241

Lee M, Kim SW (2005) Polyethylene glycol-conjugated copolymers for plasmid DNA delivery. Pharm Res 22(1):1–10

Lodmell DL, Ray NB, Ulrich JT, Ewalt LC (2000) DNA vaccination of mice against rabies virus: effects of the route of vaccination and the adjuvant monophosphoryl lipid A (MPL). Vaccine 18(11–12):1059–1066

Lv H, Zhang S, Wang B, Cui S, Yan J (2006) Toxicity of cationic lipids and cationic polymers in gene delivery. J Control Release 114(1):100–109

Mahor S, Rawat A, Dubey PK, Gupta PN, Khatri K, Goyal AK, Vyas SP (2007) Cationic transfersomes based topical genetic vaccine against hepatitis B. Int J Pharm 340(1–2):13–19

Margalith M, Vilalta A (2006) Sustained protective rabies neutralizing antibody titers after administration of cationic lipid-formulated pDNA vaccine. Genet Vaccines Ther 4:2

Martien R, Loretz B, Schnurch AB (2006) Oral gene delivery: design of polymeric carrier systems shielding toward intestinal enzymatic attack. Biopolymers 83(4):327–336

Martien R, Loretz B, Thaler M, Majzoob S, Bernkop-Schnurch A (2007) Chitosan-thioglycolic acid conjugate: an alternative carrier for oral nonviral gene delivery? J Biomed Mater Res A 82(1):1–9

Meyer M, Zintchenko A, Ogris M, Wagner E (2007) A dimethylmaleic acid-melittin-polylysine conjugate with reduced toxicity, pH-triggered endosomolytic activity and enhanced gene transfer potential. J Gene Med 9(9):797–805

Minigo G, Scholzen A, Tang CK, Hanley JC, Kalkanidis M, Pietersz GA, Apostolopoulos V, Plebanski M (2007) Poly-L-lysine-coated nanoparticles: a potent delivery system to enhance DNA vaccine efficacy. Vaccine 25(7):1316–1327

Mislick KA, Baldeschwieler JD (1996) Evidence for the role of proteoglycans in cation-mediated gene transfer. Proc Natl Acad Sci USA 93(22):12349–12354

Mounkes LC, Zhong W, Cipres-Palacin G, Heath TD, Debs RJ (1998) Proteoglycans mediate cationic liposome-DNA complex-based gene delivery in vitro and in vivo. J Biol Chem 273(40):26164–26170

Oster CG, Kim N, Grode L, Barbu-Tudoran L, Schaper AK, Kaufmann SH, Kissel T (2005) Cationic microparticles consisting of poly(lactide-co-glycolide) and polyethylenimine as carriers systems for parental DNA vaccination. J Control Release 104(2):359–377

Ott G, Singh M, Kazzaz J, Briones M, Soenawan E, Ugozzoli M, O'Hagan DT (2002) A cationic sub-micron emulsion (MF59/DOTAP) is an effective delivery system for DNA vaccines. J Control Release 79(1–3):1–5

Perrie Y, McNeil S, Vangala A (2003) Liposome-mediated DNA immunisation via the subcutaneous route. J Drug Target 11(8–10):555–563

Pichon C, Goncalves C, Midoux P (2001) Histidine-rich peptides and polymers for nucleic acids delivery. Adv Drug Deliv Rev 53(1):75–94

Ribeiro S, Rijpkema SG, Durrani Z, Florence AT (2007) PLGA-dendron nanoparticles enhance immunogenicity but not lethal antibody production of a DNA vaccine against anthrax in mice. Int J Pharm 331(2):228–232

Rogers JV, Hull BE, Fink PS, Chiou HC, Bigley NJ (2000) Murine response to DNA encoding herpes simplex virus type-1 glycoprotein D targeted to the liver. Vaccine 18(15):1522–1530

Ruponen M, Yla-Herttuala S, Urtti A (1999) Interactions of polymeric and liposomal gene delivery systems with extracellular glycosaminoglycans: physicochemical and transfection studies. Biochim Biophys Acta 1415(2):331–341

Sasaki S, Sumino K, Hamajima K, Fukushima J, Ishii N, Kawamoto S, Mohri H, Kensil CR, Okuda K (1998) Induction of systemic and mucosal immune responses to human immunodeficiency virus type 1 by a DNA vaccine formulated with QS-21 saponin adjuvant via intramuscular and intranasal routes. J Virol 72(6):4931–4939

Sedegah M, Rogers WO, Belmonte M, Belmonte A, Banania G, Patterson NB, Rusalov D, Ferrari M, Richie TL, Doolan DL (2010) Vaxfectin enhances both antibody and in vitro T cell responses to each component of a 5-gene *Plasmodium falciparum* plasmid DNA vaccine mixture administered at low doses. Vaccine 28(17):3055–3065

Singh M, Vajdy M, Gardner J, Briones M, O'Hagan D (2001) Mucosal immunization with HIV-1 gag DNA on cationic microparticles prolongs gene expression and enhances local and systemic immunity. Vaccine 20(3–4):594–602

Smith KA (1980) T-cell growth factor. Immunol Rev 51:337–357

Smith LR, Wloch MK, Ye M, Reyes LR, Boutsaboualoy S, Dunne CE, Chaplin JA, Rusalov D, Rolland AP, Fisher CL, Al-Ibrahim MS, Kabongo ML, Steigbigel R, Belshe RB, Kitt ER, Chu AH, Moss RB (2010) Phase 1 clinical trials of the safety and immunogenicity of adjuvanted plasmid DNA vaccines encoding influenza A virus H5 hemagglutinin. Vaccine 28(13):2565–2572

Somavarapu S, Bramwell VW, Alpar HO (2003) Oral plasmid DNA delivery systems for genetic immunisation. J Drug Target 11(8–10):547–553

Tang DC, DeVit M, Johnston SA (1992) Genetic immunization is a simple method for eliciting an immune response. Nature 356(6365):152–154

Thanou M, Florea BI, Geldof M, Junginger HE, Borchard G (2002) Quaternized chitosan oligomers as novel gene delivery vectors in epithelial cell lines. Biomaterials 23(1):153–159

Thomsen LL, Topley P, Daly MG, Brett SJ, Tite JP (2004) Imiquimod and resiquimod in a mouse model: adjuvants for DNA vaccination by particle-mediated immunotherapeutic delivery. Vaccine 22(13–14):1799–1809

van den Berg JH, Nuijen B, Schumacher TN, Haanen JB, Storm G, Beijnen JH, Hennink WE (2010) Synthetic vehicles for DNA vaccination. J Drug Target 18(1):1–14

Verbaan FJ, Klein Klouwenberg P, van Steenis JH, Snel CJ, Boerman O, Hennink WE, Storm G (2005) Application of poly(2-(dimethylamino)ethyl methacrylate)-based polyplexes for gene transfer into human ovarian carcinoma cells. Int J Pharm 304(1–2):185–192

Wang S, Kennedy JS, West K, Montefiori DC, Coley S, Lawrence J, Shen S, Green S, Rothman AL, Ennis FA, Arthos J, Pal R, Markham P, Lu S (2008) Cross-subtype antibody and cellular immune responses induced by a polyvalent DNA prime-protein boost HIV-1 vaccine in healthy human volunteers. Vaccine 26(8):1098–1110

Wolff JA, Malone RW, Williams P, Chong W, Acsadi G, Jani A, Felgner PL (1990) Direct gene transfer into mouse muscle in vivo. Science 247(4949 Pt 1):1465–1468

Yang X, Yuan X, Cai D, Wang S, Zong L (2009) Low molecular weight chitosan in DNA vaccine delivery via mucosa. Int J Pharm 375(1–2):123–132

Zhang A, Jin H, Zhang F, Ma Z, Tu Y, Ren Z, Zhang X, Zhu K, Wang B (2005) Effects of multiple copies of CpG on DNA vaccination. DNA Cell Biol 24(5):292–298

Rational Design of Formulated DNA Vaccines: The DermaVir Approach

6

Eszter Nátz and Julianna Lisziewicz

DermaVir features three key technological elements of a rational vaccine design: a single plasmid DNA immunogen to express 15 HIV antigens, a synthetic pDNA nanomedicine formulation and a topical dendritic cell-targeting vaccine administration. Its novel mechanism of action has been consistently demonstrated in mice, rabbits, primates and human subjects: DermaVir nanomedicine is naturally transported by epidermal Langerhans cells to the lymph nodes to express the plasmid DNA-encoded HIV antigens and induce precursor/memory T cells with high proliferation capacity. Safety, immunogenicity and preliminary efficacy of DermaVir have been clinically demonstrated in HIV-infected human subjects. DC-based therapeutic vaccination might offer a new treatment paradigm for cancer and infectious diseases.

Background and Rationale for the Development of DermaVir Therapeutic Vaccine Against HIV/AIDS

In the eighteenth century Edward Jenner developed the first prophylactic vaccine for protection against smallpox (*Variola major*). He used skin scarification to deliver a live whole pathogen, the cowpox vaccinia virus (VACV). While he didn't know it at the time, Jenner's technology induced durable and fully protective antibodies and cytotoxic T cell responses leading to the prevention and later to the eradication of smallpox infection. It has been recently demonstrated that not only the cross-protective antigen and the live virus formulation but also the vaccine administration via skin scarification was essential for the exceptional efficacy of VACV vaccine (Liu et al. 2010).

J. Lisziewicz (✉)
Genetic Immunity,
Berlini u. 47-49, 1045, Budapest, Hungary
e-mail:lisziewj@geneticimmunity.com

J. Thalhamer et al. (eds.), *Gene Vaccines*,
DOI 10.1007/978-3-7091-0439-2_6, © Springer-Verlag/Wien, 2012

A decade later in 1885 Louis Pasteur developed the first therapeutic vaccine against rabies virus. The cross-reactive antigen and the live virus formulation mirrored Jenner's vaccine but, instead of using a related virus, this vaccine contained a live attenuated version of the rabies virus. Pasteur then went on to replace the single vaccine administration via skin scarification with multiple injections. Since Pasteur, needle injections are widely used for the administration of vaccines.

For the past 200 years vaccine development was based on empirical science. Recent vaccine products contain antigens, generally a single protein of the target pathogen capable of eliciting humoral immune responses (Donnelly et al. 1997; Ada 2005). Compared to live-attenuated vaccines these protein-based vaccinations are much safer, decreasing the risk of potential infection; however, they are less effective immunogens in inducing antibodies and cytotoxic T cell responses even when formulated with adjuvants. Recently, rational vaccine design has replaced the empirical approaches with three key elements (Douek et al. 2006; Rappuoli 2000). (1) Safety is one of the most important features of modern vaccines since they are historically intended to be used in healthy individuals including children. For this reason, there are strict safety restrictions on live attenuated pathogen formulations despite their proven efficacy. (2) Vaccine efficacy has three essential elements: (a) a cross-reactive antigen pool, (b) antigen formulation, and (c) vaccine administration. (3) Scalable manufacturing technology and a predictive immunodiagnosis are additional, but equally important, elements in the development of new vaccines.

The development of DNA vaccines began in the early 1990s following the observations that injected plasmid DNA (pDNA) is taken up and expressed by muscle cells in mice and that the pDNA encoded antigens can elicit both antibody and cytotoxic T cell responses in vivo (Wolff et al. 1990; Tang et al. 1992). However, the preclinical immunogenicity demonstrated in small animals did not correlate with the immunogenicity seen in larger animals or during human studies (Babiuk et al. 2003). Likely reasons for the weak efficacy are a poor antigen repertoire, low antigen expression, and suboptimal antigen delivery to the lymphoid organs where immune responses are generated. Importantly, as pDNA does not replicate or cause disease, its excellent safety profile provides a major advantage over traditional live vaccines. An important feature of pDNA is that it can be designed to express several antigens. This represents significant manufacturing and regulatory benefits compared to the use of multiple protein antigens, in which case every single protein must be manufactured and quality controlled separately. In addition, essentially any type of protein can be encoded and expressed from a pDNA, including some that would otherwise be difficult or impossible to recombinantly express and purify in their naturally occurring conformation. Moreover, the intracellularly expressed, structurally authentic protein antigens are processed and presented on the host MHC molecules. These features, combined with recently improved large-scale manufacturing capabilities, make pDNA vaccines attractive candidates for product development.

DNA-based vaccines have been developed as both preventive and therapeutic vaccines against a wide range of infectious diseases and different kinds of cancer

6 Rational Design of Formulated DNA Vaccines: The DermaVir Approach

(Abdulhaqq and Weiner 2008; Anderson and Schneider 2007; Fioretti et al. 2010; Stevenson et al. 2010). Since its discovery in the early 1980s, HIV/AIDS has become one of the most widely researched diseases. Current antiretroviral therapy (ART) options consist of combinations of at least three antiretroviral drugs (ARVs) belonging to at least two classes of antiretroviral agents. Current ART does not cure the disease and requires lifelong use to achieve and maintain complete suppression of virus replication. Therefore, the new objective of treating HIV disease is to achieve a "functional cure" through immune mediated control of HIV-associated disease progression. Novel approaches to treat HIV and reconstitute the immune system include therapeutic vaccines. The immune control of HIV replication could improve survival, decrease HIV transmission and has the potential to achieve a "functional cure."

The discovery leading to DermaVir began with a clinical observation and extensive investigation of one exceptional HIV-infected subject (Lisziewicz et al. 1999). This individual demonstrated for the first time that induction of long-term immune control is achievable, and antiviral T cells can successfully control HIV replication. This patient was treated with ARVs shortly after infection followed by two ART interruptions, each resulting in a controlled HIV RNA rebound. In 1996, although the patient permanently discontinued therapy, his HIV did not rebound. For years, he did not receive ART because his immune system suppressed viral replication and controlled his disease. With time, his immune control diminished and HIV became detectable in his blood. Analyses revealed that the controlled virus rebound occurred early after infection and the induced HIV-specific T cells were capable of achieving a "functional cure." Later we confirmed and extended this observation demonstrating that T cell-mediated immune control can be induced with controlled rebound of the wild type virus only during primary infection (Lori et al. 2000). These results suggested that HIV antigens must be redirected from T cells to dendritic cells (DCs) to boost therapeutically effective HIV-specific T cell responses and provided the rationale and objectives for the DermaVir therapeutic vaccine development: (1) the antigen composition of DermaVir should safely mimic the naturally-occurring virus, (2) DermaVir must employ DCs (and not somatic cells) for antigen presentation, and (3) boosting of HIV-specific cellular immunity in HIV+ individuals could control virus replication and lead to a "functional cure."

DermaVir represents the first rationally designed therapeutic HIV vaccine that combines three essential elements: a novel single pDNA immunogen, a synthetic pDNA nanoformulation and a DC targeting delivery system reviewed in detail here. The active pharmaceutical ingredient (API) of DermaVir is a single pDNA immunogen expressing the broadest HIV antigen repertoire constructed to date for HIV vaccination. The medicinal product, DermaVir, consists of the pDNA formulated with a cationic polymer to form pathogen-like synthetic nanoparticles that support gene expression and antigen presentation in DCs (Toke et al. 2010). The DermaPrep needle-free transdermal vaccine administration device specifically targets DermaVir nanomedicine into epidermal Langerhans cells (LCs), the antigen presenting cells (APCs) of the skin. After topical vaccination with DermaPrep, LCs transport the DermaVir nanoparticles to the lymph nodes where they express the pDNA-encoded

HIV antigens and induce HIV-specific precursor/memory T cells with high proliferation capacity (Lisziewicz et al. 2005a).

The goal of DermaVir therapeutic vaccination is to enhance the effectiveness and durability of current antiretroviral drugs and to protect HIV-infected individuals from disease progression and the development of AIDS. The technology developed for DermaVir also represents a new vaccine platform that has application for inducing cellular immune responses against a wide range of pathogens and chronic conditions. The core platform of DermaPrep administration of the pDNA nanomedicine is the same for all vaccine candidates and ready to be used with novel pDNA antigens to address various disease conditions. In the following sections, we use the example of DermaVir to introduce all the elements of this vaccination platform technology, describing its major features and pointing out some of the differences from presently used or developed technologies.

DermaVir's pDNA Immunogen for the Expression of 15 HIV Antigens Forming VLP+

The first objective of the HIV therapeutic vaccine antigen design was to preserve the structure and the epitope content of the wild-type virus and create a safe immunogen. We constructed a single pDNA expressing 15 HIV proteins that form replication-, reverse transcription-, and integration-defective complex virus like particles (VLP+). A superscripted plus-sign (+) is used to distinguish this complex VLP+ containing most HIV proteins from a conventional VLP that only contains one or two self-assembling proteins. This immunogen is inherently safe because molecular modifications at the genetic level make it impossible for the expressed VLP+ to replicate or cause disease. It is interesting to note that the discovery and the use of VLP as antigen was essential for the development of effective prophylactic vaccines against the human papillomavirus (Garland et al. 2007; Paavonen et al. 2009).

Antigen selection has typically been based on epidemiological, phylogenic and genomic analyses of the targeted disease (Rappuoli 2000). With an ever-growing amount of experimental data being generated, this approach is commonly used to determine the most immunogenic antigens for eliciting immune responses. One recent advance in rational antigen selection is the utilization of *in silico* antigen design tools that utilize different databases for the determination of the most immunogenic proteins of various pathogens and cancers. In case of DermaVir, our goal was to retain the broadest HIV antigen repertoire and meet the highest safety requirements of regulatory agencies (Somogyi et al. 2010). To achieve these objectives, specific mutations were introduced into a cloned wild type HIV-1 sequence. These mutations completely inactivated integration, irreversibly impaired reverse transcription and the function of Nef. Additionally, truncation of the Nef protein might improve the immunogenicity of all antigens expressed by pLWXu1 as the truncated Nef cannot down-regulate the expression of MHC molecules, a mechanism that HIV has developed to escape from immune recognition (Le Gall et al. 1998; Yang et al. 2002).

To enhance antigen expression, the regions encoding the beginning and termination of protein synthesis must be optimized. Commonly used potent constitutive promoters in mammalian cells are derived from the simian virus 40 (SV40) and, preferably, human cytomegalovirus (CMV). One of the advantages of these promoters is that they are not species-specific; therefore the same constructs can be studied from preclinical animal models to human subjects. The inclusion of additional enhancers and transcription transactivators might also improve promoter activity in the target cells. For DermaVir, the 5′ HIV-LTR was used as promoter because it ensures potent and regulated expression of the HIV protein antigens in several cell types including professional APCs (Piccinini et al. 2002). The resulting pDNA immunogen (pLWXu1) encodes thirteen complete and two genetically impaired non-functional HIV-1 proteins: five functional regulatory proteins (Tat-p14, Rev-p19, Vpr-p12, Vpu-p16, Vif-p23), eight complete structural proteins, namely Gag polyprotein comprising matrix (p17), capsid (p24) and nucleocapsid (p7); Pol proteins: protease (p15), reverse transcriptase (p51) and RNase (p15); Env proteins: surface glycoprotein (gp120) and transmembrane glycoprotein (gp41); a non-functional mutant Integrase (wild type: p31) and a truncated non-functional Nef (wild type: p27).

HIV-specific CD8[+] cytotoxic T cells are elicited by 8–11 amino acid length epitopes presented on MHC I molecules. HIV-specific CD4[+] Th1 helper cells that support the CD8[+] T cell responses are elicited by the presentation of a different epitope repertoire of 13–25 amino acid length on MHC II. The expression of 15 HIV proteins from the pDNA of DermaVir within the same cell supports the presentation of the highest number of HIV epitopes and the induction of HIV-specific T cell responses with the broadest specificity. To highlight the importance of encoding both structural and regulatory proteins, we developed and validated an *in silico* high-affinity T cell epitope prediction method to analyze the immunological potential of DermaVir (Somogyi et al. 2010). DermaVir's immunogen can potentially present 933 high-affinity MHC I restricted epitopes to CD8[+] T cells and 2,330 high-affinity MHC II restricted epitopes to CD4[+] T cells, predicted for all available human MHC I alleles (n = 57) and MHC II alleles (n = 63). This potential to induce HIV-specific CD4[+] and CD8[+] T cells represents the broadest specificity reported to date among HIV vaccine candidates (Sandstrom et al. 2008; Ellenberger et al. 2005; Fischer et al. 2007).

The expressed 15 HIV proteins of DermaVir are able to self-assemble to a complex virus-like particle (VLP+) (Quan et al. 2008; Somogyi et al. 2010). The expressed VLP+ is assembled similarly and is structurally authentic to the wild-type HIV (Fig. 6.1). Beyond inducing T cell responses, this antigen might also be suitable for inducing neutralizing antibodies against viral and cellular antigens naturally occurring on the surface of HIV or structures present only during budding or entry (Mouquet et al. 2010). Such a multi-faceted immune response is a unique feature of pDNA vaccines expressing an authentic-looking HIV.

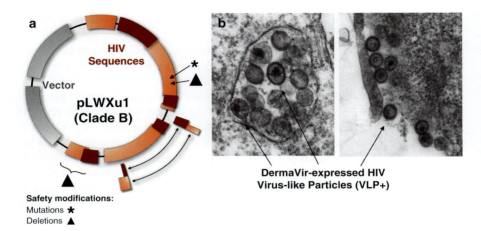

Fig. 6.1 Design of DermaVir pDNA (pLWXu1) (Somogyi et al. 2010). Features: (**a**) **1.** The pDNA has multiple molecular safety features including irreversible mutations in integration, reverse transcription and Nef. **2.** HIV-LTR promoter drives the regulated expression of 15 HIV protein antigens. **3.** A single pDNA serves as the active pharmaceutical ingredient (API). (**b**) **4.** Production of complex virus-like particles (VLP+) mimicking the structure, release and entry of the naturally occurring HIV

DermaVir's Synthetic pDNA Nanomedicine Formulation for Antigen Expression in Dendritic Cells

The next objective of the HIV therapeutic vaccine design was to express pDNA-encoded antigens in DCs to induce and boost T cell immunity. However, pDNA delivery to DCs is a complex problem involving DC binding, antigen uptake, expression, processing and presentation to naive T cells (Reddy et al. 2006). Viral vectors have been commonly used for vaccine delivery because they evolved to deliver foreign genetic material into cells. However, therapeutic vaccines require repeated boosting of T cell responses that have already been induced by the wild-type HIV in infected people. Therefore, to avoid vector-induced immunity, we needed to develop a synthetic pDNA formulation. DermaVir is a "pathogen-like" nanomedicine in which the pDNA is encapsulated within a mannobiosylated polyethylenimine (PEIm) (Fig. 6.2). The nanomedicine enters DCs via endocytosis and induces both maturation of DCs and IL-12 production favoring the induction of Th1 type cellular immunity (Lisziewicz et al. 2005a; Lisziewicz et al. 2001).

Linear PEIm is a synthetic vector developed to formulate pDNA (and other antigens) into pathogen-like nanoparticles (Toke et al. 2010). The interaction between the positively charged PEIm backbone and negatively charged pDNA leads to the spontaneous formation of nano-size complexes required for the protection of the pDNA from extra- and intracellular degradation. The pDNA/PEIm complexes are 70–300 nm nanoparticles mimicking the size, appearance and several features of viral vectors. The nanoparticles maintain their stability prior to cellular uptake by endocytosis and the buffering capacity of the PEIm allows escape from the

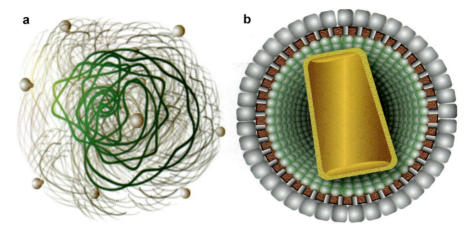

Fig. 6.2 Nanotechnology employed in DermaVir vaccine. According to the classification of nanomaterials both nano-elements belong to the soft nanoparticle (S) category (Tomalia 2009). (**a**) The DermaVir vaccine product is a synthetic nanoparticle (S3: polymeric micelles) consisting of a single pDNA and a mannosylated polyethylenimine (PEIm). This pathogen-like nanoformulation facilitates cellular entry and the expression of the pDNA-encoded antigens. (**b**) The pDNA immunogen expresses in the human body an HIV VLP+, a natural nanoparticle (S5: viruses) (Lisziewicz et al. 2001)

endosomal compartment within the cell, facilitating the release of pDNA from the nanoparticle in the proximity of the nucleus (Boussif et al. 1995). This novel "pathogen-like" nanoparticle formulation not only supports the efficient targeting of DCs but also facilitates efficient expression of antigens from the encapsulated pDNA inside the cells.

Compared to viral vectors, DermaVir and other polymeric pDNA formulation technologies are attractive for pDNA-based vaccine development due to the absence of vector-directed immune responses, enhanced antigen expression and excellent safety features (Choosakoonkriang et al. 2003; von Harpe et al. 2000). However, as DermaVir together with other pDNA- and polymer-based products approach pharmaceutical reality a number of issues need to be comprehensively addressed beyond clinical efficiency and safety such as stable formulations and scalable manufacturing that make them suitable for the global market (Ohana et al. 2004).

DermaPrep Vaccine Administration for Targeted Antigen Delivery to Dendritic Cells In Vivo

The third objective of HIV therapeutic vaccine design was to deliver DermaVir to the lymph node DCs. For cancer vaccines it has been feasible to manufacture ex vivo cultured DCs for personalized treatment (Kantoff et al. 2010). However, an ex vivo approach as a therapeutic HIV vaccine would be too costly and logistically

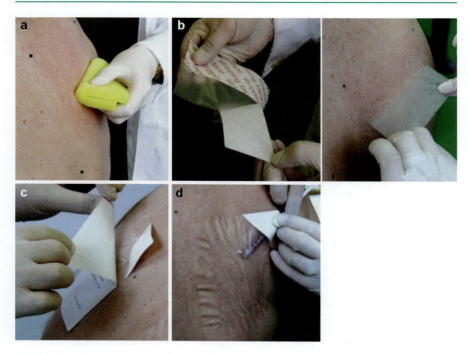

Fig. 6.3 Vaccine administration procedure using DermaPrep. (**a**) A rough sponge is used to exfoliate the skin and generate a "danger" signal. (**b**) The skin is cleansed with medical tape to remove the dead cells. (**c**) A semi-occlusive skin patch is applied to the prepared skin. (**d**) The liquid vaccine is administered under the patch using a needle-free syringe

cumbersome to successfully compete on the market. To find an alternative approach that targets DermaVir to DCs in vivo, we investigated many experimental and marketed medical devices designed for vaccine administration and found none that could efficiently target vaccines to DCs (Peachman et al. 2003). None of the devices were suitable to replace the ex vivo immunizations with cultured DCs for two main reasons: (1) DCs represented only a very small portion of the targeted cells, most of the vaccine was delivered non-specifically to the bystander somatic cells, and (2) none of the vaccine delivery devices provided an appropriate "danger" signal which is required to stimulate the DCs to maturation and migration to the lymph nodes, the organ where immune responses are initiated (Zinkernagel 2000; Steinman 1991; Matzinger 2002). These findings encouraged us to find a novel mechanism to deliver the vaccine to the lymph node DCs in vivo (Fig. 6.3). As a result, we developed DermaPrep, the first DC targeting vaccine administration device. DermaPrep employs a skin preparation method that interrupts the stratum corneum facilitating vaccine penetration and providing the essential "danger" signal to the LCs residing just below this protective layer (Matzinger 2002; Nicolas and Guy 2008). Once activated, LCs naturally look for pathogens and capture the pathogen-like DermaVir nanomedicine applied to the prepared skin surface under a semi-occlusive patch.

Once the pDNA nanomedicine has been captured, LCs mature to DCs and travel to the local lymph nodes. Here DCs express pDNA-encoded antigens and present most HIV epitopes to the passing naïve T cells. HIV-specific precursor/memory T cells primed by DCs further differentiate into HIV-specific effector T cells circulating out of the lymph node to seek virus-infected targets. Each killer effector cell can destroy several HIV-infected cells.

The DermaPrep device uses a combination of shaving, tape-stripping and exfoliation with a rough body sponge as a pre-treatment for the activation of epidermal LCs and disruption of the stratum corneum to facilitate the penetration of DermaVir nanoparticles. After the pre-treatment, an 80 cm^2 semi-occlusive patch is applied to the skin and the liquid DermaVir vaccine is administered under the empty skin patch. After 3 h the patch is removed and discarded. The main advantage of DermaPrep compared to other vaccine administration technologies is the targeting of a large number of LCs (8 million) that form a horizontal 900–1,800 cells/mm^2 network under the skin surface (Bauer et al. 2001). For example, in nonhuman primates approximately 20,000 DCs expressed the pDNA-encoded antigens of DermaVir in the draining lymph node (Lisziewicz et al. 2005a). In striking contrast, only 50–100 pDNA-expressing cells were found in the lymph nodes of mice after DNA-containing particle bombardment by gene gun (Porgador et al. 1998).

Preclinical and Clinical Development of the DermaVir HIV Therapeutic Vaccine Product

Current first-line ART is simple (often a single pill) and fully suppressive (>80% of patients achieve undetectable HIV RNA). A battery of drugs inhibiting different parts of the HIV life cycle is available to provide effective second-, third- and later-lines of therapies in case of toxicity or the emergence of resistance. However, these drugs will neither cure the disease nor reconstitute HIV-specific immunity. The absence of immune reconstitution results in rapid virus rebound after interruption of ART, development of drug resistance in case of adherence problems and significant increase of non-AIDS-defining cancers in people on fully suppressive therapy (Powles et al. 2009). Incorporating therapeutic vaccinations into patient management would improve the body's natural defense mechanisms against the virus. Initial vaccine products are not expected to fully suppress HIV RNA as monotherapy; therefore, to compete with approved drugs, it is anticipated that they will be used in combination with ARVs. However, after the approval of several therapeutic vaccines and immune modulatory drugs, the combination of these approaches could result in a "functional cure" of HIV/AIDS.

Prior to initiation of human trials with a new medicinal product, regulatory agencies require the demonstration of their quality, safety and efficacy initially in appropriate animal models. We have designed DermaVir to express the pDNA-derived antigens specifically in the DCs of the lymph nodes to prime and boost HIV-specific T cells in infected hosts (Fig. 6.4). To demonstrate the mechanism of action first we established in human primary cells in vitro and in macaques ex vivo that

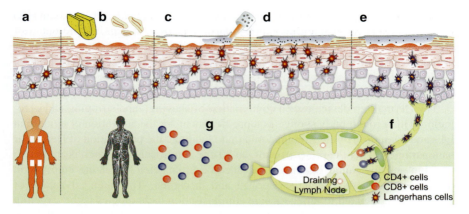

Fig. 6.4 Mechanism of action of DermaVir vaccination. (**a**) Skin sites are selected; (**b**) skin preparation using DermaPrep; (**c**) patch applied and DermaVir administered for 3 h; (**d**) activated Langerhans cells (LC) capture DermaVir nanoparticles; (**e**) LCs migrate to lymph nodes, mature to DCs; (**f**) DCs present DermaVir-encoded epitopes to naïve CD4$^+$ and CD8$^+$ T-cells; (**g**) HIV-specific CD4$^+$ and CD8$^+$ precursor/memory T-cells proliferate and search for HIV-infected cells throughout the body

DermaVir-expressing DCs prime naïve T cells and induce both HIV-specific helper and cytotoxic T cells (Lisziewicz et al. 2001). Preclinical animal studies conducted in mice, rabbits and macaques consistently demonstrated that in vivo DermaVir immunization targets the pDNA immunogen to the DCs of the lymph nodes that express the pDNA-encoded antigens. Importantly, immune responses following in vivo DermaVir immunization were shown to be similar to ex vivo immunization with cultured DCs (Lisziewicz et al. 2005a). Both ex vivo and in vivo DermaVir immunizations employed lymph node DCs to express similar amounts of pDNA-derived antigens and both induced Th1-type antigen-specific CD4$^+$ T helper and CD8$^+$ cytotoxic T cells. These Th1-type T cells were also confirmed by delayed-type hypersensitivity skin reaction (DTH) tests. Additional experiments showed that in vivo DermaVir immunization leads to the induction of antigen-specific memory/precursor T cells (Calarota et al. 2007; Cristillo et al. 2007; Lisziewicz et al. 2005a). Recent studies have demonstrated that generation of highly protective immunity against smallpox required skin scarification in combination with the live virus (Liu et al. 2010). For DermaVir we used three technologies that resulted in the modern version of the smallpox vaccination approach by employing a pDNA nanomedicine expressing complex VLP+ instead of the live VACV and using DermaPrep administration instead of skin scarification.

To study the safety of DermaVir vaccination, repeated immunization studies were performed in swine and rabbits. These preclinical studies demonstrated that the major side effect of DermaVir vaccination was erythema caused primarily by the skin preparation procedure. The erythema was transient and provided a mild inflammation ("danger signal") which is a desired side effect resulting in the activation of the LCs to seek and capture DermaVir nanoparticles applied under the patch.

6 Rational Design of Formulated DNA Vaccines: The DermaVir Approach

To assess the immunological efficacy of DermaVir immunizations in human subjects, we have developed an immunodiagnostic biomarker to quantify human precursor/memory cells with high proliferation capacity, PHPC (Calarota et al. 2008). We have demonstrated in two independent HIV-infected cohorts that high PHPC counts, but not ELISpot counts, correlated with low viral load (Calarota et al. 2008; Buchbinder et al. 2008). A similar correlation was found to be associated with spontaneous clearance of hepatitis C virus and protection against malaria (Keating et al. 2005; Schnuriger et al. 2009). Consequently, the PHPC count might be one of the relevant biomarkers for therapeutic vaccine candidates being developed for HIV-infected individuals to protect them against progression to AIDS.

Proof of concept efficacy studies in chronically SIV251-infected macaques, some of them with AIDS, suggested that repeated DermaVir immunizations, alone or in combination with antiretroviral drugs, result in viral load reduction and survival benefit (Lisziewicz et al. 2005b). DermaVir administered in combination with ART boosted SIV-specific T cells that possessed significant antiretroviral activity in both chronically-infected and late stage macaques (Fig. 6.5). These primate experiments provided the rationale to investigate repeated DermaVir immunizations in combination with ART in HIV-infected human subjects.

As DermaVir associated clinical benefits were first seen in primates receiving ART, the first two human studies were designed for the treatment of HIV-infected subjects receiving stable, fully suppressive ART. The Phase I clinical study conducted in Hungary investigated the safety and immunogenicity of a single dose (0.1, 0.4 or 0.8 mg pDNA) DermaVir in nine HIV+ subjects. DermaVir was found to be safe and well tolerated at all doses. DermaVir vaccination did not affect HIV RNA (all subjects remained <50 copies/mL) and $CD4^+$ counts. However, this therapeutic vaccination broadened and significantly increased the HIV-specific memory/precursor T cell pool, measured as the PHPC count, in a dose-dependent manner. The durability of vaccine-induced T cell responses was demonstrated after 1 year following a single vaccination in all treated individuals, albeit in significantly lower quantities (Lisziewicz et al. 2008). These findings suggest that DermaVir boosted HIV-specific T cells similarly to that seen in primates. A Phase I/II clinical trial conducted by the AIDS Clinical Trials Group (ACTG) in several USA clinical centers has used multiple administrations of escalating DermaVir doses (0.2 or 0.4 mg pDNA three times or 0.4 mg pDNA six times) or placebo on 26 HIV-infected adults receiving fully suppressive ART. The primary endpoint was any possibly or definitely vaccine-related grade ≥ 3 adverse event (AE) appearing up to 28 days after the final study vaccination. No primary safety endpoints or AE-related study treatment changes/discontinuations have occurred. AE incidence was similar across groups (Rodriguez et al. 2010). Immunogenicity data of this study has not yet been released. This trial further confirmed the safety of DermaVir vaccinations in combination with ART.

Repeated DermaVir immunizations in chronically SIV251-infected macaques in the absence of ART transiently suppressed virus replication leading to improvement of median survival time from 18 to 38 weeks compared to no treatment (Lisziewicz et al. 2005b). These primate experiments provided the rationale to investigate repeated DermaVir immunizations prior to initiation of ART in HIV-infected individuals

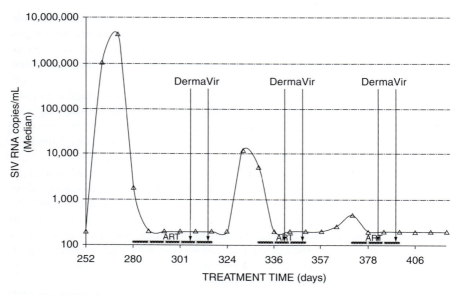

Fig. 6.5 DermaVir immunizations administered in combination with ART decreased SIV RNA rebound in late stage SIV$_{251}$-infected macaque (Lisziewicz et al. 2005b). During the first therapy interruption following DermaVir treatment, the median SIV RNA rebound dropped from 4,292,260 to 12,000 copies/mL. During the next interruption it further decreased from 12,000 to 460 copies/mL. Finally, during the last treatment interruption the median viral load remained under the limit of detection (<200 copies/mL). The animals survived longer (47, 40 and 31 months post infection) than expected as such animals typically die within 14 months after infection. Intermittent ART+DermaVir-boosted SIV-specific CD8$^+$ T cells

(NCT00711230; NCT00270205; NCT00918840). As DermaVir immunizations in combination with ART did not show any product- or administration-related AE higher than grade 2, we developed a Phase II protocol to evaluate the safety and to test the immunogenicity and antiviral efficacy of repeated DermaVir immunizations. Thirty-six HIV-infected adults (CD4>400/mm^3 and HIV RNA 5,000–150,000 copies/mL) were randomized to receive one of three DermaVir doses (0.2, 0.4 or 0.8 mg pDNA) or placebo at weeks 0, 6, 12, and 18. The primary endpoint of the trial was safety at week 24 and secondary endpoints were HIV RNA and immunogenicity (van lunzen et al. 2010). No subject stopped vaccinations due to an AE and only one subject initiated ART. Only one Grade 2 AE occurred in the 0.2 mg DermaVir group judged to be possibly related to treatment. Based on secondary analyses the 0.4 mg DermaVir dose was superior to the others. In this group, the HIV-specific memory/precursor T cells measured by PHPC increased from 5,055 to 9,978 cells/million PBMC (P=0.07) and the median log10 HIV-RNA decreased from 4.5 to 4.0, significantly different from the placebo (P=0.045). Viral load suppression by DermaVir vaccinations occurs slowly, as predicted by its mechanism of action, similarly to cancer vaccines (Kantoff et al. 2010). Consistent with the primate results, DermaVir immunizations alone did not suppress viral load to an undetectable level and did not increase CD4$^+$ T cell counts.

6 Rational Design of Formulated DNA Vaccines: The DermaVir Approach 139

These results suggested that repeated DermaVir immunization boosted HIV-specific precursor/memory T cells and the improved immunity contributed to the preservation of the health of HIV-infected individuals. Larger and longer studies are required to demonstrate that boosting of HIV-specific memory/precursor T cells slows disease progression in HIV-infected individuals.

Future of Formulated pDNA Vaccines

Recently (between 2005 and 2007) four pDNA vaccines have been approved for veterinary use. Preventive vaccines for horses against West Nile Virus, for salmon against infectious hematopoietic necrosis virus, for swine targeting growth hormone releasing hormone (GHRH), and a therapeutic vaccine for dogs against canine melanoma (Davis et al. 2001; Garver et al. 2005; Thacker et al. 2006). The canine melanoma vaccine is the first licensed therapeutic vaccine for cancer and the first product to be delivered through electroporation (Bergman et al. 2006). The successful approval of pDNA vaccines for both preventive and therapeutic use in animals suggests that similar approaches may lead to the future success of DNA vaccines in human subjects.

In April 2010 Provenge®, the first ex vivo DC-based therapeutic vaccine was approved by the US Food and Drug Administration for the treatment of metastatic castration resistant prostate cancer. Provenge® uses the patient's own immune cells to create a therapeutic vaccine following exposure to antigen and GM-CSF (Kantoff et al. 2010). This is the first therapeutic vaccine to demonstrate a significant efficacy (40% survival benefit) sufficient to obtain regulatory approval. Similar treatments are being developed to treat other cancers (breast, colon, ovarian) and viral infections.

DermaVir and Provenge® are both DC targeting therapeutic vaccines designed to boost antigen-specific Th1-type cellular immune responses in diseased hosts. Provenge® validated the long-awaited efficacy of therapeutic vaccines and provides an entirely new treatment paradigm for patients suffering from chronic neoplastic diseases. Safety and preliminary efficacy results obtained with DermaVir offer a hope for a new treatment paradigm to HIV+ individuals. DermaVir is a modern formulated pDNA vaccine version of Jenner's successful smallpox vaccine technology that used a live virus in combination with skin scarification (Liu et al. 2010). Other technological advances for formulated DNA vaccines are also expanding rapidly providing improved expression, different formulations, adjuvants and delivery technologies suitable for converting research data into viable vaccine products.

Therapeutic vaccines offer a promising solution, like the "functional cure," to the HIV epidemic sooner than do prophylactic vaccines. Initiation of therapy early in the course of HIV infection preserves immune functions and improves long-term outcomes (Kitahata et al. 2009). DermaVir is suitable for early treatment because of its safety and administration features. Although a repeated administration schedule will be necessary as the half-life of precursor/memory T cells are between 28 and 100 days depending on the plasma viral load (Ladell et al. 2008; Lisziewicz et al. 2005b), DermaVir immunizations do not require daily adherence. Therapeutic vaccinations like DermaVir could provide an effective and accessible treatment option since the present infrastructure built for treatment and prophylactic vaccinations could well serve all HIV+ individuals worldwide.

Acknowledgments This work was supported by the Research Institute for Genetic and Human Therapy (RIGHT), the European Union FP6 Marie Curie Excellence Chair Programme, and the Hungarian National Office for Research and Technology (NKTH) (HIKC05 and DVCLIN01). We are grateful for DAIDS, NIAID, NIH for several preclinical and clinical studies. We thank for the Hungarian, German, Italian, Swedish and US clinical study teams, DermaVir treated patients, L. Molnár, Z. Lisziewicz for the IT support, E.Tőke, E. Somogyi, M. Stevens and J. Chafouleas for the critical review of the manuscript.

References

Abdulhaqq SA, Weiner DB (2008) DNA vaccines: developing new strategies to enhance immune responses. Immunol Res 42(1–3):219–232

Ada G (2005) Overview of vaccines and vaccination. Mol Biotechnol 29(3):255–272

Anderson RJ, Schneider J (2007) Plasmid DNA and viral vector-based vaccines for the treatment of cancer. Vaccine 25(Suppl 2):B24–B34

Babiuk LA, Pontarollo R, Babiuk S, Loehr B, van Drunen Littel-van den Hurk S (2003) Induction of immune responses by DNA vaccines in large animals. Vaccine 21(7–8):649–658

Bauer J, Bahmer FA, Worl J, Neuhuber W, Schuler G, Fartasch M (2001) A strikingly constant ratio exists between Langerhans cells and other epidermal cells in human skin. A stereologic study using the optical disector method and the confocal laser scanning microscope. J Invest Dermatol 116(2):313–318

Bergman PJ, Camps-Palau MA, McKnight JA, Leibman NF, Craft DM, Leung C, Liao J, Riviere I, Sadelain M, Hohenhaus AE, Gregor P, Houghton AN, Perales MA, Wolchok JD (2006) Development of a xenogeneic DNA vaccine program for canine malignant melanoma at the animal medical center. Vaccine 24(21):4582–4585

Boussif O, Lezoualc'h F, Zanta MA, Mergny MD, Scherman D, Demeneix B, Behr JP (1995) A versatile vector for gene and oligonucleotide transfer into cells in culture and in vivo: polyethylenimine. Proc Natl Acad Sci USA 92(16):7297–7301

Buchbinder SP, Mehrotra DV, Duerr A, Fitzgerald DW, Mogg R, Li D, Gilbert PB, Lama JR, Marmor M, Del Rio C, McElrath MJ, Casimiro DR, Gottesdiener KM, Chodakewitz JA, Corey L, Robertson MN (2008) Efficacy assessment of a cell-mediated immunity HIV-1 vaccine (the step study): a double-blind, randomised, placebo-controlled, test-of-concept trial. Lancet 372(9653):1881–1893

Calarota SA, Weiner DB, Lori F, Lisziewicz J (2007) Induction of HIV-specific memory T-cell responses by topical DermaVir vaccine. Vaccine 25(16):3070–3074

Calarota SA, Foli A, Maserati R, Baldanti F, Paolucci S, Young MA, Tsoukas CM, Lisziewicz J, Lori F (2008) HIV-1-specific T cell precursors with high proliferative capacity correlate with low viremia and high CD4 counts in untreated individuals. J Immunol 180(9):5907–5915

Choosakoonkriang S, Lobo BA, Koe GS, Koe JG, Middaugh CR (2003) Biophysical characterization of PEI/DNA complexes. J Pharm Sci 92(8):1710–1722

Cristillo AD, Lisziewicz J, He L, Lori F, Galmin L, Trocio JN, Unangst T, Whitman L, Hudacik L, Bakare N, Whitney S, Restrepo S, Suschak J, Ferrari MG, Chung HK, Kalyanaraman VS, Markham P, Pal R (2007) HIV-1 prophylactic vaccine comprised of topical DermaVir prime and protein boost elicits cellular immune responses and controls pathogenic R5 SHIV162P3. Virology 366(1):197–211

Davis BS, Chang GJ, Cropp B, Roehrig JT, Martin DA, Mitchell CJ, Bowen R, Bunning ML (2001) West Nile virus recombinant DNA vaccine protects mouse and horse from virus

6 Rational Design of Formulated DNA Vaccines: The DermaVir Approach

challenge and expresses in vitro a noninfectious recombinant antigen that can be used in enzyme-linked immunosorbent assays. J Virol 75(9):4040–4047

Donnelly JJ, Ulmer JB, Shiver JW, Liu MA (1997) DNA vaccines. Annu Rev Immunol 15:617–648

Douek DC, Kwong PD, Nabel GJ (2006) The rational design of an AIDS vaccine. Cell 124(4): 677–681

Ellenberger D, Wyatt L, Li B, Buge S, Lanier N, Rodriguez IV, Sariol CA, Martinez M, Monsour M, Vogt J, Smith J, Otten R, Montefiori D, Kraiselburd E, Moss B, Robinson H, McNicholl J, Butera S (2005) Comparative immunogenicity in rhesus monkeys of multi-protein HIV-1 (CRF02_AG) DNA/MVA vaccines expressing mature and immature VLPs. Virology 340(1):21–32

Fioretti D, Iurescia S, Fazio VM, Rinaldi M (2010) DNA vaccines: developing new strategies against cancer. J Biomed Biotechnol 2010:174378

Fischer W, Perkins S, Theiler J, Bhattacharya T, Yusim K, Funkhouser R, Kuiken C, Haynes B, Letvin NL, Walker BD, Hahn BH, Korber BT (2007) Polyvalent vaccines for optimal coverage of potential T-cell epitopes in global HIV-1 variants. Nat Med 13(1):100–106

Garland SM, Hernandez-Avila M, Wheeler CM, Perez G, Harper DM, Leodolter S, Tang GW, Ferris DG, Steben M, Bryan J, Taddeo FJ, Railkar R, Esser MT, Sings HL, Nelson M, Boslego J, Sattler C, Barr E, Koutsky LA (2007) Quadrivalent vaccine against human papillomavirus to prevent anogenital diseases. N Engl J Med 356(19):1928–1943

Garver KA, LaPatra SE, Kurath G (2005) Efficacy of an infectious hematopoietic necrosis (IHN) virus DNA vaccine in Chinook Oncorhynchus tshawytscha and sockeye O. nerka salmon. Dis Aquat Organ 64(1):13–22

Kantoff PW, Higano CS, Shore ND, Berger ER, Small EJ, Penson DF, Redfern CH, Ferrari AC, Dreicer R, Sims RB, Xu Y, Frohlich MW, Schellhammer PF (2010) Sipuleucel-T immunotherapy for castration-resistant prostate cancer. N Engl J Med 363(5):411–422

Keating SM, Bejon P, Berthoud T, Vuola JM, Todryk S, Webster DP, Dunachie SJ, Moorthy VS, McConkey SJ, Gilbert SC, Hill AV (2005) Durable human memory T cells quantifiable by cultured enzyme-linked immunospot assays are induced by heterologous prime boost immunization and correlate with protection against malaria. J Immunol 175(9):5675–5680

Kitahata MM, Gange SJ, Abraham AG, Merriman B, Saag MS, Justice AC, Hogg RS, Deeks SG, Eron JJ, Brooks JT, Rourke SB, Gill MJ, Bosch RJ, Martin JN, Klein MB, Jacobson LP, Rodriguez B, Sterling TR, Kirk GD, Napravnik S, Rachlis AR, Calzavara LM, Horberg MA, Silverberg MJ, Gebo KA, Goedert JJ, Benson CA, Collier AC, Van Rompaey SE, Crane HM, McKaig RG, Lau B, Freeman AM, Moore RD (2009) Effect of early versus deferred antiretroviral therapy for HIV on survival. N Engl J Med 360(18):1815–1826

Ladell K, Hellerstein MK, Cesar D, Busch R, Boban D, McCune JM (2008) Central memory CD8+ T cells appear to have a shorter lifespan and reduced abundance as a function of HIV disease progression. J Immunol 180(12):7907–7918

Le Gall S, Erdtmann L, Benichou S, Berlioz-Torrent C, Liu L, Benarous R, Heard JM, Schwartz O (1998) Nef interacts with the mu subunit of clathrin adaptor complexes and reveals a cryptic sorting signal in MHC I molecules. Immunity 8(4):483–495

Lisziewicz J, Rosenberg E, Lieberman J, Jessen H, Lopalco L, Siliciano R, Walker B, Lori F (1999) Control of HIV despite the discontinuation of antiretroviral therapy. N Engl J Med 340(21):1683–1684

Lisziewicz J, Gabrilovich DI, Varga G, Xu J, Greenberg PD, Arya SK, Bosch M, Behr JP, Lori F (2001) Induction of potent human immunodeficiency virus type 1-specific T-cell-restricted immunity by genetically modified dendritic cells. J Virol 75(16):7621–7628

Lisziewicz J, Trocio J, Whitman L, Varga G, Xu J, Bakare N, Erbacher P, Fox C, Woodward R, Markham P, Arya S, Behr JP, Lori F (2005a) DermaVir: a novel topical vaccine for HIV/AIDS. J Invest Dermatol 124(1):160–169

Lisziewicz J, Trocio J, Xu J, Whitman L, Ryder A, Bakare N, Lewis MG, Wagner W, Pistorio A, Arya S, Lori F (2005b) Control of viral rebound through therapeutic immunization with DermaVir. AIDS 19(1):35–43

Lisziewicz J, Calarota S, Banhegyi D, LIsziewicz Z, Ujhelyi E, Lori F (2008) Single DermaVir patch treatment of HIV+ individuals induces long-lasting, high-magnitude, and broad HIV-specific T cell responses. Paper presented at the 15th conference on retroviruses and opportunistic infections, Boston, MA, 3–6 Feb 2008

Liu L, Zhong Q, Tian T, Dubin K, Athale SK, Kupper TS (2010) Epidermal injury and infection during poxvirus immunization is crucial for the generation of highly protective T cell-mediated immunity. Nat Med 16(2):224–227

Lori F, Lewis MG, Xu J, Varga G, Zinn DE Jr, Crabbs C, Wagner W, Greenhouse J, Silvera P, Yalley-Ogunro J, Tinelli C, Lisziewicz J (2000) Control of SIV rebound through structured treatment interruptions during early infection. Science 290(5496):1591–1593

Matzinger P (2002) The danger model: a renewed sense of self. Science 296(5566):301–305

Mouquet H, Scheid JF, Zoller MJ, Krogsgaard M, Ott RG, Shukair S, Artyomov MN, Pietzsch J, Connors M, Pereyra F, Walker BD, Ho DD, Wilson PC, Seaman MS, Eisen HN, Chakraborty AK, Hope TJ, Ravetch JV, Wardemann H, Nussenzweig MC (2010) Polyreactivity increases the apparent affinity of anti-HIV antibodies by heteroligation. Nature 467(7315):591–595

NCT00270205 Safety and tolerability of and immune response to LC002, an experimental therapeutic vaccine, in adults receiving anti-HIV treatment. http://clinicaltrials.gov/ct2/show/NCT00270205. Accessed July 2011

NCT00711230 DermaVir patch (LC002) in HIV-1 infected treatment-naïve patients. http://clinicaltrials.gov/ct2/show/NCT00711230. Accessed July 2011

NCT00918840 antiretroviral-sparing concept: investigate the effect of therapeutic immunization with DermaVir patch. http://clinicaltrials.gov/ct2/show/NCT00918840. Accessed July 2011

Nicolas JF, Guy B (2008) Intradermal, epidermal and transcutaneous vaccination: from immunology to clinical practice. Expert Rev Vaccines 7(8):1201–1214

Ohana P, Gofrit O, Ayesh S, Al-Sharef W, Mizrahi A, Birman T, Schneider T, Matouk I, de Groot N, Tavdy E, Sidi A, Hochberg A (2004) Regulatory sequences of the H19 gene in DNA based therapy of bladder cancer. Gene Ther Mol Biol 8:181–192

Paavonen J, Naud P, Salmeron J, Wheeler CM, Chow SN, Apter D, Kitchener H, Castellsague X, Teixeira JC, Skinner SR, Hedrick J, Jaisamrarn U, Limson G, Garland S, Szarewski A, Romanowski B, Aoki FY, Schwarz TF, Poppe WA, Bosch FX, Jenkins D, Hardt K, Zahaf T, Descamps D, Struyf F, Lehtinen M, Dubin G, Greenacre M (2009) Efficacy of human papillomavirus (HPV)-16/18 AS04-adjuvanted vaccine against cervical infection and precancer caused by oncogenic HPV types (PATRICIA): final analysis of a double-blind, randomised study in young women. Lancet 374(9686):301–314

Peachman KK, Rao M, Alving CR (2003) Immunization with DNA through the skin. Methods 31(3):232–242

Piccinini G, Foli A, Comolli G, Lisziewicz J, Lori F (2002) Complementary antiviral efficacy of hydroxyurea and protease inhibitors in human immunodeficiency virus-infected dendritic cells and lymphocytes. J Virol 76(5):2274–2278

Porgador A, Irvine KR, Iwasaki A, Barber BH, Restifo NP, Germain RN (1998) Predominant role for directly transfected dendritic cells in antigen presentation to CD8+ T cells after gene gun immunization. J Exp Med 188(6):1075–1082

Powles T, Robinson D, Stebbing J, Shamash J, Nelson M, Gazzard B, Mandelia S, Moller H, Bower M (2009) Highly active antiretroviral therapy and the incidence of non-AIDS-defining cancers in people with HIV infection. J Clin Oncol 27(6):884–890

Quan FS, Steinhauer D, Huang C, Ross TM, Compans RW, Kang SM (2008) A bivalent influenza VLP vaccine confers complete inhibition of virus replication in lungs. Vaccine 26(26):3352–3361

Rappuoli R (2000) Reverse vaccinology. Curr Opin Microbiol 3(5):445–450

Reddy ST, Swartz MA, Hubbell JA (2006) Targeting dendritic cells with biomaterials: developing the next generation of vaccines. Trends Immunol 27(12):573–579

Rodriguez B, Asmuth D, Matining R, Spritzler J, Li X, Jacobson J, Read S, Lisziewicz J, Lori F, Pollard R, Team AS (2010) Repeated-dose transdermal administration of DermaVir, a candidate plasmid DNA-based therapeutic HIV vaccine, is safe and well-tolerated: a 61-week analysis of ACTG study 5176. Paper presented at the XVIII international AIDS conference, Vienna, Austria

Sandstrom E, Nilsson C, Hejdeman B, Brave A, Bratt G, Robb M, Cox J, Vancott T, Marovich M, Stout R, Aboud S, Bakari M, Pallangyo K, Ljungberg K, Moss B, Earl P, Michael N, Birx D, Mhalu F, Wahren B, Biberfeld G (2008) Broad immunogenicity of a multigene, multiclade HIV-1 DNA vaccine boosted with heterologous HIV-1 recombinant modified vaccinia virus Ankara. J Infect Dis 198(10):1482–1490

Schnuriger A, Dominguez S, Guiguet M, Harfouch S, Samri A, Ouazene Z, Slama L, Simon A, Valantin MA, Thibault V, Autran B (2009) Acute hepatitis C in HIV-infected patients: rare spontaneous clearance correlates with weak memory CD4 T-cell responses to hepatitis C virus. AIDS 23(16):2079–2089

Somogyi E, Xu J, Gudics A, Tóth J, Kovács A, Lori F, Lisziewicz J (2011) A plasmid DNA immunogen expressing fifteen protein antigens and complex virus-like particles (VLP+) mimicking naturally occurring HIV. Vaccine 29(4):744-53 doi:10.1016/j.vaccine.2010.11.019

Steinman RM (1991) The dendritic cell system and its role in immunogenicity. Annu Rev Immunol 9:271–296

Stevenson FK, Ottensmeier CH, Rice J (2010) DNA vaccines against cancer come of age. Curr Opin Immunol 22(2):264–270

Tang DC, DeVit M, Johnston SA (1992) Genetic immunization is a simple method for eliciting an immune response. Nature 356(6365):152–154

Thacker EL, Holtkamp DJ, Khan AS, Brown PA, Draghia-Akli R (2006) Plasmid-mediated growth hormone-releasing hormone efficacy in reducing disease associated with *Mycoplasma hyopneumoniae* and porcine reproductive and respiratory syndrome virus infection. J Anim Sci 84(3):733–742

Toke ER, Lorincz O, Somogyi E, Lisziewicz J (2010) Rational development of a stable liquid formulation for nanomedicine products. Int J Pharm 392(1–2):261–267

Tomalia DA (2009) In quest of a systematic framework for unifying and defining nanoscience. J Nanopart Res 11:1251–1310

van Lunzen J, Pollard R, Stellbrink HJ, Plettenberg A, Natz E, Lisziewicz Z, Freese R, Molnar L, Calarota SA, Lori F, Lisziewicz J (2010) DermaVir for initial treatment of HIV-infected subjects demonstrates preliminary safety, immunogenicity and HIV-RNA reduction versus placebo immunization. Paper presented at the XVIII international AIDS conference, Vienna, Austria

von Harpe A, Petersen H, Li Y, Kissel T (2000) Characterization of commercially available and synthesized polyethylenimines for gene delivery. J Control Release 69(2):309–322

Wolff JA, Malone RW, Williams P, Chong W, Acsadi G, Jani A, Felgner PL (1990) Direct gene transfer into mouse muscle in vivo. Science 247(4949 Pt 1):1465–1468

Yang OO, Nguyen PT, Kalams SA, Dorfman T, Gottlinger HG, Stewart S, Chen IS, Threlkeld S, Walker BD (2002) Nef-mediated resistance of human immunodeficiency virus type 1 to antiviral cytotoxic T lymphocytes. J Virol 76(4):1626–1631

Zinkernagel RM (2000) Localization dose and time of antigens determine immune reactivity. Semin Immunol 12(3):163–171; discussion 257–344

Improvement of DNA Vaccines by Electroporation

7

Arielle A. Ginsberg, Xuefei Shen, Natalie A. Hutnick, and David B. Weiner

DNA vaccines have been on the scientific horizon since 1992, yet the past decade of clinical study has been precarious, with most trials exhibiting excellent safety, yet poor immune responses in humans. Despite the initial disappointments of immunogenicity observed in early clinical trials, the advantageous properties of plasmid DNA as a vaccine strategy over existing technologies continued to drive the field forward. Recently, non- human primate preclinical models as well as data generated in a few clinical trials have suggested that there are significant improvements in immunogenicity by the renewed enhanced DNA platform. This is due to a host of new technological improvements that together have improved vaccine antigen expression, delivery, and formulation resulting in improved immune potency. Improvements in plasmid delivery by modalities including the gene gun, biojector and most recently electroporation (EP) in particular, in combination with other technological developments such as species-specific codon optimization, improved RNA structural design, incorporation of novel leader sequences, novel formulations and adjuvant strategies have had a significant effect on immune outcome in relevant primate models and now humans. This new generation of DNA vaccines will likely have a more prominent role in vaccine clinical research.

Introduction

In vivo gene delivery dates back to the discovery of the functions of DNA (Yin et al. 2008). Early experiments documented the ability of cells within a live animal to take up recombinant DNA and express the gene of interest (Neumann et al. 1982;

D.B. Weiner (✉)
Department of Pathology and Laboratory Medicine,
University of Pennsylvania,
Philadelphia, PA, USA
e-mail: dbweiner@mail.med.upenn.edu

J. Thalhamer et al. (eds.), *Gene Vaccines*,
DOI 10.1007/978-3-7091-0439-2_7, © Springer-Verlag/Wien, 2012

145

Fig. 7.1 Vectors used in gene therapy clinical trials. Clinical trials of plasmid DNA account for approximately 18% of all clinical trials utilizing gene therapy vector delivery technologies. These data support the overall preclinical success, phase I safety, and continued improvement of the platform. Previous to 1998, DNA plasmid vectors constituted an average of only 4% of all gene-therapy platform trials. (This data is adapted from *Gene Therapy Trials Worldwide* provided by the *Journal of Gene Medicine* and represents clinical trials from phase I through phase III and is current as of March, 2011.)

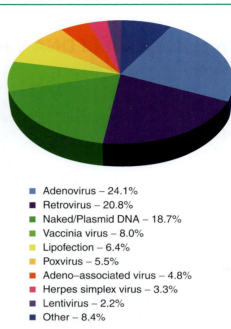

- Adenovirus – 24.1%
- Retrovirus – 20.8%
- Naked/Plasmid DNA – 18.7%
- Vaccinia virus – 8.0%
- Lipofection – 6.4%
- Poxvirus – 5.5%
- Adeno–associated virus – 4.8%
- Herpes simplex virus – 3.3%
- Lentivirus – 2.2%
- Other – 8.4%

Dubensky and Campbell 1984; Benvenisty and Reshef 1986; Okino and Mohri 1987; Wolff et al. 1990). By the fall of 1992, three independent reports presented at the annual Cold Spring Harbor (CSH) vaccine meeting described the use of plasmid encoded DNA vectors to induce humoral and cellular immune responses against pathogen and tumor antigens in pre-clinical animal models (Thomas 2001; Ferraro et al. 2011).

The years following this CSH meeting witnessed a surge in the preclinical development of the DNA platform. Much data, generated in small animal models, demonstrated that successful in vivo antigen expression after vaccination with plasmid DNA, drove humoral and cellular immunity, and conferred protection (Fynan et al. 1993; Tang and DeVit 1992; Ulmer et al. 1993; Wang et al. 1993). The surge of resulting publications opened the door for DNA vaccines to enter the clinic in the mid-1990s (Belshe et al. 1993; Ciccarelli et al. 1998). A number of clinical trials have since taken place utilizing plasmid DNA for the treatment and prevention of diseases such as HIV, malaria, influenza, hepatitis B, hepatitis C, and cancer (Fig. 7.1). The conclusion from early trials was that DNA is both very well tolerated and immunogenic in humans. The low level immunity generated by the first generation of DNA vaccines was below that induced by competing vaccine platforms, including several recombinant vector systems. The limited DNA driven responses observed in these initial clinical studies relegated the DNA platform to a mainly supportive role in the field of vaccine development over the past decade, utilizing DNA as a part of the priming component in prime boost vaccination strategies. DNA as a stand-alone technology was viewed as too weak to drive effective and consistent protective levels of immune responses against a majority of important human pathogens.

Accordingly there has been an extensive focus on improving the immune potency of DNA over the last decade. The increase in the immunogenicity of DNA vaccination observed in both the clinical and pre-clinical arenas has contributed greatly to the growth of the field and can be attributed to the several innovative strategies implemented in the past 20 years, including codon and plasmid optimization, the use of molecular adjuvants, and the development of novel delivery systems. The continual development of improved delivery platform technologies combined with increasing knowledge of cellular and humoral immune mechanisms are positive indicators of a future for DNA vaccines. An important aspect of new delivery includes the impressive in vivo delivery of plasmid vaccines by electroporation.

Basic Principles of Electroporation

The use of electroporation, defined here as the application of controlled electrical fields to facilitate permeabilization of the cellular membrane, began in the 1960s (Coster 1965). These early experiments were designed to explore the electrically induced breakdown of the cell membrane. In 1982, Neumann et al. published findings first demonstrating the ability of electroporation to increase transfection efficiency of DNA into eukaryotic cells (Neumann and Kakorin 1999; Neumann et al. 1982). They hypothesized that electroporation made the cellular membrane "transiently more permeable by the action of short electric impulses above a certain field strength, without damaging the membrane structure." Since that time, the mechanism by which electroporation works has been extensively explored and optimized. During the early experiments of the 1960s, it was established that extracellular molecules gain entry into cells after being treated with an electrical pulse. These pulses induce the formation of "pores" in the cellular membrane through which the injected plasmid, diffusing across the concentration gradient, may pass into a cell. Over a very short period of time, these "pores" naturally close, leaving the plasmid inside where transgene encoded antigens become integrated into host transcription process, where they can be expressed, processed by intracellular machinery, and presented within the context of MHC class I or II on the cell surface. In addition, these novel antigens can be shed from the transfected cell and be picked up by the antigen receptor on B cells thus allowing for the induction of humoral immunity. At higher voltages there is low level of transient damage done to the cell as a result of electroporation, which may send a "danger signal" stimulating the recruitment of increased numbers of professional antigen presenting cells along with modest CD4+ T-cells to the site of vaccination (Chiarella et al. 2008). However, newer lower voltage delivery can also stimulate strong immune responses without clear evidence of cellular damage. Electroporation also significantly increases the number of locally transfected mononuclear cells (MNCs), which can include immature DC, which can then mature into efficient antigen presenting cells (APC). Studies have also shown that MHC II positive cells accumulate around transfected MNC suggesting transfer of antigen from the transfected MNCs to additional antigen presenting cells, further contributing to the immune response (Grønevik et al. 2003). Furthermore, EP can deliver plasmid in sufficient amounts with a large degree of flexibility in the size of the desired gene insert. This is in contrast to methods such as ballistic delivery, where only µg amounts of DNA can be delivered and viral vectors, where gene size constraints, reactogenicity, as well as cost and complexity issues limit vector delivery (Chiarella et al. 2008; Dubensky and Campbell 1984; Fu et al. 1997; Raz et al. 1993).

The ability of EP to induce cellular transfection can be described in terms of basic physics, a model that clarifies the mechanism of enhanced antigen uptake. Cellular membranes that are subjected to electrical pulses can be thought of as capacitors subjected to an applied voltage. A capacitor is an electrical component consisting of a pair of conductors, each holding opposite electrical charges that are separated by an insulator, known as a dielectric, which is a nonconductive substance. The application of voltage, or a potential difference, across the conductors induces the formation of a static electrical field in the dielectric that stores energy and can produce a mechanical force between the two conductors. In the case of in vivo electroporation, the bipolar lipid membrane mimics the behavior of a capacitor with the neutrally charged lipid acting as the dielectric placed between the cellular cytoplasm and extracellular fluid, both of which are conductive, ionic fluids. When an electrical field is applied to the membrane, these membrane capacitors build up a transmembrane potential until the ability of the dielectric, or lipid, to hold charge is exceeded, resulting in mechanical force that causes an opening in the membrane.

While this model is useful in providing a conceptual understanding of the principles of electroporation, it does not adequately incorporate many factors of the in vivo environment of electroporation. The extracellular environment is filled with water, salts, lipids and proteins that may act as conductors, resistors, or capacitors themselves. The complexity of the extracellular milieu impedes accurate modeling. Likewise, applications need to be modified depending on the site of delivery, as the extracellular environment in the muscle and dermis differ. An additional challenge in clinical application is maintaining consistent electrical parameters in patients with different body compositions, which causes differences in the resulting applied electrical forces. Thus, the potential clinical applications of these fundamental concepts also rely on empirical data for development and optimization.

Development of Electroporation for In Vivo Application

In comparison to other delivery technologies, electroporation appears to be a highly efficient gene delivery platform which relies on development strategies based on physical parameters (membrane properties and electrical parameters) that are relatively constant among species, rather than complex biological processes such as receptor mediated uptake that may vary from species to species. The ease of administration to multiple target tissues, such as muscle and skin is also a benefit for

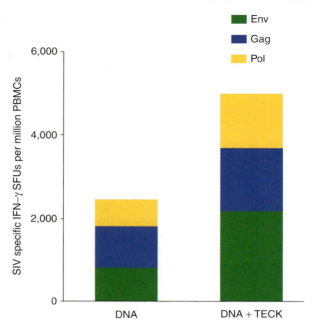

Fig. 7.2 Increased immunogenicity with EP + molecular adjuvant. This figure shows the results study in the macaque model that compares administration of plasmid DNA encoding Macaque HIV antigens gag, pol and env delivered by EP with and without the molecular adjuvant CCL28 (TECK). Although combination of EP with the administration of DNA vaccines has greatly increased the immunogenicity of these vaccines, adjuvants, as well as other technologies, continue to improve the immune response of the DNA platform

clinical applications, allowing for multiple different treatment sites and diverse plasmid delivery strategies.

Dramatic improvements in the immune responses driven by DNA vaccines co-administered with electroporation have been observed in non-human primate preclinical models. A study of HIV-1 plasmids demonstrated that when administered with EP, animals vaccinated with one fifth the amount of DNA (1.7 mg in comparison to 8.5 mg) showed a significant increase in their cellular immune response, as measured by IFN-γ ELISpot assay. After three vaccinations, a mean response of ~8000 IFN-γ spot forming units per million (SFU × 10^6) was observed in comparison to a mean response of ~900 IFN-γ SFU × 10^6 observed in the group of primates that received a much higher dose of plasmid without electroporation. This same study showed a similar trend for humoral immune responses, when HIV specific IgG antibody production was measured by ELISA assay. All macaques receiving the DNA vaccine with EP seroconverted by week 10, 2 weeks after the final pDNA immunization whereas no detectable antibodies were present in macaques that did not receive EP (Luckay et al. 2007; Hirao et al. 2008). The use of adjuvant strategies in combination with EP has been shown to further improve vaccine immunity. Other studies in NHPs have shown that after a single injection with pDNA alone, cellular immune responses can be detected. Results shown in Fig. 7.2 demonstrate that while co-administration of pDNA and electroporation gives a better response than pDNA alone, these responses can be significantly increased through use of a molecular adjuvant (Ginsberg et al. 2011).

Optimization of EP conditions can also significantly impact the immunogenicity of DNA vaccines. There are several factors that contribute to the process of determining optimal conditions for electroporation, including duration of electrical pulse administration, electrode shape, number, and spacing as well as the size and force of the resulting electrical field, and also (to some extent), the dose and volume of the DNA delivered (Niidome and Huang 2002).

Penetrating needle electrodes have proven the most effective and consistent means for EP application in subdermal tissues. Standard intramuscular EP utilizes a number of electrodes which penetrate into skeletal muscle. DNA can be delivered via a separate intramuscular (IM) injection, or via the devices that utilize penetrating needle arrays that serve a dual role for both DNA injection into muscle and also functioning as electrodes after injection. This results in co-localization of the injected DNA and the generated electrical field causing high efficiency of transfection. Electrical field uniformity and coverage of tissue can be improved by using multi-electrode arrays although these improvements are limited by the practicality of clinical application, such as cost of applicators and tolerance. One limitation of successful intramuscular vaccination is patient variability. The thickness of subdermal adipose tissue and patient size affects the depth of needle required for optimal intramuscular delivery. Vaccine efficacy therefore is partially dependent on proper delivery by clinicians and precludes the use of a standard "one size fits all" device. It is likely that in the future application specific platforms will provide advantages due to inherent system complexity.

Compared to intramuscular EP, intradermal EP has the potential to result in generation of a unique immune phenotype due to the presence of professional antigen presenting cells such as Langerhans cells and dermal dendritic cells in the target tissue. This is an important issue for future studies. To specifically achieve dermal delivery of vaccine vectors, investigators have recently explored a variety of devices. Novel dermal electroporation devices explored include microneedle arrays, such as the EasyVax applicator (Cytopulse), a device which utilizes multiple microneedles coated with DNA designed to penetrate the stratum corneum resulting in intradermal delivery of the plasmid. One approach has been the development of a minimally invasive EP device, which is administered at low voltage parameters. By using non-penetrating electrode needle array and lower voltage, this device is not only more tolerable, but is able to drive protective immunity without indications of tissue specific stress (Fig. 7.3) (Broderick et al. 2011). In the future, non-invasive devices may offer a safe, tolerable, and efficient method to administer DNA vaccines in a clinical, prophylactic setting. Further investigation of such minimal or non-invasive devices are worthy of additional attention.

A contactless electropermeabilization method to deliver DNA plasmids to dermal tissue in vivo was reported recently. This process has the advantage of eliminating the insertion of additional needles that serve as electrodes to facilitate the application of electric pulses in conventional electroporation processes. This eliminates the need for disposable needle arrays, thereby decreasing the cost and safety of use. Importantly, this device successfully facilitates increased expression of antigen and immune responses (Broderick et al. 2011). Importantly, this array also improved transfection efficiencies as well as increased immune responses.

7 Improvement of DNA Vaccines by Electroporation

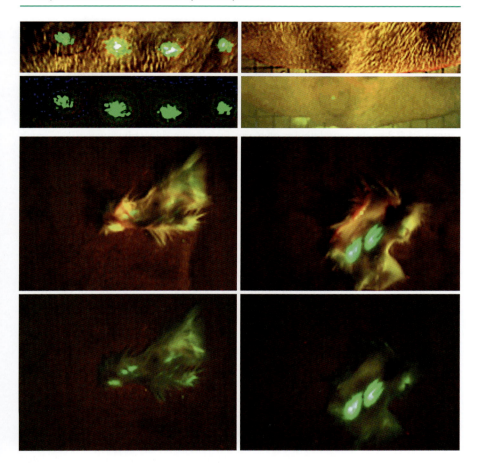

Fig. 7.3 Transfection efficiency of a novel EP device. The above panel highlights the efficacy of GFP plasmid delivery using a targeted EP device, which utilizes a four by four electrode array. This device is designed to simultaneously administer DNA based vaccines intradermally. The top panel of images shows the efficacy of the device in a guinea pig model. The images on the left show tissue samples after vaccination with plasmid encoding the GFP protein was administered with EP and the images on the right show tissue samples after vaccination with the plasmid alone. The bottom panel shows the device's transfection efficacy in the mouse model. The images on the left both show tissue samples after two successful vaccinations with the DNA-GFP construct administered with EP and the images on the right show vaccination with the construct alone. Note differences in efficiency with DNA alone in guinea pig vs. mouse. Also note large increase in transfection efficiency with the EP delivery

Other novel techniques have been developed for selected applications. These include electroporation catheters for the delivery of DNA and drugs into blood vessel walls to treat vascular diseases. Transfection of the ciliary muscle of the eye has also been successfully demonstrated using eye electrodes. In addition arrays that target different tissues simultaneously have recently been reported (Lin et al. 2011).

The continued development of specific delivery arrays and devices represents an important contribution to the DNA vaccine field.

Clinical Applications of Electroporation

There are 29 ongoing clinical trials, in all phases of development, utilizing a wide range of EP devices as a delivery platform for a range of biopharmaceuticals, such as chemotherapeutic agents, antigen specific DNA vaccines and gene-therapy strategies. These trials are summarized in Table 7.1. Following a seminal EP clinical trial in 1987 (Okino and Mohri 1987) for delivery of chemotherapeutic agents, approximately 1/3 of the current studies utilize EP in the context of improving electrochemotherapy strategies, targeting a wide range of cancers, including head and neck cancer, pancreatic cancer, melanoma, rectal cancer, and breast cancer.

In addition to the electrochemotherapy field, a major area of focus for ongoing clinical trials is the use of DNA plasmids as gene-based vaccines, immune modulation and gene therapy treatments. The testing of the same device in many different applications is an essential part of optimizing the clinical applications of electroporation in the context of plasmid delivery, as each combination approach likely will bring different strengths to the clinical table and provide a wealth of guidance for future plasmid vaccine enhancement (Lin et al. 2011).

Of the 16 ongoing antigen-specific clinical trials that are assessing the immunogenicity of DNA vaccines, eight utilize the CELLECTRA intramuscular EP device (Inovio Pharmaceuticals). This device employs a five-needle electrode array that inserts the plasmid into skeletal muscle using an injection needle built into the center of the array. To ensure maximal electric field coverage, the electrodes are fired in pairs in a rotating pattern. Phase I trials of DNA vaccines being assessed for immunogenicity following EP with the CELLECTRA device target influenza, HIV (preventive and therapeutic), and a therapeutic HPV. A phase II trial of Inovio's HPV vaccine has recently been approved and is scheduled to begin enrolling patients in mid-2011. Another recently approved trial of a preventive HIV vaccine will test the administration of a DNA prime followed by MVA vector boost with two devices, the CELLECTRA device, and a second delivery system, the Biojector, a needle-free injection system approved for the delivery of vaccines and other injected medications. The results of this clinical trial will highlight the strengths and weaknesses of all three methods of DNA delivery within the context of this prime boost vaccine model, information which can be used to further define the optimal circumstances for utilization of each device in future clinical applications.

The TriGrid delivery system (Ichor Medical Systems) is another EP device that is currently being evaluated in clinical trials. This device has a triangular pulsing pattern created by the shape of the array, consisting of two needles of same polarity and one needle of opposite polarity set in triangular pattern. A phase I/II clinical trial to test the efficacy of DNA plus EP in treatment of melanoma with a DNA plasmid, SCIB1, encodes an antibody designed to express a common melanoma antigen (tyrosinase related protein 2, TRP2) as well as two CD4 T cell epitopes.

7 Improvement of DNA Vaccines by Electroporation

Table 7.1 Clinical trials involving electroporation

Phase	Condition	Biological	Device
Antigen specific DNA vaccines (16)			
I	Avian influenza	VGX-3400X	CELLECTRA® (Inovio Pharmaceuticals), IM
I	Melanoma (skin), intraocular melanoma	Xenogeneic tyrosinase DNA Vaccine	TriGrid Delivery System (Ichor Medical Systems), IM
I	HIV infections	PENNVAX-B	CELLECTRA® (Inovio Pharmaceuticals), IM
I	Avian influenza	VGX-3400	CELLECTRA® (Inovio Pharmaceuticals), IM
I	Papillomavirus infections	VGX-3100	CELLECTRA® (Inovio Pharmaceuticals), IM
I	HIV infections	ADVAX	TriGrid Delivery System (Ichor Medical Systems), IM
I	*Plasmodium falciparum* malaria	EP-1300	Electroporation, IM
I	Human papillomavirus (HPV)	VGX-3100	CELLECTRA® (Inovio Pharmaceuticals), IM
I	HIV infections	Profectus HIV MAG pDNA vaccine; IL-12	Electroporation, IM
I	HIV infections	PENNVAX-B; IL-12 DNA plasmids	CELLECTRA® (Inovio Pharmaceuticals), IM
I	HIV infections	PENNVAX-G DNA Vaccine; MVA-CMDR Vaccine	Biojector 2000; CELLECTRA® (Inovio Pharmaceuticals), IM
II	Human papillomavirus (HPV)	VCX-3100	CELLECTRA® (Inovio Pharmaceuticals), IM
I/II	Colorectal cancer	tetwtCEA DNA (wt CEA with tetanus toxoid Th epitope); GM-CSF; Cyclophosphamide	Derma Vax (Cyto Pulse Sciences), ID
I/II	Prostate cancer	pVAXrcPSAv531 (DNA encoding rhesus PSA);	DERMA VAX™ (Cyto Pulse Sciences), ID
I/II	Hepatitis C virus infection	CHRONVAC-C®	MedPulser (Inovio Pharmaceuticals), IM
I/II	Malignant melanom	SCIB1	TriGrid Delivery System (Ichor Medical Systems), IM
II	Human papillomavirus (HPV)	VGX-3100	CELLECTRA® (Inovio Pharmaceuticals), IM
Immune modulation and gene therapy (4)			
I	Metastatic melanoma	VCL-IM01 (encoding IL-2)	MedPulser® (Inovio Pharmaceuticals), intratumor
I	Malignant melanoma	IL-12pDNA	Electroporation, intratumor
I	Melanoma	DNA coding for protein AMEP	Electrotransfer, intratumor
I	Advanced metastatic carcinoma	Autologous cancer cells transfected with a TGFβ2 antisense//GMCSF expression vector	In vitro electroporation of cancer cells

(continued)

Table 7.1 (continued)

Phase	Condition	Biological	Device
Electrochemotherapy (9)			
I	Pancreatic cancer	Bleomycin sulfate	Electroporation, pancreas
I	Melanoma (skin)	Bleomycin sulfate	Electroporation, melanoma tumors
I	Rectal cancer	Bleomycin	Intratumor endoVe endoscopic electroporation
II	Ulcerated cutaneous metastases	Bleomycin	Electrochemotherapy, intratumor
II	Breast cancer	Bleomycin	Cliniporator, intratumor
III	Head and neck cancer	Bleomycin	MedPulser® (Inovio Pharmaceuticals), IM
III	Head and neck cancer	Bleomycin	MedPulser® (Inovio Pharmaceuticals), IM
IV	Head and neck cancer	Bleomycin	MedPulser® (Inovio Pharmaceuticals), IM
IV	Cutaneous and subcutaneous cancer	Bleomycin	MedPulser® (Inovio Pharmaceuticals), IM

Information is based on ClinicalTrials.gov, which is a registry of federally and private supported clinical trials conducted both in the United States and around the world

Once expressed, the antibody will be processed by professional APCs resulting in a targeted immune response against tumorous cells expressing the TRP2 antigen. The efficacy of the TriGrid device is also being explored in three additional phase I clinical trials. They all test antigen-specific DNA vaccines, one a therapeutic melanoma vaccine and two prophylactic vaccines for prevention of HIV-1 infection and malaria. These are all exciting studies that will add greatly to our knowledge of the strengths and weaknesses of these approaches. More detailed information about this device is provided in Chap. 8 in this book.

In January 2011, a phase II clinical trial to evaluate a DNA vaccine to treat chronic myeloid leukemia and acute myeloid leukemia was approved that will be utilizing an automated vaccine delivery device, requiring only the push of a button to deliver the vaccine and electrical pulses, an ease of administration that may provide important simplification for this delivery strategy. Though the initial studies examining in vivo applications of electroporation were published in 1987, the technology continues to advance in the clinic today.

Other Technologies

In addition to optimal delivery platforms, design of the DNA plasmids themselves is an essential component for inducing maximal expression of the encoded antigen of interest, and to improve immunogenicity as well as breadth and longevity of response.

Consensus Sequences

Many targets of DNA vaccines such as viral diseases and cancers demonstrate high genomic variability, causing a challenge in the selection of genes to be utilized in DNA vaccines. A familiar example is influenza, a virus that can mutate so quickly and dramatically that a vaccine may be rendered ineffective within a single season (Fauci 2006). HIV-1 is also highly diverse with nine clades in group M strain and an ever changing number of circulating recombinant forms (CRFs). Another target of DNA vaccination, hepatitus C virus (HCV) demonstrates similar variability, with over 50 subtypes (Elmowalid et al. 2007). Constructs are therefore designed with the goal of inducing a wide breadth of antigen specific immunity with the goal of protecting against both homologous and heterologous challenge. This is achieved through the use of consensus immunogens, which encode the amino acid sequences of the regions most highly conserved across the various strains of the pathogenic target of interest (Abdulhaqq and Weiner 2008). Consensus sequences are also edited to exclude sequences of antigenic targets that have evolved to evade the effector arm of the immune system, such as glycosylation sites. These changes interfere with the naturally occurring peptide processing and presentation in order to cause interference to the relatively low avidity binding between the TCR and the peptide-MHC class I complex (Yewdell and Bennink 1999).

Mosaic Sequences

An alternative method for enhancing the immunogenicity of DNA vaccines involves generating mosaic sequences. Mosaic sequences are designed by identifying 9-mer amino acid sequences within a pathogen which are likely to be T-cell epitopes. These 9-mer sequences are then combined to create a synthetic protein with natural recombination breakpoints. This strategy was shown to effectively increase the breadth and depth of vaccine induced immune responses for a HIV-1 vaccine compared with a vaccine utilizing native viral sequences (Barouch et al. 2010). Unlike consensus vaccines, mosaic vaccines lack the secondary protein structure necessary to induce humoral immunity and rely on cellular responses only. In addition, center of tree strategies as well as ancestral antigen sequence design represent interesting approaches to improve the targeting of the host immune responses (Santra et al. 2008).

Codon Optimization

Although all organisms share the basic commonality of a genetic language as expressed through codons, the levels of transfer RNA (tDNA) present in cells of a certain species to express those codon sequences varies, resulting in negative selection against specific codons on a species to species basis (Rocha 2004). In order to enhance expression of an antigen, the antigenic sequence may be custom tailored for the target species by using codons that are present in tRNA at higher frequencies in the target species, leading to more efficient antigenic translation. The resultant increased expression may stimulate increased immunogenicity to the protein being expressed (Ko 2005; Nagata 1999). RNA optimization is another aspect of plasmid optimization taking into account many factors such as RNA tertiary structure, high CG values, splice sites, and other factors that may contribute to premature destruction of messenger RNA (mRNA) inhibiting antigenic expression. Inclusion of a highly efficient leader sequence is also an effective strategy to promote improved expression of the target antigen resulting in improved immune potency of the gene vaccine.

Molecular Adjuvants

In addition to optimization strategies that target the DNA plasmid itself, another common approach utilized to enhance the immunogenicity of DNA vaccines is the inclusion of molecular adjuvants. Unlike traditional adjuvants that enhance the immune response through innate inflammatory pathways, molecular adjuvants aim to specifically modulate vaccine induced adaptive immunity to generate a protective response. Additionally, molecular adjuvants are encoded on a separate plasmid and co-delivered with the vaccine vectors. The majority of molecular adjuvants can be divided into three main classes; cytokine, chemokine and activating receptors.

Cytokine molecular adjuvants can be generally classified by whether they are involved in Th1 or Th2 immunity. Th1 adjuvants include IL-2, IL-12, IL15 and IFN-g and are included to promote cellular immunity (Boyer et al. 2005; Kim et al. 1997; Kim et al. 2000a; Halwani et al. 2008; Valentin et al. 1998). In contrast, common Th2 adjuvants include granulocyte-macrophage cell stimulating factor (GM-CSF), IL-1, and IL-4 and are included to promote humoral immunity (Chu et al. 2006; Zhao et al. 2009; Pasquini et al. 1997; Xiang and Ertl 1995; Okada et al. 1997; Kim et al. 2000b). Pre-clinical evaluation is critical for the use of cytokine molecular adjuvants as the activation of either the Th1 or Th2 pathway can result in inhibition of the other pathway and ultimately reduced immunity (Yin et al. 2008). Interestingly, IL-15 has been shown to enhance both cellular and humoral immune responses in both mouse and non-human primate models (Perera et al. 2007; Morris et al. 2006; Li et al. 2010; Ramanathan et al. 2011; Gagnon et al. 2008).

Chemokine molecular adjuvants are designed to target responses induced by a systemic DNA vaccine to the site of infection where protective responses are required. In non-human primates, the inclusion of a CCL27 (CTACK) plasmid increased mucosal homing of antigen specific cells following an HIV-1 DNA vaccination in non-human primates (Kraynyak et al. 2010). Likewise, co-delivery of CCL27 or CCL28 (MECK) with a DNA flu vaccine protected mice from lethal influenza challenge (Kutzler et al. 2010). Though research into the use of chemokine adjuvants is limited compared to cytokine adjuvants, these studies suggest that co-delivery of chemokine adjuvants can modify cellular trafficking.

7 Improvement of DNA Vaccines by Electroporation

Both cytokine and chemokine adjuvants aim to skew the quality of the vaccine induced response. In contrast, co-stimulatory adjuvants aim to increase the immunity of cellular responses. A resting T-cell requires signaling through binding of the T-cell receptor and MHC class I complex as well as CD80 or CD86 ligands binding to CD28 in order to become activated. Transduced muscle cells are unable to express the co-stimulatory molecules making them unable to directly activate T-cells through the traditional pathway of peptide presentation in the context of MHC class I or II molecules. To address this issue, researchers are exploring the inclusion of vectors encoding co-stimulatory molecules as a way to increase the magnitude of DNA vaccine immune responses. Though both CD86 and CD80 were found to enhance cellular immunity in cows receiving a bovine tuberculosis DNA vaccine, only CD86 was shown to improve HIV-1 or influenza vaccination in mice (Agadjanyan et al. 1999; Iwasaki et al. 1997; Maue et al. 2004; Tsuji et al. 1997). Immunologic pathways are often redundant and may differ significantly between animal models, highlighting the need for extensive pre-clinical testing, and possibly the inclusion of several molecular adjuvants in order to elicit the appropriate immune response. In this regard, studies have used heat shock proteins to improve immunity to DNA vaccines. These adjuvants drive Th1 cellular immunity and improved protection in tumor model systems. The use of these adjuvants in the context of electroporation or other improved delivery strategies will be informative (Zheng et al. 2007; Long et al. 2005).

Conclusion

In 1994, the first DNA vaccine was awarded Investigation New Drug (IND) approval from the federal government. The vaccine targeted the recently emergent HIV virus as a therapeutic approach. Shortly after, the same vaccine was approved in 1995 as a prophylactic intervention strategy and then an influenza prophylactic approach was also initiated. Since then, the field has expanded considerably, with 319 DNA vaccines (preventive and therapeutic) currently in human trials that span all phases of clinical development. These studies target conditions such as cancer (61%), cardiovascular diseases (17%), infectious diseases (6%), neurological diseases (3%), and genetic disorders (1%) (Edelstein et al. 2007).

Although DNA vaccines have yet to reach their final stage of development for application in human diseases, the recent approval of several DNA vaccines and therapeutics for veterinary application demonstrates the success of the method (Table 7.2). The approval of the LifeTide®, a gene therapy treatment delivered via electroporation for breeding sows that increases offspring survival, marks a significant advancement of DNA vaccines as the target species is part of the human food chain and is therefore held to a more stringent set of standards than other veterinary pharmaceutical products. Other antigens targeted by veterinary DNA vaccines include melanoma, West Nile Virus, and Infectious haematopoietic necrosis virus. The widespread usage of these plasmids in a veterinary setting will provide a unique opportunity to expand the

Table 7.2 Currently licensed DNA vaccines

Year	Indication	Name	Company	Species	Genes delivered	Immune response
2005	West Nile Virus (WNV)	West Nile-Innovator®	Fort Dodge Animal Health, Fort Dodge, IA, USA	Horses	PreM-E	Generation of neutral-izing antibodies
2005	Infectious haematopoi-etic necrosis virus	Apex-IHN®	Novartis Animal Health, Basel, Switzerland	Salmon	Glycoprotein	Induction of innate and adaptive immune responses
2008	Increase survival for litters of breeding sows	LifeTide® SW 5	VGX Animal Health, Inc., The Woodlands, TX, USA	Pigs (food animals)	Growth hormone releasing hormone	NA
2010	Melanoma	Oncept™	Merial, Lyon, France	Dogs	Human tyrosine	Generation of antibodies

To date, three DNA vaccines have been successfully licensed for veterinary use and fourth DNA therapeutic has been approved as a way to regulate growth hormone in pigs, utilizes EP delivery. The success and efficacy of these plasmid DNA products is important and supports further clinical development of human therapies

current understanding of pDNA and use that knowledge to better inform future vaccine design.

This novel non-live approach to vaccine design is also an attractive alternative in consideration of the safety concerns associated with many other current vaccine technologies. Early clinical use of live attenuated vaccines in the Salk polio vaccine development resulted in Iatrogenic disease, causing spread of polio in areas where OPV administration coverage was low (Offit 2005). The exploration of HIV live attenuated vaccines has been largely abandoned by the research community as a result of several studies conducted using live attenuated strains of the simian immunodeficiency virus (SIV) as a model system of HIV vaccines with little success. While considerable efficacy was observed in many cases, particularly in delta-nef strains of the SIV virus where protective immunity against both homologous and heterologous viral challenges was observed for over 2 years after last immunization (Ruprecht 1999), these encouraging results were eclipsed by safety concerns as reversion back to pathogenic strains was observed over time. Attempts to cripple the replication competency of these delta-nef strains have also resulted in decreased immunogenicity. Efforts in vaccine development using whole killed viruses have also presented serious safety concerns. Errors in the production of Sabin's formalin inactivated vaccine resulted in product contamination with live virus. The use of viral vectors, a strategy utilized for targeted gene delivery, was shown to have serious complications during the Merck sponsored STEP trial where the use of an adenovirus vector to delivery HIV genes may have resulted in increased susceptibility to HIV infection in individuals with pre-existing immunity to the adenovirus vector. These situations highlight the need for the expedient development of an inexpensive, safe, and immunogenic addition to the current repertoire of vaccine development strategies. These issues as well as a host of others, including the ability to rapidly combine different antigens in a single universal formulation, the ability to customize the immunogen, and the ability to have the immunogen naturally processed in the host served to keep interest focused on improving the DNA platform through the past 20 years research.

DNA vaccines have several clear advantages over traditional approaches; however their clinical success will ultimately hinge on increasing antigen-specific immunogenicity. Plasmid co-delivery with in vivo electroporation has enhanced cellular and humoral immune responses in both pre-clinical and clinical settings. Continued engineering and development of in vivo electroporation technology has had a positive impact on the technology in several ways. By lowering the amount of DNA needed per vaccination, this likely will improve the cost of the vaccine, by improving the immune potency of the platform, immune responses can be generated with a more limited injection volume as well as immunization regime, improving the efficacy is likely to improve the ability of this platform to result in the generation of a successful product. Accordingly, the combined strategies, including and in particular focusing on electroporation provide an important new tool for vaccine research and development. Building on the early successes of the combined platforms will be an important focus for the field over the next several years.

Acknowledgements D.B.W. and the D.B.W. laboratory would like to note several commercial relationships for purposes of disclosure. These relations may include the provision of board or committee service, consultations, stock ownership, S.R.A., royalties, etc. on the part of one or both parties as a result of collaborative work with commercial entities including but not limited to Novartis, Inovio, VGXi, BMS, Medarex, Pfizer, Virxsys, Ichor, Merck, and Althea.

References

Abdulhaqq SA, Weiner DB (2008) DNA vaccines: developing new strategies to enhance immune responses. Immunol Res 42(1–3):219–232

Agadjanyan MG, Kim JJ, Trivedi N, Wilson DM, Monzavi-Karbassi B, Morrison LD, Nottingham LK, Dentchev T, Tsai A, Dang K, Chalian AA, Maldonado MA, Williams WV, Weiner DB (1999) CD86 (B7-2) can function to drive MHC-restricted antigen-specific CTL responses in vivo. J Immunol (Baltimore, MD: 1950) 162(6):3417–3427

Barouch DH, O'Brien KL, Simmons NL, King SL, Abbink P, Maxfield LF, Sun Y-H, La Porte A, Riggs AM, Lynch DM, Clark SL, Backus K, Perry JR, Seaman MS, Carville A, Mansfield KG, Szinger JJ, Fischer W, Muldoon M, Korber B (2010) Mosaic HIV-1 vaccines expand the breadth and depth of cellular immune responses in rhesus monkeys. Nat Med 16(3):319–323

Belshe R, Clements M, Dolin R (1993) Safety and immunogenicity of a fully glycosylated recombinant gp160 human immunodeficiency virus type 1 vaccine in subjects at low risk of infection. J Infect Dis 168:1387–1395

Benvenisty N, Reshef L (1986) Direct introduction of genes into rats and expression of the genes. Proc Natl Acad Sci USA 83(24):9551

Boyer J, Robinson T, Kutzler M (2005) SIV DNA vaccine co-administered with IL-12 expression plasmid enhances CD8 SIV cellular immune responses in cynomolgus macaques. J Med Primatol 34(5–6):262–270

Broderick KE, Shen X, Soderholm J, Lin F, McCoy J, Khan AS, Yan J, Morrow MP, Patel A, Kobinger GP, Kemmerrer S, Weiner DB, Sardesai NY (2011) Prototype development and preclinical immunogenicity analysis of a novel minimally invasive electroporation device. Gene Ther 18(3):258–265

Broderick K, Kardos T, McCoy J, Fons M (2011) Piezoelectric permeabilization of mammalian dermal tissue for in vivo DNA delivery leads to enhanced protein expression and increased immunogenicity. Hum Vaccines 7:22–28

Chiarella P, Massi E, De Robertis M, Sibilio A, Parrella P, Fazio VM, Signori E (2008) Electroporation of skeletal muscle induces danger signal release and antigen-presenting cell recruitment independently of DNA vaccine administration. Expert Opin Biol Ther 8(11):1645–1657

Chu Y, Xia M, Lin Y, Li A, Wang Y, Liu R, Xiong S (2006) Th2-dominated antitumor immunity induced by DNA immunization with the genes coding for a basal core peptide PDTRP and GM-CSF. Cancer Gene Ther 13(5):510–519

Coster HG (1965) A quantitative analysis of the voltage-current relationships of fixed charge membranes and the associated property of "punch-through". Biophys J 5(5):669–686

Dubensky T, Campbell B (1984) Direct transfection of viral and plasmid DNA into the liver or spleen of mice. Proc Natl Acad Sci USA 81(23):7529–7533

Edelstein ML, Abedi MR, Wixon J (2007) Gene therapy clinical trials worldwide to 2007 – an update. J Gene Med 9(10):833–842

Elmowalid GA, Qiao M, Jeong SH, Borg BB, Baumert TF, Sapp RK, Hu Z, Murthy K, Liang TJ (2007) Immunization with hepatitis C virus-like particles results in control of hepatitis C virus infection in chimpanzees. Proc Natl Acad Sci USA 104(20):8427–8432

Fauci AS (2006) Pandemic influenza threat and preparedness. Emerg Infect Dis 12(1):73–77

Ferraro B, Morrow MP, Hutnick NA, Shin TH, Lucke CE, Weiner DB (2011) Clinical applications of DNA vaccines: current progress. Clin Infect Dis 53(3):296–302

Fu T, Ulmer J, Caulfield M, Deck R, Friedman A, Wang S, Liu X, Donnelly J, Liu M (1997) Priming of cytotoxic T lymphocytes by DNA vaccines: requirement for professional antigen presenting cells and evidence for antigen transfer from myocytes. Mol Med 3(6):362

Fynan EF, Webster RG, Fuller DH, Haynes JR, Santoro JC, Robinson HL (1993) DNA vaccines: protective immunizations by parenteral, mucosal, and gene-gun inoculations. Proc Natl Acad Sci USA 90(24):11478–11482

Gagnon J, Ramanathan S, Leblanc C, Cloutier A, McDonald PP, Ilangumaran S (2008) IL-6, in synergy with IL-7 or IL-15, stimulates TCR-independent proliferation and functional differentiation of CD8+ T lymphocytes. J Immunol 180(12):7958–7968

Grønevik E, Tollefsen S, Sikkeland LIB, Haug T, Tjelle TE, Mathiesen I (2003) DNA transfection of mononuclear cells in muscle tissue. J Gene Med 5(10):909–917

Halwani R, Boyer JD, Yassine-Diab B, Haddad EK, Robinson TM, Kumar S, Parkinson R, Wu L, Sidhu MK, Phillipson-Weiner R, Pavlakis GN, Felber BK, Lewis MG, Shen A, Siliciano RF, Weiner DB, Sekaly RP (2008) Therapeutic vaccination with simian immunodeficiency virus (SIV)-DNA+IL-12 or IL-15 induces distinct CD8 memory subsets in SIV-infected macaques. J Immunol 180(12):7969–7979

Hirao LA, Wu L, Khan AS, Hokey DA, Yan J, Dai A, Betts MR, Draghia-Akli R, Weiner DB (2008) Combined effects of IL-12 and electroporation enhances the potency of DNA vaccination in macaques. Vaccine 26(25):3112–3120

Iwasaki A, Stiernholm BJ, Chan AK, Berinstein NL, Barber BH (1997) Enhanced CTL responses mediated by plasmid DNA immunogens encoding costimulatory molecules and cytokines. J Immunol 158(10):4591–4601

Kim JJ, Ayyavoo V, Bagarazzi ML, Chattergoon MA, Dang K, Wang B, Boyer JD, Weiner DB (1997) In vivo engineering of a cellular immune response by coadministration of IL-12 expression vector with a DNA immunogen. J Immunol 158(2):816–826

Kim J, Yang J, Montaner L, Lee D (2000a) Coimmunization with IFN-gamma or IL-2, but not IL-13 or IL-4 cDNA can enhance Th1-type DNA vaccine-induced immune responses in vivo. J Interferon Cytokine Res 20(3):311–319

Kim JJ, Yang JS, VanCott TC, Lee DJ, Manson KH, Wyand MS, Boyer JD, Ugen KE, Weiner DB (2000b) Modulation of antigen-specific humoral responses in rhesus macaques by using cytokine cDNAs as DNA vaccine adjuvants. J Virol 74(7):3427–3429

Ko HJ, Ko SY, Kim YJ, Lee EG, Cho SN, Kang CY (2005) Optimization of codon usage enhances the immunogenicity of a DNA vaccine encoding mycobacterial antigen Ag85B. Infect Immun 73(9):5666–5674

Kraynyak KA, Kutzler MA, Cisper NJ, Khan AS, Draghia-Akli R, Sardesal NY, Lewis MG, Yan J, Weiner DB (2010) Systemic immunization with CCL27/CTACK modulates immune responses at mucosal sites in mice and macaques. Vaccine 28(8):1942–1951

Kutzler MA, Kraynyak KA, Nagle SJ, Parkinson RM, Zharikova D, Chattergoon M, Maguire H, Muthumani K, Ugen K, Weiner DB (2010) Plasmids encoding the mucosal chemokines CCL27 and CCL28 are effective adjuvants in eliciting antigen-specific immunity in vivo. Gene Ther 17(1):72–82

Nagata T, Uchijima M, Yoshida A, Kawashima M, Koide Y (1999) Codon optimization effect on translational efficiency of DNA vaccine in mammalian cells: analysis of plasmid DNA encoding a CTL epitope derived from microorganisms. Biochem Biophys Res Commun 261(2):445–451

Li S, Qi X, Gao Y, Hao Y, Cui L, Ruan L, He W (2010) IL-15 increases the frequency of effector memory CD8+ T cells in rhesus monkeys immunized with HIV vaccine. Cell Mol Immunol 7(6):491–494

Lin F, Shen X, McCoy JR, Mendoza JM, Yan J, Kemmerrer SV, Khan AS, Weiner DB, Broderick KE, Sardesai NY (2011) A novel prototype device for electroporation-enhanced DNA vaccine delivery simultaneously to both skin and muscle. Vaccine

Long ZY, Niu PY, Gong ZY, Duan YY, Chen YW, Wang J, Tan H, Yuan J, Wu TC (2005) Role of heat shock protein 70 expression in DNA damage induced by 7, 8-dihydrodiol-9, 10-epoxide-benzo(a)pyrene. Zhonghua Lao Dong Wei Sheng Zhi Ye Bing Za Zhi 23(6):454–456

Luckay A, Sidhu MK, Kjeken R, Megati S, Chong SY, Roopchand V, Garcia-Hand D, Abdullah R, Braun R, Montefiori DC, Rosati M, Felber BK, Pavlakis GN, Mathiesen I, Israel ZR, Eldridge JH, Egan MA (2007) Effect of plasmid DNA vaccine design and In vivo electroporation on the resulting vaccine-specific immune responses in rhesus macaques. J Virol 81(10): 5257–5269

MacGregor RR, Boyer JD, Ugen KE, Lacy KE, Gluckman SJ, Bagarazzi ML, Chattergoon MA, Baine Y, Higgins TJ, Ciccarelli RB, Coney LR, Ginsberg RS, Weiner DB (1998) First human trial of a DNA-based vaccine for treatment of human immunodeficiency virus type 1 infection: safety and host response. J Infect Dis 178(1):92–100

Maue AC, Waters WR, Palmer MV, Whipple DL, Minion FC, Brown WC, Estes DM (2004) CD80 and CD86, but not CD154, augment DNA vaccine-induced protection in experimental bovine tuberculosis. Vaccine 23(6):769–779

Morris JC, Janik JE, White JD, Fleisher TA, Brown M, Tsudo M, Goldman CK, Bryant B, Petrus M, Top L, Lee CC, Gao W, Waldmann TA (2006) Preclinical and phase I clinical trial of blockade of IL-15 using Mikbeta1 monoclonal antibody in T cell large granular lymphocyte leukemia. Proc Natl Acad Sci USA 103(2):401–406

Neumann E, Kakorin S (1999) Fundamentals of electroporative delivery of drugs and genes. Bioelectrochem Bioenerg 48(1):3–16

Neumann E, Schaefer-Ridder M, Wang Y (1982) Gene transfer into mouse lyoma cells by electroporation in high electric fields. EMBO J 1(7):841–845

Niidome T, Huang L (2002) Gene therapy progress and prospects: nonviral vectors. Gene Ther 9(24):1647–1652

Offit P (2005) The cutter incident: how America's first polio vaccine led to the growing vaccine crisis. Yale University Press, New Haven

Okada E, Sasaki S, Ishii N, Aoki I, Yasuda T, Nishioka K, Fukushima J, Miyazaki J, Wahren B, Okuda K (1997) Intranasal immunization of a DNA vaccine with IL-12- and granulocyte-macrophage colony-stimulating factor (GM-CSF)-expressing plasmids in liposomes induces strong mucosal and cell-mediated immune responses against HIV-1 antigens. J Immunol 159(7):3638–3647

Okino M, Mohri H (1987) Effects of a high-voltage electrical impulse and an anticancer drug on in vivo growing tumors. Jpn J Cancer Res (Gann) 78(12):1319

Pasquini S, Xiang Z, Wang Y, He Z, Deng H, Blaszczyk-Thurin M, Ertl HC (1997) Cytokines and costimulatory molecules as genetic adjuvants. Immunol Cell Biol 75(4):397–401

Perera LP, Waldmann TA, Mosca JD, Baldwin N, Berzofsky JA, Oh SK (2007) Development of smallpox vaccine candidates with integrated interleukin-15 that demonstrate superior immunogenicity, efficacy, and safety in mice. J Virol 81(16):8774–8783

Ramanathan S, Dubois S, Chen XL, Leblanc C, Ohashi PS, Ilangumaran S (2011) Exposure to IL-15 and IL-21 enables autoreactive CD8 T cells to respond to weak antigens and cause disease in a mouse model of autoimmune diabetes. J Immunol 186(9):5131–5141

Raz E, Watanabe A, Baird SM, Eisenberg RA, Parr TB, Lotz M, Kipps TJ, Carson DA (1993) Systemic immunological effects of cytokine genes injected into skeletal muscle. Proc Natl Acad Sci U S A 90(10):4523–4527

Rocha EPC (2004) Codon usage bias from tRNA's point of view: redundancy, specialization, and efficient decoding for translation optimization. Genome Res 14(11):2279–2286

Ruprecht R (1999) Live attenuated AIDS viruses as vaccines: promise or peril? Immunol Rev 170:135–149

Santra S, Korber BT, Muldoon M, Barouch DH, Nabel GJ, Gao F, Hahn BH, Haynes BF, Letvin NL (2008) A centralized gene-based HIV-1 vaccine elicits broad cross-clade cellular immune responses in rhesus monkeys. Proc Natl Acad Sci USA 105(30):10489–10494

Tang D, DeVit M (1992) Genetic immunization is a simple method for eliciting an immune response. Nature 356(6365):152–154

Thomas P (2001) Big shot: passion, politics, and the struggle for an AIDS vaccine. PublicAffairs, New York, p 515

Tsuji T, Hamajima K, Ishii N, Aoki I (1997) Immunomodulatory effects of a plasmid expressing B7-2 on human immunodeficiency virus-1-specific cell-mediated immunity induced by a plasmid encoding the virel antigen. Eur J Immunol 27(3):782–787

Ulmer J, Donnelly J, Parker S, Rhodes G (1993) Heterologous protection against influenza by injection of DNA encoding a viral protein. Science (New York)

Valentin A, Lu W, Rosati M, Schneider R, Albert J, Karlsson A, Pavlakis GN (1998) Dual effect of interleukin 4 on HIV-1 expression: implications for viral phenotypic switch and disease progression. Proc Natl Acad Sci USA 95(15):8886–8891

Wang B, Ugen K, Srikantan V (1993) Gene inoculation generates immune responses against human immunodeficiency virus type 1. Proc Natl Acad Sci USA 90(9):4156–4160

Weiner DB, Kutzler MA, Kraynyak KA, Sylvester AJ, Ginsberg AA, Carnathan D, Kathuria N, Khan AS, Pahar B, Moldoveanu Z, Mestecky J, Betts MR, Marx P, Weiner DB (2011) Co-delivery of mucosal chemokine plasmids in a systemically administered DNA vaccine elicits systemic and mucosal immune responses in rhesus macaques. Oral presentation in: ICMI 2011. 15th International Congress of Mucosal Immunology. Paris, France 5–8.

Wolff J, Malone R, Williams P, Chong W (1990) Direct gene transfer into mouse muscle in vivo. Science (New York)

Xiang Z, Ertl HC (1995) Manipulation of the immune response to a plasmid-encoded viral antigen by coinoculation with plasmids expressing cytokines. Immunity 2(2):129–135

Yewdell JW, Bennink JR (1999) Mechanisms of viral interference with MHC class I antigen processing and presentation. Annu Rev Cell Dev Biol 15:579–606

Yin J, Dai A, Kutzler MA, Shen A, Lecureux J, Lewis MG, Waldmann T, Weiner DB, Boyer JD (2008) Sustained suppression of SHIV89.6P replication in macaques by vaccine-induced CD8+ memory T cells. AIDS 22(14):1739–1748

Zhao J, Lai L, Amara RR, Montefiori DC, Villinger F, Chennareddi L, Wyatt LS, Moss B, Robinson HL (2009) Preclinical studies of human immunodeficiency virus/AIDS vaccines: inverse correlation between avidity of anti-Env antibodies and peak postchallenge viremia. J Virol 83(9):4102–4111

Zheng JP, Sun JY, Guo L, Liang HS, Tian FJ, Wu TC (2007) Relationship between heat shock protein 72 and DNA genetic damage in peripheral blood lymphocytes of coke oven workers. Zhonghua Lao Dong Wei Sheng Zhi Ye Bing Za Zhi 25(7):394–397

Electroporation Based TriGrid™ Delivery System (TDS) for DNA Vaccine Administration

8

Drew Hannaman

Electroporation (EP) is a promising device based method for increasing the delivery of genetic vaccines to their intracellular site of action. This is achieved through the brief application of electrical fields at the target tissue site in the presence of the vaccine candidate. Non-clinical studies comparing EP mediated delivery with conventional injection methods have demonstrated 10–1,000 fold increases in antigen expression and subsequent cellular and humoral immune responses. Prompted by this promising data, multiple groups have developed EP device technologies to support translation of this delivery modality into the clinical setting. Among these is the TriGrid™ Delivery System (TDS) platform developed by Ichor Medical Systems. TDS devices are characterized by the integration of the means for agent administration and EP application into a single automated device which controls the site, rate, and timing of agent administration relative to the application of EP. This design ensures co-localization of the electrical fields with the site of genetic vaccine distribution and facilitates consistent procedure application independent of operator skill or experience. Device configurations for genetic vaccine delivery into either skeletal muscle or skin have been developed and are being evaluated in both non-clinical and clinical studies for delivery of a wide range of vaccine applications.

Introduction

Electroporation (EP) is a physical, non-viral delivery method currently under investigation as a method for DNA vaccine administration. EP is based on the propagation of brief, high amplitude electrical fields to living cells (either in culture or in tissue). This process induces a transient state of membrane destabilization/

D. Hannaman
Ichor Medical Systems, Inc., San Diego, CA, USA
e-mail: dhannaman@ichorms.com

J. Thalhamer et al. (eds.), *Gene Vaccines*,
DOI 10.1007/978-3-7091-0439-2_8, © Springer-Verlag/Wien, 2012

permeability, during which time exogenous substances present in the extracellular space are taken up into the affected cells. Shortly after application of the EP inducing electrical fields is completed, the membranes re-stabilize and the cells resume normal function (subject to the biological activity of the exogenous substances delivered to the cells).

EP has its origins in research on the effects of electrical fields on biological membranes leading to the identification of electrical conditions that were capable of transiently and reversibly increasing the permeability of cell membranes (Crowley 1973; Zimmermann et al. 1976). The first application for *in vivo* EP was to increase the uptake of chemotherapeutic agents in experimental solid tumors in rodents (Okino and Mohri 1987). Shortly thereafter, it was demonstrated that the technique could also be adapted for *in vivo* DNA delivery; first in skin (Nomura et al. 1996; Titomirov et al. 1991), tumor (Nishi et al. 1996), skeletal muscle (Nomura et al. 1996), and liver (Heller et al. 1996), followed by a wide range of other tissue types (reviewed in Mir et al. (2005); Somiari et al. (2000)).

With the basic feasibility of EP mediated DNA delivery established, multiple groups initiated systematic reporter gene studies in order to optimize EP conditions for *in vivo* DNA delivery. Due to their ready accessibility for DNA administration and because they offered potential to support a wide range of product applications (including DNA vaccine delivery) skeletal muscle and skin were the target tissues of primary interest (Aihara and Miyazaki 1998; Mir et al. 1998; Mathiesen 1999; Drabick et al. 2001; Glasspool-Malone et al. 2000). Using refined administration conditions, EP mediated DNA delivery was capable not only of increasing expression of encoded proteins by multiple orders of magnitude compared to conventional DNA injection, but also to decrease the inter-subject variability (Mir et al. 1998). When utilized for DNA vaccine administration, the dramatic increase in DNA expression achievable with EP correlated with improvements in both humoral and cell mediated immune responses against encoded antigens (Drabick et al. 2001; Dupuis et al. 2000; Kadowaki et al. 2000; Selby et al. 2000; Widera et al. 2000; Zucchelli et al. 2000). Importantly, the EP mediated enhancements in DNA vaccine delivery were maintained even as the procedure was applied in larger animal species (Babiuk et al. 2002, 2003, 2007; van Drunen Littel-van den Hurk et al. 2004; Laddy et al. 2008; Otten et al. 2004).

When juxtaposed with the suboptimal potency demonstrated in multiple clinical trials of DNA vaccines administered by conventional injection (reviewed in Donnelly et al. (2003); Ulmer et al. (2006)), the encouraging non-clinical findings with EP mediated DNA immunization delivery provided a strong rationale for the continued development of EP technology for DNA vaccine delivery.

Development of the TriGrid Delivery System™ for DNA Vaccine Delivery

Based on the promising non-clinical studies demonstrating dramatic enhancements in DNA vaccine potency with EP delivery, Ichor Medical Systems, Inc. (San Diego, CA, USA) was one of several entities to initiate development of EP technology for

8 Electroporation Based TriGrid™ Delivery System (TDS)

DNA vaccine delivery in the clinical setting (reviewed in Luxembourg et al. (2007)). The premise guiding Ichor's technology development efforts was that the long term commercial viability of this approach is contingent on the development of EP devices capable of safe, effective, reproducible application across heterogenous target populations. Moreover, devices should be simple and cost effective to use, comply with guidelines for medical device design, and be acceptable for both vaccine recipients and healthcare workers.

Ichor has sought to achieve this objective with the development of its platform for EP mediated DNA vaccine administration, called the TriGrid Delivery System (TDS). Design of the TDS was guided by several key technical issues relevant to EP mediated DNA delivery. These included:

- The increased DNA delivery characteristic of EP occurs only in cells where the electrical fields are applied in the presence of the exogenous DNA. Specifically, the DNA must be distributed into the tissue prior to EP application (not after) (Mathiesen 1999). Therefore, EP devices should be designed to consistently achieve spatial and temporal "co-localization" of the administered DNA and EP inducing electrical fields within the target tissue.
- The magnitude of antigen expression and resulting immunological response is determined not only by the dose of DNA vaccine administered, but also by the volume of injection in which it is delivered (which correlates with the number of cells transfected) (Dupuis et al. 2000; Gardiner et al. 2006). Therefore, EP devices should be designed not only to accommodate varying DNA doses, but also a range of injection volumes.
- The level of discomfort perceived by the recipient during EP application is correlated with the volume of tissue exposed to EP and the duration of electrical stimulation (Tjelle et al. 2008; Wong et al. 2006; Rabussay 2008). In order to minimize the discomfort associated with the procedure, EP devices should be configured to efficiently induce the EP effect while avoiding electrical stimulation of tissue regions where DNA is not present during EP application.
- The time interval between DNA injection and EP application can affect the efficiency of delivery (Khan et al. 2003). To minimize inter-subject and inter-operator variability, EP devices should control this interval in a user independent fashion.
- Humans exhibit wide variation in skin and subcutaneous tissue thickness which can affect intramuscular administration procedures (Cook et al. 2006; Poland et al. 1997). Since improperly injected vaccines can exhibit suboptimal immunogenicity, EP devices designed for intramuscular DNA delivery should provide simple means to ensure that intramuscular distribution of DNA can be achieved across a heterogeneous target population.
- Activation of electrodes in tissue can result in unwanted electrochemical reactions at the electrode tissue interface which can lead to deposition of metal ions in the local tissue (Greatbatch 1981). To avoid potential safety issues, the surfaces of electrodes for EP should comprise electrochemically stable materials.
- Existing U.S. and European guidelines require that the use of novel injection devices include an evaluation/consideration of means for the prevention or reduction of sharps injuries (Daley 2000; Mooney 2009).

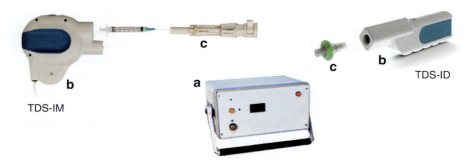

Fig. 8.1 Components of a TDS device. Each TDS device comprises a Pulse Stimulator (**a**), Integrated Applicator (**b**), and a single use Administration Cartridge (**c**)

Taking into consideration these key technical requirements, Ichor has designed its TDS for safe, effective, and reproducible DNA vaccine administration in the clinical setting. This is achieved with the TDS platform by integrating the means for DNA delivery and electrical field propagation into a single, automated device. In a TDS device, the site, rate, and timing of the DNA injection and subsequent EP application are controlled in a consistent, user independent fashion. The TDS electrode arrays used to propagate the EP inducing electrical fields are configured to correspond to the pattern of DNA distribution characteristic of the target tissue. By combining automated injection control with appropriately configured electrode arrays the TDS is designed so that the application of the EP inducing electrical fields is consistently confined to the tissues where DNA has been distributed. The use of an integrated, automated device also enables the entire administration to be completed in less than 10 s. Taken together, the TDS platform is designed for effective and reproducible application of the administration procedure across heterogeneous recipient populations with minimal operator training.

In order to support the routes of administration relevant for DNA vaccine delivery, the TDS platform has been adapted to produce devices for administration into either skeletal muscle (TDS-IM) or skin (TDS-ID) (Fig. 8.1). Each of these integrated, automated application systems consists of four components: a **Pulse Stimulator**, an **Integrated Applicator** and a single use **Application Cartridge** containing a **TriGrid electrode array**. A detailed description of each system component is provided below.

TDS Pulse Stimulator

The TDS Pulse Stimulator is an electronic apparatus compatible with both the TDS-IM and TDS-ID devices. The Pulse Stimulator controls the administration procedure sequence, generates the electrical signals necessary to enhance the intracellular delivery of the agent, and monitors the administration sequence for potential safety hazards. It connects to either the TDS-IM or TDS-ID Integrated Applicator through an incorporated cable. Upon start up, a comprehensive self diagnostic routine is performed to ensure proper device function. Device outputs include low voltage control signals for the Integrated Applicators as well as high voltage signals required for propagation of the EP inducing electrical fields.

Multiple safety systems have been incorporated into the Pulse Stimulator to prevent excessive energy from being delivered to the tissue of the recipient. These include continuous monitoring circuitry to ensure that the current, voltage, and total energy of the EP signals remain within prescribed limits. Detection of one or more fault conditions at any time during procedure application will result in immediate disconnection of the patient from the voltage supply and notification of the user that a fault condition has occurred.

TDS-IM and TDS-ID Integrated Applicators

The TDS Integrated Applicators are reusable, hand-held electromechanical devices that contain mechanisms to deploy the electrodes into the target tissue, administer the biologic agent, and relay the EP signals from the Pulse Stimulator to the electrodes. Tissue distribution studies were performed to identify the best method of DNA injection for each route of administration. Based on the ability to achieve consistent distribution in the target tissue across heterogeneous sites, the TDS-IM device utilizes a needle injection to distribute the DNA in the target tissue whereas the TDS-ID device is based on needle-free jet injection. Notwithstanding the differences in injection technique, the TDS-IM and TDS-ID Integrated Applicators are both configured so that, after the user activates the device, the electrodes are automatically deployed into the target tissue site with the rate and timing of the DNA injection, and subsequent EP application controlled in a user independent fashion. This ensures that the key administration parameters will be implemented for every recipient in a uniform fashion, thereby decreasing the potential for variation in the administration procedure and reducing the need for operator training to ensure consistent procedure application.

TDS-IM and TDS-ID Single Use Application Cartridges

The TDS Application Cartridge and the enclosed TriGrid electrode array (see section "TDS-IM and TDS-ID TriGrid Electrode Arrays") are the only component of a TDS device that contacts the recipient during the administration procedure. Each TDS-IM and TDS-ID Application Cartridge is packaged sterile for single use. The current device configurations interface with an "off the shelf" syringe (TDS-IM) or a needle free jet injection cartridge (TDS-ID) that are loaded with the DNA vaccine candidate prior to delivery. The TDS-IM cartridge utilizes a 3.0 cc syringe and has an injection capacity of up to 1.2 mL per intramuscular administration site. The TDS-ID Application Cartridge utilizes a needle free jet injection cartridge and is capable of delivering up to 200 µL per skin administration site. Multiple TDS Cartridge sizes have been designed to accommodate the range of injection volumes

Fig. 8.2 TDS Integrated Applicators with Application Cartridges

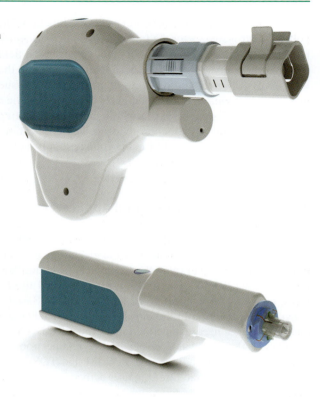

in non-clinical and clinical use (see section "TDS-IM and TDS-ID TriGrid Electrode Arrays").

The current TDS device configurations are designed for use in early phase clinical trials where the dose and formulation of the DNA vaccine candidates have not been specified. The standard "off the shelf" components utilized as the means for agent administration can readily accommodate changes in DNA dose and/or formulation that may be required during initial clinical testing. Once the specifications for the biologic have been finalized, a functionally identical TDS device accommodating a pre-filled cartridge or syringe at a dose level specific for that product can be implemented for late stage clinical studies and eventual commercial deployment.

Prior to each administration procedure, the syringe (for TDS-IM) or needle free cartridge (for TDS-ID) containing the agent of interest is loaded into an Application Cartridge. Once loaded with the agent for delivery, the Application Cartridge is attached to the relevant Integrated Applicator for administration to the recipient (Fig. 8.2). A safety cap located on the tip of the Application Cartridge protects the operator from accidental sharps injury and ensures that the recessed electrodes remain sterile during handling.

In order to ensure intramuscular administration in recipients with differences in skin and subcutaneous tissue thickness, the TDS-IM Application Cartridge incorporates an adjustable gauge to control injection depth. Prior to administration, the thickness of the recipient's skin at the administration site is evaluated using a pinch test in order to select one of three depth settings for administration. This procedure is comparable to that which is used for selection of needle length prior to intramuscular administration by conventional injection methods. According to published surveys of deltoid anatomy conducted in United States subpopulations, the depth range encompassed by the TDS-IM will accommodate deltoid administration in >99% of adult U.S. males and >95% of adult U.S. females (Cook et al. 2006; Poland et al. 1997).

Once the device is placed at the target tissue site and activated by the operator, the electrodes are deployed into the tissue to the prescribed depth. A brief impedance check is performed to ensure that the electrodes have been inserted to the target depth and that they have the proper orientation along their length (i.e., the electrodes have not deflected). By ensuring that the electrodes are properly deployed into the tissue prior to delivery of the agent, the device reduces the potential that the agent could be administered without subsequent EP. Once the impedance check is passed, the DNA is administered to the target tissue site at a controlled rate of injection. Immediately after the completion of the injection, the EP inducing electrical fields are propagated at the site of DNA distribution.

At the conclusion of the procedure, the device is withdrawn from the recipient, automatically activating sharps protection measures incorporated into the Application Cartridges. For the TDS-IM device, a spring loaded stick shield locks over the electrodes and injection needle. For the TDS-ID device, the electrodes are retracted within the Application Cartridge following completion of EP application. These measures facilitate safe disposal and compliance with current guidelines for sharps injury prevention. These designs are also favorable from a tolerability/acceptability perspective since the sharps are never visible to the recipient.

TDS-IM and TDS-ID TriGrid Electrode Arrays

Electrode Array Design

As described above, EP mediated DNA vaccine delivery is dependent on the propagation of threshold level electrical fields in the target tissue in the presence of the DNA vaccine candidate. This spatial and temporal "co-localization" is essential for the increased intracellular uptake characteristic of EP. However, because the discomfort perceived by the recipient is correlated with the volume of tissue exposed to EP it is not feasible to simply apply EP to large volumes of tissue around the injection site. From a cost-benefit perspective, the optimal approach for EP mediated delivery is to ensure that the electrical fields are applied only in tissue where DNA has been distributed prior to the application of EP.

To achieve this objective, the TDS devices utilize an array of penetrating electrodes configured in a pattern of interlocking triangles (hence the name "TriGrid"). Each TriGrid array is designed so that the electrical fields propagated by the array correspond to the pattern of vaccine distribution characteristic of the target tissue.

Fig. 8.3 TriGrid electrode array configurations for DNA delivery in muscle (TDS-IM) and skin (TDS-ID). Top view schematic diagram of the relationship between the electrodes and injection orifice in the TDS-IM and TDS-ID devices (**a**) and the DNA distribution patterns characteristic of the relevant tissue targets (**b**)

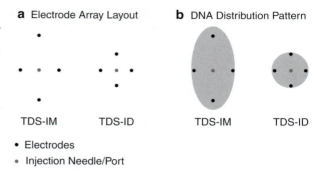

During the EP application, all of the electrodes are activated simultaneously to enhance the uniformity of the electrical fields at the site of application, thereby providing consistent induction of the EP effect while minimizing the risk of focal tissue damage. This approach also enables the EP effect to be induced using a relatively short duration of electrical stimulation (e.g., 40 mS stimulation over a 400 mS interval) which is favorable from a tolerability perspective.

For intramuscular delivery, the TriGrid array consists of four electrodes arranged in two adjoining equilateral triangles forming a diamond shape around the central injection needle (Figs. 8.3a and 8.4a). With the long axis of the diamond placed in parallel with the direction of the muscle fibers this configuration corresponds with the ellipsoid fluid distribution characteristic of an intramuscular injection (Figs. 8.3b and 8.4b). In order to confine the EP application to the desired depth within the muscle, each electrode is coated with a biocompatible insulation material above the level of the injection site. A range of electrode array sizes have been developed in order to accommodate the range of injection volumes typically used for DNA vaccine delivery as well as testing in different animal species.

The TDS-ID electrodes are arranged in two isosceles triangles around the central jet injection port (Fig. 8.3a) in order to accommodate the raised circular bleb characteristic of DNA administration in skin (Figs. 8.3b and 8.5a). The electrodes can be inserted to a maximum depth of 3 mm. As with the TDS-IM device, the range of injection volumes utilized for DNA vaccine delivery to skin in the non-clinical and clinical settings is accommodated with multiple array sizes.

Electrode Array Scaling

In order to support procedure application across a range of injection volumes and target species, multiple TDS-IM and TDS-ID electrode array sizes have been developed (Fig. 8.6). The electrical fields generated by the array can be scaled consistently across the size range by preserving the geometric relationship of the electrodes within the array and maintaining a consistent relationship between their diameter and spacing. In this way, the EP administration devices can be scaled up from small animals (2.5–4.8 mm TDS-IM devices, 2.5 mm TDS-ID device) for use in larger species and/or the human clinical setting (6.0–10.0 mm TDS-IM device, 4.5 mm TDS-ID device) without a loss in efficiency.

8 Electroporation Based TriGrid™ Delivery System (TDS)

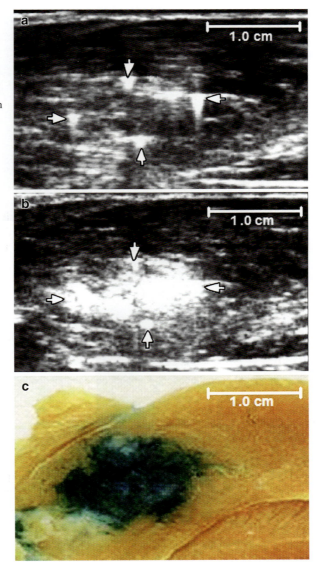

Fig. 8.4 DNA distribution and gene expression following TDS-IM delivery. Longitudinal ultrasound images of TDS-IM electrode array deployment in rabbit muscle (electrodes denoted by *arrows*) (**a**), administration of a 0.5 mL β-galactosidase DNA injection (**b**), and detection of β-galactosidase expression at the administration site 7 days after administration (**c**)

Scalability of the TriGrid array system was verified in a study of intramuscular delivery of a reporter gene in a range of species, including mice, rats, and rabbits. DNA encoding human secreted alkaline phosphatase (SeAP) was administered to each species at a dose of 0.1 mg DNA/kg mean body mass either by conventional intramuscular injection or using the TDS-IM device. The TDS-IM array sizes used were 2.5 mm in mice, 3.0 mm in rats, and 6.0 mm in rabbits. All electrode arrays were activated using the same EP conditions adjusted for electrode size (250 V/cm

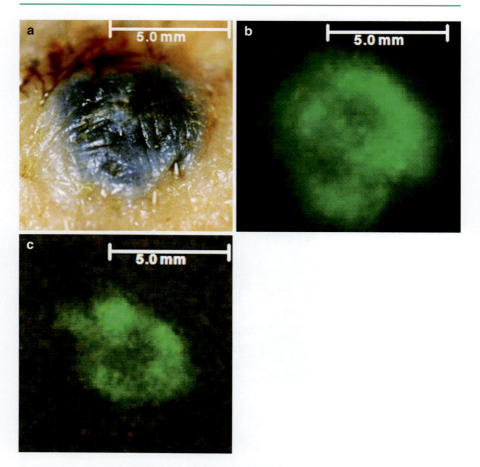

Fig. 8.5 DNA distribution and gene expression following TDS-ID delivery. Images of weal formation following TDS-ID distribution of DNA (mixed with Evan's blue dye for visualization) in pig skin (**a**). GFP expression detected 24 h after TDS-ID mediated administration of a 100 μL GFP DNA injection in pig skin (**b**). GFP expression detected 24 h after administration of a 100 μL GFP DNA injection in pig skin using the TDS-ID device without EP application (**c**)

of electrode spacing; stimulation of 40 mS duration over a 400 mS interval). Injection volumes were 10 μL in mice, 20 μL in rats, and 300 μL in rabbits. SeAP levels were analyzed in serum samples obtained prior to administration and then 7 days after plasmid DNA administration. The results of the study are depicted in Fig. 8.7. Consistent with the increased DNA delivery achievable with EP, the serum SeAP levels observed in the TDS EP groups were at least 100 fold higher than conventional intramuscular injection for all species tested. Importantly, unlike with conventional intramuscular injection, expression levels were largely maintained as the TDS-IM devices for rodent administration were scaled to a size appropriate for use in the human clinical setting. In mice, mean serum SeAP levels were 250 ng/mL. The mean

8 Electroporation Based TriGrid™ Delivery System (TDS) 173

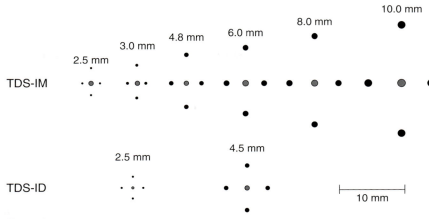

Fig. 8.6 TriGrid electrode array sizes. A scaled representation of the electrode array sizes available for the TDS-IM and TDS-ID devices. Size labels indicate the distance between adjacent electrodes. A wider range of TDS-IM electrode sizes are available to accommodate the larger injection volumes that can be administered via intramuscular injection

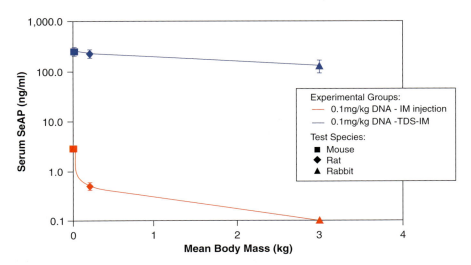

Fig. 8.7 Scalability of the TDS-IM Administration Procedure. DNA encoding human secreted alkaline phosphatase (SeAP) was administered at a dose of 0.1 mg DNA/kg body weight in multiple animal species (mouse, rat, and rabbit) using either conventional intramuscular injection or scaled versions of the TDS-IM device. The concentration of SeAP was measured in serum 7 days after administration. Across all species, DNA delivered by TDS-IM resulted in mean serum SeAP levels over 100-fold higher compared to conventional intramuscular injection

Table 8.1 Effect of electrode coating on metal ion discharge and biocompatibility

Test method	Electrode type			
	304 Stainless steel (uncoated)		304 Stainless steel (coated)	
Plasma spectroscopy	Element	Concentration (ppm)	Element	Concentration (ppm)
	Iron	2.16	Iron	Not detected
	Chromium	1.36	Chromium	Not detected
	Manganese	0.09	Manganese	Not detected
	Nickel	0.85	Nickel	Not detected
Cell cytotoxicity (grade 0–4)	1 (Slight toxicity)		0 (No toxicity)	

serum SeAP levels in rats were not significantly different at 230 ng/mL. Rabbits exhibited mean serum SeAP levels of 130 ng/mL. Although significantly lower than that observed in mouse (p < 0.05 Student's t test), the SeAP level in rabbits was not significantly different from that in rat, representing an overall decrease of less than 50%. Taken together, these results indicate that the TDS delivery device and administration procedure can be predictably scaled between species and that the levels of DNA delivery and antigen expression observed in small animal models can be extrapolated into species of larger body mass.

Electrode Composition

The electrodes used in the TDS-IM and TDS-ID arrays are comprised of 300 series surgical grade stainless steel. To minimize undesirable electrochemical reactions at the electrode tissue interface, TDS devices utilize electrodes that are coated in a titanium alloy that has previously been used in implantable electrode applications (ASM International 2009; Schaldach et al. 1989, 1990). An extract study (Ichor, unpublished) was performed to assess the effect of electrode coating on the potential for discharge of metal ions and cell cytotoxicity associated with EP application. The test devices were two 10 mm TriGrid electrode arrays comprised of 300 series stainless steel electrodes that were either uncoated or coated with the titanium alloy. The test devices were inserted into 20 mL of physiologic saline solution. The electrode arrays were then activated with two consecutive applications of the standard EP parameters for that array (250 V for a total duration of 40 ms ×2).

The saline extracts were analyzed for the presence of metallic elements by plasma spectroscopy and for biocompatibility using the *in vitro* cell cytotoxicity study (agarose overlay method). As depicted in Table 8.1, metallic elements present in 300 series stainless steel were detected in the uncoated electrode extract with accompanying cell cytotoxicity. In contrast, there were no metallic elements or cell cytotoxicity detected with the coated electrode extract. Although the *in vivo* significance of these findings is currently unknown, exposure to the metal species comprising stainless steel can have adverse consequences in susceptible individuals (Forte et al. 2008; Hsu et al. 2010). These findings indicate that the safety of EP could be enhanced through the use of electrodes designed to reduce electrochemical reactions at the electrode-tissue interface.

8 Electroporation Based TriGrid™ Delivery System (TDS)   175

Table 8.2 Published non-clinical studies of EP mediated DNA vaccine delivery with the TriGrid delivery system

Pathogen/antigen	Antigen(s)	Animal species	References
Bacillus anthracis	Protective antigen lethal factor	Mouse, rat, rabbit, non-human primate	NCT00471133 (2009), Livingston et al. (2010), Luxembourg et al. (2007, 2008a)
Hepadnavirus	Surface antigen core antigen	Mouse, rabbit, cattle	Luxembourg et al. (2006), van Drunen Littel-van den Hurk et al. (2008), Luxembourg et al. (2008b)
Severe acute respiratory syndrome virus	S glycoprotein	Mouse	Liu et al. (2007), Yi et al. (2005)
Clostridium difficile	Toxin A	Mouse	Gardiner et al. (2009)
Human immunodeficiency virus	gag, pol, nef, tat, env	Mouse, rat, rabbit	Dolter et al. (2011), Nchinda et al. (2008)
Influenza virus	Hemagglutinin antigen (H5N1 and H1N1) conserved CD4+ T cell epitopes	Mouse	Alexander et al. (2010), Chen et al. (2008), Tenbusch et al. (2010)
Human papillomavirus	E7 antigen (serotype 16)	Mouse	Best et al. (2009), Kang et al. (2010), Ohlschlager et al. (2010)
Bovine viral diarrhea virus	E2 antigen (type 1 and type 2)	Cattle	van Drunen Littel-van den Hurk et al. (2010)
Plasmodium falciparum	Pfs-25 antigen	Mouse	LeBlanc et al. (2008)

TDS Based DNA Vaccine Delivery: Non-Clinical Evaluation

The TDS platform has been used extensively for delivery of DNA vaccines encoding viral, bacterial, and tumor associated antigens in a wide range of animal species (Table 8.2). EP mediated delivery with the TDS has demonstrated the capacity to enhance gene expression and/or DNA vaccine potency by multiple orders of magnitude compared to conventional DNA injection across a range of species, including rodents (Best et al. 2009; LeBlanc et al. 2008), rabbits (Luxembourg et al. 2006, 2008b), non-human primates (Livingston et al. 2010), and cattle (van Drunen Littel-van den Hurk et al. 2008). The device does not require use of any species DNA formulations and, although most commonly used for delivery of DNA vaccines encoding whole antigen sequences, the TDS platform has also demonstrated the capacity to deliver DNA vaccines encoding polyepitopes strings (Alexander et al. 2010) as well as fusion proteins (Best et al. 2009; Nchinda et al. 2008).

The enhanced potency observed with the TDS can confer improved dose efficiency as well as significant improvements in the magnitude of cellular and humoral immune responses against the encoded antigen(s). Moreover, EP mediated delivery with the TDS has also been associated with enhanced functional characteristics and protection against pathogen challenge (Chen et al. 2008; Livingston et al. 2010; van Drunen Littel-van den Hurk et al. 2010). Recent comparative testing of DNA vaccines delivered with the TDS indicates that this approach also compares favorably to the immunological responses that can be induced following DNA vaccine delivery by gene gun (Best et al. 2009) or by the administration of a currently licensed adjuvanted subunit vaccine (Livingston et al. 2010). Favorable results from toxicological analysis as well as studies to characterize the biodistribution, persistence, and integrative potential of TDS EP mediated DNA vaccine delivery have provided the basis to advance the TDS technology into clinical testing, including for application in healthy subjects (Dolter et al. 2011).

TDS Based DNA Vaccine Delivery: Clinical Evaluation

As of the end of 2010, the TDS-IM has been used as the means of DNA vaccine administration in four clinical trials. A summary of these studies is provided in Table 8.3. Formal non-clinical safety evaluation of the TDS-ID device is underway with the first clinical study expected to be initiated in 2011.

The four TDS-IM clinical studies include two completed studies: a xenogeneic tyrosinase DNA vaccine candidate in patients with Stage IIB–IV melanoma and a randomized placebo controlled comparison of a HIV-1 subtype C/B' DNA vaccine candidate delivered in healthy subjects by either TDS-IM or conventional intramuscular injection. Two ongoing TDS-IM studies include a poly-epitope vaccine containing multiple CD8+ and CD4+ T-cell epitopes derived from antigens expressed in the pre-erythrocytic stages of *Plasmodium falciparum* infection and a DNA based vaccine candidate encoding an antibody with embedded CD8+ and CD4+ epitopes from the TRP-2 and gp100 melanosomal differentiation antigens.

In clinical studies to date, the TDS-IM administration procedure has been used to deliver regimens of up to five administrations and DNA doses of up to 4.0 mg. The most common adverse responses reported in association with use of the device have included acute discomfort during procedure application, minor, transient cutaneous bleeding immediately after procedure application at the sites of injection needle and/ or electrode penetration, and transient injection site soreness for 24–72 h following administration. Encouraging results from questionnaire based tolerability assessments indicate the potential feasibility of TDS-IM even for application in prophylactic immunization (van Drunen Littel-van den Hurk and Hannaman 2010).

Analysis of immune responses in the randomized, placebo controlled comparative HIV DNA vaccine delivery study indicates significant improvement in the frequency, magnitude, breadth, and duration of responses associated with TDS-IM based delivery versus conventional intramuscular injection ((Vasan et al. 2009), reviewed in van Drunen Littel-van den Hurk and Hannaman (2010)). These findings not only verify that the EP effect can be induced in humans, but also demonstrate that the TDS-IM procedure can be effectively extrapolated for use in the clinical

Table 8.3 Human clinical evaluation of EP mediated DNA vaccine delivery with the TriGrid delivery system

Vaccine candidate	Disease indication	Clinical phase and study design	Study population	Initiation date	Route of administration	Study status (2010)	Additional information/References
DNA vaccine encoding a xenogeneic form (murine) of the tyrosinase antigen	Melanoma	Phase Ia/Ib; dose escalation study for safety and immunogenicity analysis	Stage IIB–IV melanoma patients	2007	Intramuscular	Completed	NCT00471133 (2009)
DNA vaccine encoding multiple HIV-1 subtype C antigens (env, gag, pol, nef, tat)	HIV infection (preventive)	Phase I; placebo controlled, randomized comparison of TDS-IM delivery vs. conventional IM injection	Healthy subjects	2007	Intramuscular	Completed	NCT00545987 (2009), Vasan et al. (2009)
DNA vaccine encoding an antibody embedded with CD4+ and CD8+ T cell epitopes from the melanosomal antigens TRP-2 and gp-100	Melanoma	Phase I/II; dose escalation for safety and immunogenicity analysis	Stage IV melanoma (Phase I) Stage IIIB–IV melanoma (Phase II)	2010	Intramuscular	Ongoing	NCT01138410 (2010)
DNA vaccine encoding CD4+ and CD8+ T cell epitopes derived from multiple pre-erythrocytic *Plasmodium falciparum* antigens	Malaria (preventative)	Phase I; placebo controlled, dose escalation study for safety and immunogenicity analysis	Healthy subjects	2010	Intramuscular	Ongoing	NCT01169077 (2010)

setting. By the end of 2011, data is expected from the additional clinical studies of TDS DNA vaccine delivery described in Table 8.3. With four or more additional DNA vaccines scheduled to begin clinical testing with TDS delivery during this time frame (including the first study of the TDS-ID device) there will be substantial data available within the next 12–24 months to assess the long term potential of the TDS platform as a means for DNA vaccine delivery.

Acknowledgements The author would like to thank the current and former colleagues at Ichor Medical Systems, Inc. who contributed to the work described herein including R. Bernard, B. Ellefsen, B. Bernard, S. Masterson, R. Betts, A. Ubach, G. Hague, C. Yih, C. Evans, K. Dolter, J. Song, and L. Chau. Work described herein was supported in part by a grant from the NIH SBIR program (GM064909).

References

Aihara H, Miyazaki J (1998) Gene transfer into muscle by electroporation in vivo. Nat Biotechnol 16(9):867–870

Alexander J, Bilsel P, del Guercio MF, Stewart S, Marinkovic-Petrovic A, Southwood S, Crimi C, Vang L, Walker L, Ishioka G, Chitnis V, Sette A, Assarsson E, Hannaman D, Botten J, Newman MJ (2010) Universal influenza DNA vaccine encoding conserved CD4+ T cell epitopes protects against lethal viral challenge in HLA-DR transgenic mice. Vaccine 28(3):664–672

ASM-International (2009) *Materials and coatings for medical devices: cardiovascular*. Materials and Processes for Medical Devices, ASM International

Babiuk S, Baca-Estrada ME, Foldvari M, Storms M, Rabussay D, Widera G, Babiuk LA (2002) Electroporation improves the efficacy of DNA vaccines in large animals. Vaccine 20(27–28):3399–3408

Babiuk S, Baca-Estrada ME, Foldvari M, Baizer L, Stout R, Storms M, Rabussay D, Widera G, Babiuk L (2003) Needle-free topical electroporation improves gene expression from plasmids administered in porcine skin. Mol Ther 8(6):992–998

Babiuk S, Tsang C, van Drunen Littel-van den Hurk S, Babiuk LA, Griebel PJ (2007) A single HBsAg DNA vaccination in combination with electroporation elicits long-term antibody responses in sheep. Bioelectrochemistry 70(2):269–274

Best SR, Peng S, Juang CM, Hung CF, Hannaman D, Saunders JR, Wu TC, Pai SI (2009) Administration of HPV DNA vaccine via electroporation elicits the strongest CD8+ T cell immune responses compared to intramuscular injection and intradermal gene gun delivery. Vaccine 27(40):5450–5459

Chen MW, Cheng TJ, Huang Y, Jan JT, Ma SH, Yu AL, Wong CH, Ho DD (2008) A consensus-hemagglutinin-based DNA vaccine that protects mice against divergent H5N1 influenza viruses. Proc Natl Acad Sci USA 105(36):13538–13543

Cook IF, Williamson M, Pond D (2006) Definition of needle length required for intramuscular deltoid injection in elderly adults: an ultrasonographic study. Vaccine 24(7):937–940

Crowley JM (1973) Electrical breakdown of bimolecular lipid membranes as an electromechanical instability. Biophys J 13(7):711–724

Daley K (2000) Needlestick Prevention Bill unanimously passes Senate. Ohio Nurses Rev 75(3):7–8

Dolter KE, Evans CF, Ellefsen B, Song J, Boente-Carrera M, Vittorino R, Rosenberg TJ, Hannaman D, Vasan S (2011) Immunogenicity, safety, biodistribution and persistence of ADVAX, a prophylactic DNA vaccine for HIV-1, delivered by in vivo electroporation. Vaccine 29(4):795–803

Donnelly J, Berry K, Ulmer JB (2003) Technical and regulatory hurdles for DNA vaccines. Int J Parasitol 33(5–6):457–467

Drabick JJ, Glasspool-Malone J, King A, Malone RW (2001) Cutaneous transfection and immune responses to intradermal nucleic acid vaccination are significantly enhanced by in vivo electropermeabilization. Mol Ther 3(2):249–255

Dupuis M, Denis-Mize K, Woo C, Goldbeck C, Selby MJ, Chen M, Otten GR, Ulmer JB, Donnelly JJ, Ott G, McDonald DM (2000) Distribution of DNA vaccines determines their immunogenicity after intramuscular injection in mice. J Immunol 165(5):2850–2858

Forte G, Petrucci F, Bocca B (2008) Metal allergens of growing significance: epidemiology, immunotoxicology, strategies for testing and prevention. Inflamm Allergy Drug Targets 7(3):145–162

Gardiner DF, Huang Y, Basu S, Leung L, Song Y, Chen Z, Ho DD (2006) Multiple-site DNA vaccination enhances immune responses in mice. Vaccine 24(3):287–292

Gardiner DF, Rosenberg T, Zaharatos J, Franco D, Ho DD (2009) A DNA vaccine targeting the receptor-binding domain of *Clostridium difficile* toxin A. Vaccine 27(27):3598–3604

Glasspool-Malone J, Somiari S, Drabick JJ, Malone RW (2000) Efficient nonviral cutaneous transfection. Mol Ther 2(2):140–146

Greatbatch W (1981) Metal electrodes in bioengineering. Crit Rev Bioeng 5(1):1–36

Heller R, Jaroszeski M, Atkin A, Moradpour D, Gilbert R, Wands J, Nicolau C (1996) In vivo gene electroinjection and expression in rat liver. FEBS Lett 389(3):225–228

Hsu JW, Matiz C, Jacob SE (2010) Nickel allergy: localized, Id, and systemic manifestations in children. Pediatr Dermatol

Kadowaki S, Chen Z, Asanuma H, Aizawa C, Kurata T, Tamura S (2000) Protection against influenza virus infection in mice immunized by administration of hemagglutinin-expressing DNAs with electroporation. Vaccine 18(25):2779–2788

Kang TH, Chung JY, Monie A, Pai SI, Hung CF, Wu TC (2010) Enhancing DNA vaccine potency by co-administration of xenogenic MHC class-I DNA. Gene Ther 17(4):531–540

Khan AS, Smith LC, Abruzzese RV, Cummings KK, Pope MA, Brown PA, Draghia-Akli R (2003) Optimization of electroporation parameters for the intramuscular delivery of plasmids in pigs. DNA Cell Biol 22(12):807–814

Laddy DJ, Yan J, Kutzler M, Kobasa D, Kobinger GP, Khan AS, Greenhouse J, Sardesai NY, Draghia-Akli R, Weiner DB (2008) Heterosubtypic protection against pathogenic human and avian influenza viruses via in vivo electroporation of synthetic consensus DNA antigens. PLoS ONE 3(6):e2517

LeBlanc R, Vasquez Y, Hannaman D, Kumar N (2008) Markedly enhanced immunogenicity of a Pfs25 DNA-based malaria transmission-blocking vaccine by in vivo electroporation. Vaccine 26(2):185–192

Liu L, Fang Q, Deng F, Wang H, Yi CE, Ba L, Yu W, Lin RD, Li T, Hu Z, Ho DD, Zhang L, Chen Z (2007) Natural mutations in the receptor binding domain of spike glycoprotein determine the reactivity of cross-neutralization between palm civet coronavirus and severe acute respiratory syndrome coronavirus. J Virol 81(9):4694–4700

Livingston BD, Little SF, Luxembourg A, Ellefsen B, Hannaman D (2010) Comparative performance of a licensed anthrax vaccine versus electroporation based delivery of a PA encoding DNA vaccine in rhesus macaques. Vaccine 28(4):1056–1061

Luxembourg A, Hannaman D, Ellefsen B, Nakamura G, Bernard R (2006) Enhancement of immune responses to an HBV DNA vaccine by electroporation. Vaccine 24(21):4490–4493

Luxembourg A, Evans CF, Hannaman D (2007) Electroporation-based DNA immunisation: translation to the clinic. Expert Opin Biol Ther 7(11):1647–1664

Luxembourg A, Hannaman D, Nolan E, Ellefsen B, Nakamura G, Chau L, Tellez O, Little S, Bernard R (2008a) Potentiation of an anthrax DNA vaccine with electroporation. Vaccine 26(40):5216–5222

Luxembourg A, Hannaman D, Wills K, Bernard R, Tennant BC, Menne S, Cote PJ (2008b) Immunogenicity in mice and rabbits of DNA vaccines expressing woodchuck hepatitis virus antigens. Vaccine 26(32):4025–4033

Mathiesen I (1999) Electropermeabilization of skeletal muscle enhances gene transfer in vivo. Gene Ther 6(4):508–514

Mir LM, Bureau MF, Rangara R, Schwartz B, Scherman D (1998) Long-term, high level in vivo gene expression after electric pulse-mediated gene transfer into skeletal muscle. C R Acad Sci III 321(11):893–899

Mir LM, Moller PH, Andre F, Gehl J (2005) Electric pulse-mediated gene delivery to various animal tissues. Adv Genet 54:83–114

Mooney H (2009) E.U. laws to enforce needlestick safety. Nurs Times 105(22):1

Nchinda G, Kuroiwa J, Oks M, Trumpfheller C, Park CG, Huang Y, Hannaman D, Schlesinger SJ, Mizenina O, Nussenzweig MC, Uberla K, Steinman RM (2008) The efficacy of DNA vaccination is enhanced in mice by targeting the encoded protein to dendritic cells. J Clin Invest 118(4):1427–1436

NCT00471133 (2009) Safety and immunogenicity of a melanoma DNA vaccine delivered by electroporation. http://clinicaltrials.gov/ct2/show/NCT00471133. Accessed 30 Nov., 2009

NCT00545987 (2009) Study of a potential preventive vaccine against HIV in healthy volunteers (ADVAX-EP). http://clinicaltrials.gov/ct2/show/NCT00545987. Accessed 27 Nov., 2009

NCT01138410 (2010) Study of a DNA immunotherapy to treat melanoma. http://clinicaltrials.gov/ct2/show/NCT01138410. Accessed 30 Nov., 2010

NCT01169077 (2010) EP1300 polyepitope DNA vaccine against *Plasmodium falciparum* malaria. http://clinicaltrials.gov/ct2/show/NCT01169077. Accessed 30 Nov., 2010

Nishi T, Yoshizato K, Yamashiro S, Takeshima H, Sato K, Hamada K, Kitamura I, Yoshimura T, Saya H, Kuratsu J, Ushio Y (1996) High-efficiency in vivo gene transfer using intraarterial plasmid DNA injection following in vivo electroporation. Cancer Res 56(5):1050–1055

Nomura M, Nakata Y, Inoue T, Uzawa A, Itamura S, Nerome K, Akashi M, Suzuki G (1996) In vivo induction of cytotoxic T lymphocytes specific for a single epitope introduced into an unrelated molecule. J Immunol Methods 193(1):41–49

Ohlschlager P, Spies E, Alvarez G, Quetting M, Groettrup M (2010) The combination of TLR-9 adjuvantation and electroporation-mediated delivery enhances in vivo antitumor responses after vaccination with HPV-16 E7 encoding DNA. Int J Cancer 128(2):473–481

Okino M, Mohri H (1987) Effects of a high-voltage electrical impulse and an anticancer drug on in vivo growing tumors. Jpn J Cancer Res 78(12):1319–1321

Otten G, Schaefer M, Doe B, Liu H, Srivastava I, Otten G, Schaefer M, Doe B, Liu H, Srivastava I, zur Megede J, O'Hagan D, Donnelly J, Widera G, Rabussay D, Lewis MG, Barnett S, Ulmer JB (2004) Enhancement of DNA vaccine potency in rhesus macaques by electroporation. Vaccine 22(19):2489–2493

Poland GA, Borrud A, Jacobson RM, McDermott K, Wollan PC, Brakke D, Charboneau JW (1997) Determination of deltoid fat pad thickness. Implications for needle length in adult immunization. JAMA 277(21):1709–1711

Rabussay D (2008) Applicator and electrode design for in vivo DNA delivery by electroporation. Meth Mol Biol 423:35–59

Schaldach M, Hubmann M, Hardt R, Weikl A (1989) Titanium nitride cardiac pacemaker electrodes. Biomed Tech (Berl) 34(7–8):185–190

Schaldach M, Hubmann M, Weikl A, Hardt R (1990) Sputter-deposited TiN electrode coatings for superior sensing and pacing performance. Pacing Clin Electrophysiol 13(12 Pt 2):1891–1895

Selby M, Goldbeck C, Pertile T, Walsh R, Ulmer J (2000) Enhancement of DNA vaccine potency by electroporation in vivo. J Biotechnol 83(1–2):147–152

Somiari S, Glasspool-Malone J, Drabick JJ, Gilbert RA, Heller R, Jaroszeski MJ, Malone RW (2000) Theory and in vivo application of electroporative gene delivery. Mol Ther 2(3):178–187

Tenbusch M, Grunwald T, Niezold T, Storcksdieck Genannt Bonsmann M, Hannaman D, Norley S, Uberla K (2010) Codon-optimization of the hemagglutinin gene from the novel swine origin H1N1 influenza virus has differential effects on CD4(+) T-cell responses and immune effector mechanisms following DNA electroporation in mice. Vaccine 28(19):3273–3277

Titomirov AV, Sukharev S, Kistanova E (1991) In vivo electroporation and stable transformation of skin cells of newborn mice by plasmid DNA. Biochim Biophys Acta 1088(1):131–134

Tjelle TE, Rabussay D, Ottensmeier C, Mathiesen I, Kjeken R (2008) Taking electroporation-based delivery of DNA vaccination into humans: a generic clinical protocol. Methods Mol Biol 423:497–507

Ulmer JB, Wahren B, Liu MA (2006) Gene-based vaccines: recent technical and clinical advances. Trends Mol Med 12(5):216–222

van Drunen Littel-van den Hurk S, Hannaman D (2010) Electroporation for DNA immunization: clinical application. Expert Rev Vaccines 9(5):503–517

van Drunen Littel-van den Hurk S, Babiuk SL, Babiuk LA (2004) Strategies for improved formulation and delivery of DNA vaccines to veterinary target species. Immunol Rev 199:113–125

van Drunen Littel-van den Hurk S, Luxembourg A, Ellefsen B, Wilson D, Ubach A, Hannaman D, van den Hurk JV (2008) Electroporation-based DNA transfer enhances gene expression and immune responses to DNA vaccines in cattle. Vaccine 26(43):5503–5509

van Drunen Littel-van den Hurk S, Lawman Z, Wilson D, Luxembourg A, Ellefsen B, van den Hurk JV, Hannaman D (2010) Electroporation enhances immune responses and protection induced by a bovine viral diarrhea virus DNA vaccine in newborn calves with maternal antibodies. Vaccine 28(39):6445–6454

Vasan S, Hurley A, Schlesinger SJ, Hannaman D, Gardiner DF, Dugin DP, Boente-Carrera M, Vittorino R, Caskey M, Andersen J, Huang Y, Cox JH, Tarragona-Fiol T, Gill DK, Cheeseman H, Clark L, Dally L, Smith C, Schmidt C, Park HH, Kopycinski JT, Gilmour J, Fast P, Bernard R, Ho DD. In vivo electroporation enhances the immunogenicity of an HIV-1 DNA vaccine candidate in healthy volunteers. PLoS One 2011;6(5):e19252

Widera G, Austin M, Rabussay D, Goldbeck C, Barnett SW, Chen M, Leung L, Otten GR, Thudium K, Selby MJ, Ulmer JB (2000) Increased DNA vaccine delivery and immunogenicity by electroporation in vivo. J Immunol 164(9):4635–4640

Wong TW, Chen CH, Huang CC, Lin CD, Hui SW (2006) Painless electroporation with a new needle-free microelectrode array to enhance transdermal drug delivery. J Control Release 110(3):557–565

Yi CE, Ba L, Zhang L, Ho DD, Chen Z (2005) Single amino acid substitutions in the severe acute respiratory syndrome coronavirus spike glycoprotein determine viral entry and immunogenicity of a major neutralizing domain. J Virol 79(18):11638–11646

Zimmermann U, Pilwat G, Holzapfel C, Rosenheck K (1976) Electrical hemolysis of human and bovine red blood cells. J Membr Biol 30(2):135–152

Zucchelli S, Capone S, Fattori E, Folgori A, Di Marco A, Casimiro D, Simon AJ, Laufer R, La Monica N, Cortese R, Nicosia A (2000) Enhancing B- and T-cell immune response to a hepatitis C virus E2 DNA vaccine by intramuscular electrical gene transfer. J Virol 74(24):11598–11607

Prime Boost Regimens for Enhancing Immunity: Magnitude, Quality of Mucosal and Systemic Gene Vaccines

9

Danushka K. Wijesundara and Charani Ranasinghe

The use of therapeutic or prophylactic vaccines against numerous infectious agents has been well documented. The hallmark of most vaccine strategies is to mimic infection and induce immunological memory that has the potential to confer protection. The use of live attenuated viruses, "killed" viruses and recombinant viral proteins for vaccination are classical vaccine approaches that have successfully induced protective antibody and cell mediated immune responses (CMI) against viruses such as small pox, influenza, polio, mumps, measles, and rubella. Despite the successes of classical vaccine approaches, these have been ineffective against chronic and highly pathogenic diseases such as human immunodeficiency virus-1 (HIV-1), tuberculosis (TB) or malaria. Hence, this paved the way for the emergence of range of novel vaccine approaches. In particular, the use of recombinant vector technologies such as the use of recombinant DNA (rDNA) or recombinant live virus vectors encoding single or multiple epitopes used in prime-boost vaccination strategies have exhibited immense potential for generating excellent immunity against intracellular pathogens such as *M. tuberculosis*, HIV-1, simian immunodeficiency virus (SIV), *Plasmodium*, *Leishmania*, *S. mansoni*, hepatitis C virus, herpes simplex virus and hepatitis B virus. In this chapter, we discuss the use of gene based heterologous prime-boost immunisation strategies for improved vaccination against intracellular pathogens, particularly with respect to HIV-1, given that prime-boost vaccine strategies have been extensively tested and studied against this virus in animal models as well as in humans.

C. Ranasinghe (✉)
Department of Immunology, Molecular Mucosal Vaccine Immunology Group
The John Curtin School of Medical Research, The Australian National University,
Canberra, ACT, Australia
e-mail: Charani.Ranasinghe@anu.edu.au

J. Thalhamer et al. (eds.), *Gene Vaccines*,
DOI 10.1007/978-3-7091-0439-2_9, © Springer-Verlag/Wien, 2012

What is Heterologous Prime-Boost Immunisation?

Heterologous prime-boost immunization is a consecutive immunization strategy whereby initially antigens of interest are encoded in rDNA or recombinant live viral vectors such as pox viral vectors (Corbett et al. 2008; Coupar et al. 2006; Kent et al. 2005; Ranasinghe et al. 2006; Wright et al. 2004), influenza (Gherardi et al. 2003), or adenovirus (Xiang et al. 1999; Shiver et al. 2002; Sekaly 2008), which are used for immunization to prime an individual's immune response against the vector-encoded antigens (Fig. 9.1). Subsequently, few weeks following the prime the same antigens are delivered in genetically distinct (heterologous) vectors to boost or amplify the number of antigen-specific effector/memory lymphocytes to encoded vaccine antigens (Fig. 9.1). The use of heterologous vectors mainly circumvents the anti-vector immunity, which can dampen vector-encoded antigen processing and

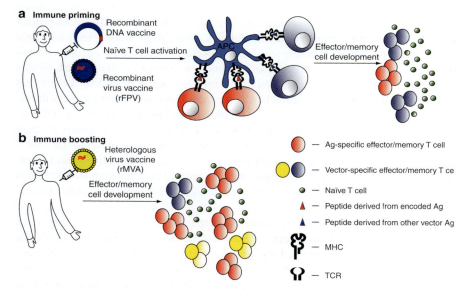

Fig. 9.1 Heterologous prime-boost immunisation. (**a**) In immune priming, antigens (Ag) of interest (red) encoded in a recombinant DNA vector or a recombinant live virus vector (i.e. fowl pox virus, rFPV) is used for immunisation of an individual. These vectors tend to infect antigen presenting cells (APCs) usually in the case of viral vectors or get taken up by APCs through phagocytic mechanisms. Peptide components of these vectors are then presented to naïve T cells via peptide-major histocompatibility complexes (pMHC), which facilitates naïve T cell activation and subsequent differentiation of activated T cells into effector/memory T cells. Following immune priming, the periphery T cell pool is expected to comprise primarily of naïve T cells (green) and relatively small proportion of effector/memory T cells specific to the encoded vaccine antigen of interest (red) or specific to vector components (blue). (**b**) In immune boosting, same vaccine antigens (red) are delivered in a heterologous viral vector such as modified vaccinia Ankara – rMVA (yellow) to minimise the anti-vector immunity. Hence, following heterologous booster immunisation the number of memory T cells against the desired vaccine antigens gets further expanded

9 Prime Boost Regimens for Enhancing Immunity

immune responses against these antigens. Recombinant proteins have also been used in booster immunisation strategies. However, if more than one booster immunisation is involved then following a vector-encoded antigen boost, usage of protein formulations of antigens have been proven to be of great value as antigens could be delivered in their native form to be immunogenic without the requirement of vector-based processing of antigens (Epstein et al. 2004; Stambas et al. 2005; Yang et al. 2008; Demberg et al. 2008). This would avert the risk of anti-vector immunity, which may occur. If genetically similar vectors were used for immune priming and boosting.

Use of rDNA and/or Recombinant Virus Prime-Boost Immunisation Against Intracellular Pathogens

The use of rDNA vaccines to induce immune responses against pathogens emerged in the early 1990s. Wolf and co-workers demonstrated that intramuscular delivery of recombinant plasmid DNA constructs could drive protein expression of the plasmid encoded reporter genes in muscle cells of mice (Wolff et al. 1990). Similarly Fuller et al. for the first time demonstrated that gene-gun delivery of plasmid containing HIV-1 gp120 gene could generate effective humoral and cytotoxic T cell (CTL) immunity in mice (Fuller and Haynes 1994). Since then many subsequent studies have demonstrated that rDNA vaccines could be delivered in various different routes (i.e. intramuscular (i.m.), intradermal (i.d.), intraperitoneal (i.p.), intravenous (i.v.)) without significantly affecting the capacity of these plasmids to drive gene expression. Furthermore, it has also been shown that rDNA vaccines after formulation with cationic lipid complexes (Klavinskis et al. 1999) or cholera toxins (Hagiwara et al. 2006; Cox et al. 2006) could be delivered via mucosal routes such as, oral, intra vaginal, intra rectal (i.r.) or intranasal (i.n.) routes to generate mucosal immunity.

There are many advantages associated with the use of rDNA vaccines: (a) safety due to plasmids being non-infectious, non-replicating and non-integrating into the host genome; (b) ability to persist prolonged periods following vaccination; (c) ability of these vaccines to be prepared large-scale in a cost-effective manner; (d) ability to clone multiple immunogens and co-express various molecular adjuvants on the same vector. Despite these numerous advantages, the sole use of rDNA vectors for immunisation against highly pathogenic intracellular organisms have proven to be ineffective. Hence, researchers have also attempted to use recombinant live virus vectors, in particular pox virus vectors (i.e. fowl pox virus (FPV), New York vaccinia (NYVAC), canary pox and modified vaccinia Ankara (MVA)) and adenoviruses (i.e. adenovirus serotype 5 (Ad5)), encoding antigens of interest to enhance antigen expression to levels that is not achievable using rDNA vaccines. Recombinant live virus vectors can infect cells unlike rDNA constructs and consist of robust promoters that can efficiently drive gene expression in mammalian cells. Most of these recombinant vectors are unable to replicate in human cells (i.e. FPV and MVA), and have been proven to be safe in humans (Moorthy et al. 2004; Kelleher et al. 2006), thus minimise adverse side effects, especially in immuno-compromised individuals. However, similar to rDNA vectors alone, the use of recombinant live virus vectors alone have also resulted in disappointing outcomes, due to their inability to generate long lasting immunity against chronic diseases like HIV and TB.

Hence, consecutive immunisation strategy, referred to as heterologous prime-boost immunisation, whereby antigens of interest are sequentially exposed to the immune system using different vectors was developed (Leong et al. 1994; Ramsay et al. 1997). Numerous studies since then have shown that heterologous prime-boost immunisation can significantly enhance the magnitude of CMI responses (i.e. CTL responses) against encoded antigens compared to homologous prime-boost immunisation (Boyer et al. 1997; Amara et al. 2001). Heterologous HIV-1, rDNA/rFPV prime-boost immunization has been shown to generate enhanced systemic and mucosal CTL responses in mice and macaques, and protection against pathogenic challenge (Kent et al. 1998, 2005). Similarly, Amara et al. also showed that an HIV rDNA prime followed by rMVA boost immunization can also generate protective immunity against a highly pathogenic HIV intra rectal (i.r.) challenge in a rhesus macaque model 7 months post booster immunization (Amara et al. 2001). These observations generated great optimism for potential human HIV-1 rDNA prime-boost vaccines. Furthermore, rDNA priming and rMVA boosting against *Plasmodium* antigens (e.g. thromobospondin-related adhesion protein or TRAP) have also been shown to confer some degree of protection against *P. falciparum* in human clinical trials and generate higher CTL responses than when either vector was used alone or when vaccine vectors were used in a homologous prime-boost manner (Hill et al. 2000; McConkey et al. 2003). Also, following rDNA/rMVA prime-boost immunization with vectors expressing TB antigen 85A (Ag85A) and a fusion protein of 6-kDa early secretory antigenic target (ESAT-6) and Ag85B, significantly higher IFN-γ secreting CD4+ T-cell responses were reported in guinea pigs and this vaccine regime offered better protection compared to BCG alone (Williams et al. 2005). rDNA prime-*Mycobacterium bovis* BCG boost vaccination strategy in cattle also has shown to induce significantly enhanced protection against bovine tuberculosis, compared to BCG alone (Skinner et al. 2003). Similarly, rDNA/BCG strategy was also shown to induce increased CD4+ T cell responses, specific antibody responses and superior protection against virulent *M. bovis* compared to the rDNA or BCG alone strategies (Cai et al. 2006). Moreover, in a *Leishmaniasis major* prime-boost study, DNA-LACK/MVA-LACK (*Leishmania* homologue of the mammalian receptor for activated C kinase) immunization was shown to generate greater IFN-γ and TNF-α expression by CD8+ T cells and protective immunity in mice (Perez-Jimenez et al. 2006). Recently, rDNA prime and Venezuelan equine encephalitis virus like-replicon particles (VRP) boost encoding the six-transmembrane epithelial antigen of the prostate (STEAP) was also shown to induce enhanced poly-functional T cells (that produced IFN-γ, TNF-α and IL-2) which significantly delayed prostate tumor growth when compared to either of the vaccine modality alone (Garcia-Hernandez Mde et al. 2007).

Overall, these observations clearly suggest that heterologous rDNA prime-boost vaccine strategies can generate enhanced immunity across various different infectious models compared to stand-alone vaccine strategies or homologous prime-boost vaccine strategies. Unfortunately, due to the poor outcomes generated in human clinical trials with rDNA prime-boost vaccination strategies (most likely due to the problems associated with dose of rDNA) (Kelleher et al. 2006), viral-viral and viral-protein prime-boost immunization strategies have also been investigated against diseases such as malaria (Anderson et al. 2004; Moorthy et al. 2004), hepatitis B (Hutchings et al. 2005), TB (Vordermeier et al. 2009) and HIV-1 (Corbett et al. 2008; Ranasinghe et al. 2006), which have been shown to generate greater magnitude of T cell immunity compared to rDNA/viral or protein prime-boost strategies. However, recently rDNA electroporation EP (Wallace et al. 2009) or nanopatch (Chen et al. 2009) delivery using minimal amount of rDNA have shown to be more effective at generating enhanced expression of the encoded vaccine antigens *in vivo*. Hence, these novel strategies have once again revived optimism of usage of rDNA prime-boost strategies for diseases such as HIV-1, TB and also cancer (Brave et al. 2010; Buchan et al. 2005).

The Importance of Cell-Mediated Immunity Against Intracellular Pathogens

The success of heterologous prime-boost immunisation in conferring protection against intracellular pathogens is largely dependent on the induction of robust type 1 (Th1) immune responses or cell-mediate immunity. Numerous prime-boost vaccination studies in the context of HIV-1, tuberculosis, *Leishmania major* and malaria have shown that CMI, even in the absence of neutralising antibodies at occasions, can confer protection against these pathogens (Robinson et al. 1999; Ramshaw and Ramsay 2000; Skinner et al. 2003; Darrah et al. 2007). Th1 immunity involves activation of CTLs, natural killer (NK) cells and the production of type 1 cytokines (e.g. interferon (IFN)-γ, interleukin (IL)-2 and tumor necrosis factor (TNF-α) whilst type 2 (Th2) immunity is more involved in the activation of B cells, production of high titres of antibodies and Th2 cytokines such as IL-4, IL-10 and IL-13 (Spellberg and Edwards 2001). TNF-α and IFN-γ can directly function to trigger apoptotic pathways on infected cells and enhance activation of immune cells such as CTLs, macrophages and NK cells. CTLs are directly involved in mediating cytolysis of cells infected with intracellular pathogens. They recognize peptide-major histocompatibility complex class one (MHC-I) complexes presented on the surface of pathogen-infected cells. This recognition triggers CTL cytotoxic machinery causing apoptosis of infected cells and secretion of cytokines that are crucial for controlling infection. Early recognition and cytolysis of virus-infected cells is important to minimize virus spread and replication.

Due to the dichotomous nature of Th1 and Th2 immunity, it is often difficult to envisage both types of immunity occurring at similar magnitudes. Hence, the type of immunity achieved following infection with a pathogen or even following vaccination tends to be biased towards Th1 or Th2 immunity. The choice of vaccine vectors used for prime-boost immunisation tends to bias the type of immunity

(Th1 versus Th2) acquired. rDNA or attenuated live virus vectors (e.g. rFPV and rMVA) have been known to bias Th1 immune responses following prime-boost immunisation (Leong et al. 1995; Estcourt et al. 2002). It is believed that plasmids used for DNA vaccination may enter MHC-I antigen presentation pathway either via direct expression of plasmid DNA in dendritic cells or through antigen cross-presentation (Gurunathan et al. 2000). Endogenous protein expression leads to presentation of expressed protein components (i.e. peptides) through the MHC-I presentation pathway, which is responsible for priming naïve CD8+ T cells. In antigen cross-presentation, dendritic cell mediated phagocytosis of secreted peptides (derived from plasmid DNA expressed in somatic cells or other antigen presenting cells), which is usually presented through the MHC-II presentation pathway, may enter the MHC-I presentation pathway. The exact mechanisms responsible for antigen cross-presentation are not yet known, but have been demonstrated in few studies (Staerz et al. 1987; Harding and Song 1994). Furthermore, rDNA vaccines are usually constructed from *E.coli* derived plasmids, which contain unmethylated CpG motifs. These motifs have been known to promote the production of pro-inflammatory Th1 cytokines such as IL-12, which enhances the development of Th1 immunity. Recombinant live viruses retain the ability to infect cells such as dendritic cells and thereby stimulate innate immune responses (Zhong et al. 1999). In contrast, recombinant proteins have been known to bias Th2 immune responses given that exogenous proteins usually enter the MHC-II antigen-processing pathway (Stambas et al. 2005).

Enhancement of Vaccine Specific Immunity by Co-Expression of Molecular Adjuvants

Co-expression of cytokines, chemokines and other molecules together with vaccine antigens have been utilised to enhance magnitude of immune responses to vaccine antigens. Adjuvants that has been used include: danger signals such as unmethylated CpG motifs, cytokines such as IFN-α/β, IFN-γ, IL-12, IL-15 and IL-18 (Boyer et al. 2005; Day et al. 2008; Gherardi et al. 2000; Kozlowski and Neutra 2003; Kutzler et al. 2005; Ranasinghe et al. 2007; Tapia et al. 2003) and chemokines CCL2, CCL3, CCL5 (Boyer et al. 1999; Lillard et al. 2001) and also lymphocyte co-stimulatory molecules CD40L, B7-1, ICAM-1, and LFA-3 (Liu et al. 2008; Oh et al. 2003). Also, molecules such as 41BBL have been used in booster vaccination to enhance magnitude of T cell immunity (Harrison et al. 2006). For instance, rDNA plasmids encoding influenza hemagglutinin (HA) and IL-6 have shown to augment anti-HA IgG and IgA responses whilst rDNA plasmids co-expressing HA and IL-12 was shown to augment CTL responses against HA (Ramsay et al. 1999). We have also found that to enhance immunity adjuvants such as IL-12 should be delivered in the priming phase rather than the booster immunisation (Ranasinghe and Ramsay unpublished observations; (Ranasinghe et al. 2006). However, even though many of these adjuvants have shown to enhance magnitude of T cell responses, we have observed that following prime-boost vaccination not many molecular adjuvants are

9 Prime Boost Regimens for Enhancing Immunity

capable of enhancing the avidity of T cell immunity (Ranasinghe and Ramshaw 2009a) (Ranasinghe, manuscript in preparation). Furthermore, we have also found that to generate high avidity CTL the molecular adjuvant should preferentially be delivered in the priming phase, not the booster immunisation (Ranasinghe, manuscript in preparation).

The Importance of T Cell Avidity Following Vaccination

Another important factor known to be crucial for control of intracellular pathogens is T cell quality or avidity. More and more studies have shown that T cell avidity (Alexander-Miller 2005) and poly-functionality or the ability of CD8+ T cells to secrete multiple cytokines such as IFN-γ, IL-2 and TNF-α are crucial for protection against intracellular pathogens (Ahmed and Gottschalk 2009; Duvall et al. 2006; Ferre et al. 2009; McCormack et al. 2008; Sekaly 2008; Imrie et al. 2007). T cell avidity can be defined as the amount of cognate peptide-MHC complexes required for T cell activation. It has been well established that high avidity T cells are more effective at recognising low concentrations of antigen and controlling virus infection than low avidity T cells which only are able to recognise high concentrations of antigen on target cells (Fig. 9.2) (Derby et al. 2001; Bihl et al. 2006). This suggests that high avidity CTLs can mediate cytolysis of virus-infected target cells early on following infection given that lower levels of viral antigens are expected to be expressed early on following infection of target cells. T cells are multipotential in nature and they have the capacity to produce numerous different Th1 and Th2 cytokines (Kelso and Groves 1997). For this reason there is a diverse functional heterogeneity amongst the T cell population of an individual. Increasing number of studies suggest that the presence of antigen-specific T cells that have the capacity to secrete multiple Th1 cytokines, especially IFN-γ, TNF-α and IL-2 better correlate with protection than antigen-specific T cells that have the capacity to produce simply IFN-γ (Seder et al. 2008).

Prime-boost immunisation of macaques against SIV has shown that SIV-specific CD8+ T cells that produce IFN-γ and TNF-α correlate with protection against SIV infection and better control of this virus (Hansen et al. 2009). Similar findings have been observed in HIV-1 infected patients in that individuals that possess higher numbers of HIV-specific CD8+ T cells that produce IFN-γ and TNF-α are better able to control HIV-1 than individuals that possess lower numbers of such polyfunctional CD8+ T cells (Almeida et al. 2007). Furthermore, CTLs that produce multiple Th1 cytokines appear to be of higher avidity than CTLs that produce Th2 cytokines, for example IL-4 and IL-13 (Kienzle et al. 2004; La Gruta et al. 2004; Ranasinghe and Ramshaw 2009b; Ranasinghe et al. 2007). We have shown that depending on the route of delivery of poxvirus vectors in a prime-boost regime, the avidity of CTLs can be vastly different. We have also shown that mucosal vaccination can generate more high avidity CTLs compared to pure systemic vaccination, and the avidity is inversely correlated to the expression of IL-4 and IL-13 by CTLs (Table 9.1). Overall, more and more studies are indicating that rather than the

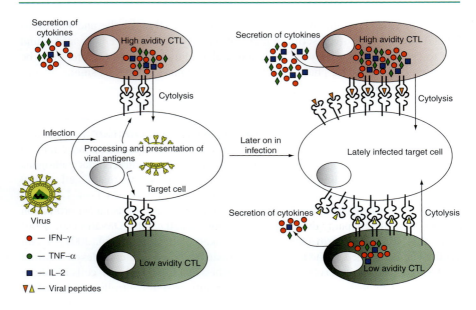

Fig. 9.2 T cell quality is defined by polyfunctionality and avidity and is an important parameter in the control of intracellular pathogens. This diagram shows the importance of T cell avidity in the context of a viral infection. Early on following viral infection of a target cell, lower levels of viral proteins are produced compared to a lately infected target cell. Therefore, presentation of viral pMHC complexes is expected to occur at low levels in early-infected target cells. These target cells are usually recognized and eliminated by high avidity CTLs given that high avidity CTLs recognise lower amounts of cognate pMHC complexes than low avidity CTLs to trigger effector functions (i.e. target cell cytolysis and secretion of cytokines). High avidity CTLs are also often poly-functional in nature and are able to secret multiple Th1 cytokines (i.e. TNF-α, IFN-γ, IL-2). Low avidity CTLs usually require much higher densities of viral pMHC complexes to be presented on target cells to trigger effector functions compared to high avidity CTLs. Therefore, low avidity CTLs mediate cytolysis of lately infected target cells. Low avidity CTLs are thought to be poorly poly-functional (i.e. may secrete only one Th1 cytokine – IFN-γ), but may produce multiple Th2 cytokines (i.e. IL-4 and IL-13; see also Table 9.2)

Table 9.1 Route dependent expression of IL-4/IL-13 cytokines and dependence of avidity and magnitude of CTL immunity following HIV-1 prime-boost vaccination

Route of delivery	Mice	Magnitude of HIV-specific CTL immunity	IL-4/IL-13 expression by HIV-specific CTLs	CTL avidity
Pure mucosal i.n./i.n.	BALB/c	+	+	High
	IL-13[-/-]	+	–	High
Combined mucosal systemic i.n./i.m.	BALB/c	+++	++	Medium
	IL-13[-/-]	+++	–	High
Pure systemic i.m./i.m.	BALB/c	+++	+++	Low
	IL-13[-/-]	+++	–	High

Mice were primed with rFPV encoding HIV-1 genes *gag, pol, env, rev and tet* and boosted with rVV encoding *gag* and *pol*. All mice were on BALB/c background, *i.n.*, intranasal, *i.m.*, intramuscular. Magnitude of response was measured by IFN-γ production

9 Prime Boost Regimens for Enhancing Immunity

magnitude of T cell responses the presence of optimal numbers of high quality (i.e. high avidity and poly-functional) antigen-specific T cells is desirable in achieving the best protective outcomes against intracellular pathogens.

Prime-Boost Vaccine Strategies to Generate Mucosal Immunity

The presence of immune responses against pathogens at sites where they are first encountered is known to be crucial to prevent or minimize the systemic spread of these pathogens. Over 90% of pathogens are first encountered in the mucosae (Ogra 1999, 2001; Kiyono and Fukuyama 2004). Hence, there is growing interest to optimise vaccine strategies for the induction of robust mucosal immunity especially against mucosal pathogens. With respect to HIV-1, the induction of robust anti-HIV mucosal immune responses is crucial mainly due to: (a) more than 80% of global HIV-1 transmissions are thought to occur through sexual exposure of the genitorectal mucosa (Musey et al. 1997); (b) the primary CD4+ depletion and HIV-1 replication predominantly occurs in the gut mucosa (Veazey et al. 1998, 2001) and (c) systemic spread of HIV-1 from the initial mucosal sites of viral entry results in the establishment of a greater pool of latent viruses and virus quasi-species (mutants), which makes it extremely difficult for an infected individual's immune system to control infection (McMichael et al. 2010). The presence of strong sustained mucosal immunity (i.e. lung immune responses) is also important for protection against diseases like influenza and TB, given that these pathogens are first encountered and spread via aerosol through the upper respiratory tract (Santosuosso et al. 2005; Kallenius et al. 2007).

Mucosal delivery (i.e. oral, intranasal, intradermal, intrarectal or intranasal) of vaccine vectors has been successful in inducing protective immune responses against influenza virus, *M. tuberculosis*, *S. typhi*, polio virus, *V. cholera*, SIV, and HIV-1. In principle, to generate effective mucosal immunity a vaccine has to be delivered to the mucosae (Ogra et al. 2001). Many studies have shown that generating "strong sustained mucosal immunity" following systemic vaccination has been a difficult task, despite some systemic (i.e. intramuscular) immunisation strategies eliciting some mucosal immunity (Pal et al. 2006; Kaufman et al. 2008). In our studies we have found that HIV-FPV i.m./HIV-VV i.m. prime-boost immunisation can generate mucosal immunity 3 days following booster vaccination but these responses were short lived (Ranasinghe et al. 2007). However, many mucosal prime-boost immunisation strategies have facilitated the development of more effective, long lasting and high avidity mucosal immune responses compared to pure systemic prime-boost immunisations in local and distal mucosa where pathogens are initially encountered (Belyakov and Ahlers 2009a; Belyakov et al. 2006; Kantele et al. 1998; Kent et al. 2005; Ranasinghe et al. 2007). This is mainly due to the existence of a common mucosal system comprised of gastrointestinal, respiratory and genital mucosae, where lymphocyte encounter of pathogens at one site could result in migration of these lymphocytes to another mucosal site via the expression of mucosal homing markers such as integrins $\alpha_4\beta_7, \alpha_4\beta_1$ and chemokine receptor (CCR) 9 on antigen-specific lymphocytes. It is well established that $\alpha_4\beta_7$ (Wagner et al. 1996) and CCR9 (Bowman et al. 2002) are required in efficient trafficking of IgA-antibody-secreting cells migrating to the gut. We have found that systemic (i.e. intramuscular) prime-boost immunisation against HIV-1 are less efficient in inducing the expression of mucosal homing markers in HIV-specific CD8+ T cells compared to mucosal (i.e. intranasal) prime-boost immunisation against HIV-1. This further supports the fact that mucosal immunisation strategies are most effective in the induction of mucosal immunity. Nonetheless, mucosal immunisation at one site may not necessarily facilitate the development of optimal universal mucosal immunity or optimal immunity at all distal mucosal sites. For instance, individuals immunised i.r. against *S. typhi* using a live attenuated *S. typhi* vaccine (Ty21a) were shown to have significantly higher levels of antibody secreting cells (IgA and IgG) in nasal secretion, rectum and tears compared to orally vaccinated individuals with Ty21a (Kantele et al. 1998). On the contrary, orally vaccinated individuals in this instance were found to possess higher numbers of antibody secreting cells in saliva and vaginal secretion compared to i.r. vaccinated individuals (Kantele et al. 1998). We have also found that HIV-FPV oral prime/HIV-VV i.m. booster immunisation was unable to generate good HIV-specific CD8+ T cell immunity in genito-rectal nodes whereas the same vaccine given i.n./i.m. was able to generate robust immunity in these sites (Ranasinghe et al. 2006). These observations clearly indicate that route of delivery is a significant factor when designing effective vaccines against mucosal pathogens such as HIV-1 and TB.

Strategies That Can Be Used to Enhance Protective Outcomes in Prime-Boost Immunisation

Optimisation of prime-boost immunisation strategies holds great promise in enhancing protection conferred against intracellular pathogens. The route of immunisation chosen for prime-boost immunisation is an important parameter for the induction of optimal immunity at desired sites (i.e. mucosae) or sites of initial pathogen encounter. To achieve this, delivery of vaccine vectors via routes that mimic natural infection appears to be most favourable. For instance, it has been shown that intranasal prime-boost immunisation strategies confer protection against respiratory pathogens that enter hosts intranasally such as influenza (Perrone et al. 2009). Similarly, it has been shown that intrarectal prime-boost immunisation of macaques against simian-human immunodeficiency virus (SHIV) confers protection against a lethal intrarectal SHIV challenge (Belyakov et al. 2001). The route for vaccine vector delivery chosen for immune priming versus the boosting is also important for the induction of optimal desired immunity. We have found in mice that were immunised using purely mucosal (i.n./i.n.) HIV-1 prime-boost vaccination significantly lower levels of HIV-specific CD8+ T cell responses compared to purely systemic (i.m./i.m.) prime-boost vaccination, but the avidity of HIV-specific CD8+ T cells generated was lower in the purely systemic compared to the purely mucosal regime (Ranasinghe et al. 2007). On the contrary, combined mucosal/systemic (i.n. HIV-FPV/i.m. HIV-VV) prime-boost immunisation was shown to facilitate the development of high numbers of HIV-specific CD8+ T cells both in the systemic and mucosal compartments without significantly compromising the avidity of the HIV-specific CD8+ T cells that had developed following immunisation (Ranasinghe et al. 2007).

Other important parameters that can significantly affect the avidity and magnitude of immunity achieved following prime-boost immunisation include the choice of vaccine vectors, the dose of vaccine vectors used, the choice of antigens and incorporation of relevant molecular adjuvants. rDNA vectors are known to express low levels of antigen persistently to the immune system and are not as efficient as recombinant live virus vectors to induce high magnitude of systemic and mucosal immunity. We have found that when compared to HIV-DNA/HIV-FPV (i.m./i.n.) immunisation, HIV-FPV/HIV-VV (i.n./i.m.) prime-boost immunisation can generate high magnitude as well as high avidity CTL (Ranasinghe and Ramsay, submitted). CD8+ T cells that recognize immunodominant epitopes are known to be of higher avidity (Dzutsev et al. 2007). Therefore, incorporation of immunodominant epitopes for T cell priming can enhance the avidity of the developing effector/memory T cells. The caveat in this instance is that viruses can in some cases mutate immunodominant epitopes to escape CTL recognition (Barouch et al. 2002; Reece et al. 2010). Therefore, it is important to select antigens that encode immunodominant epitopes that when mutated can detrimentally affect fitness of the pathogen in question.

Lessons Learnt from HIV-1 Prime-Boost Clinical Vaccine Trials

Nearly three decades after isolation of HIV-1 as the causative agent of acquired immunodeficiency syndrome (AIDS), (Barre-Sinoussi et al. 1983; Broder and Gallo 1984) a vaccine that can be used for prophylactic or therapeutic purposes is still not available. The development of an effective vaccine against HIV-1 has been difficult due to: (a) extremely high mutation rate of HIV-1, which is mainly due to high error rates of virus reverse transcriptase (Roberts et al. 1988), (b) the extraordinary diversity of HIV-1, due to divergent clades, (Osborn 1995), (c) HIV-1 envelop being heavily glycosylated conferring considerable energy barriers for B-cells to recognize neutralizing epitopes (Kwong et al. 1998), and (d) also not well understanding the immune correlates of protection in humans. Moreover, HIV-1 is also capable of integrating into the host genome and remaining latent for indefinite durations. This makes it nearly impossible to completely clear the virus from an infected host. Nonetheless vaccine strategies, that can reduce HIV-1 viral loads below the thresholds (<1000 viral RNA copies/mL blood) that may facilitate transmission of this virus is deemed to be achievable. This notion has been supported following prime-boost immunisation and SIV/SHIV challenges conducted in non-human primate models (Belyakov et al. 2001; Amara et al. 2001).

Prime-boost vaccines against HIV-1 that have shown clear protective effects in animal models have also failed in numerous human clinical trials (Kelleher et al. 2006). Despite these failures, prime-boost vaccination remains the only vaccine strategy that has shown some protective effect against HIV-1 in human clinical trials (Table 9.2). This was demonstrated recently in one of the largest HIV-1 clinical trials in Thailand, where participants in the vaccine group were primed with ALVAC-HIV or recombinant canary pox virus expressing HIV envelope, *gag* and protease sequences and boosted with AIDSVAX B/E, an HIV-1 envelope protein formulated in alum (Rerks-Ngarm et al. 2009). This trial demonstrated that the vaccine recipients had

Table 9.2 Prime-boost vaccine concepts that have been tested in phase III human clinical trials against HIV-1 and possible causes for their failure

Concept	Most likely causes for failure	Trial references
Induction of protective neutralizing antibody responses via immunisation with recombinant HIV-1 envelope glycoprotein 120 subunit vaccine	Failure to induce broadly neutralising antibodies against HIV-1 Establishment of HIV-1 quasi-species with mutated envelope proteins in infected trial participants	Flynn et al. (2005), Pitisuttithum et al. (2006)
Induction of protective T cell responses via immunisation with recombinant Ad5 encoding HIV-1 *gag*, *pol* and *nef*	The presence of pre-existing immunity against Ad5 vector in vaccines Homologous boosting with Ad5 vector used for vaccination	Priddy et al. (2008), Buchbinder et al. (2008)
Induction of protective T cell and neutralizing antibody responses via immunisation with recombinant canarypox virus (encoding HIV-1 *env*, *gag* and protease) and with protein formulation of HIV-1 envelope glycoprotein 120 subunit vaccine	Only vaccine strategy to show some protective effect (vaccine efficacy of 31%) against HIV-1 in clinical trials Protective efficacy was reduced due to the failure to induce robust CTL immunity and/or broadly neutralizing antibodies	Rerks-Ngarm et al. (2009)

higher levels of neutralizing antibodies and CD4+ T cell responses, but not CD8+ T cell responses against HIV-1 compared to the placebo group (Rerks-Ngarm et al. 2009) (Table 9.2). The weak CD8+ T cell responses in this instance is most likely due to the use of a recombinant protein composition for immune boosting, which typically bias Th2 immune responses, and also possibly the weak expression of protein by canarypox vector. The lack of protection across the majority of individuals in the vaccinated group and the inability of individuals in the vaccine group who got infected with HIV-1 to control HIV-1 viraemia also suggests that CD8+ T cell responses are crucial in controlling HIV-1 and failure to efficiently induce these responses following vaccination may significantly reduce the efficacy of the vaccine being tested.

Historically, HIV-1 prime-boost strategies that have attempted to induce neutralizing antibodies against HIV-1 have not been associated with protective outcomes in human clinical trials despite showing considerable promise in animal models (Pitisuttithum 2005). In these trials, recombinant HIV envelope proteins (i.e. glycoprotein (gp)120 and gp160) from a single clade has been incorporated in vaccine vectors in a prime-boost manner. Currently, researchers have focused on using multiple envelope proteins from different clades (up to five different clades) to account for the antigenic diversity of HIV given that antigenic diversity is the major issue in the induction of protective neutralizing antibody responses against HIV-1. This approach referred to as the cocktail approach has yielded better immune outcomes than vaccines that rely on HIV envelope proteins from a single clade (Chakrabarti et al. 2005; Rollman et al. 2005). The recently concluded human clinical trial in Thailand also implemented the cocktail approach where recombinant envelope proteins from clades B and E were used for prime-boost immunisation.

9 Prime Boost Regimens for Enhancing Immunity

Another prime-boost vaccination approaches have also shown to induce broadly neutralizing antibodies that bind to conserved CD4 binding regions of the HIV envelope protein, which is required for making viral entry into host CD4+ T cells (Mascola and Montefiori 2010). These antibodies are not known to occur at high enough frequency to be protective or are deleted through clonal deletion mechanisms in the course of a natural HIV-1 infection. Despite this, a recently described broadly neutralizing antibody, VRC01, is known to occur at higher frequency than other known broadly neutralizing antibodies against HIV-1 in humans and is capable of neutralizing about 90% of the circulating HIV-1 isolates (Zhou et al. 2010). Thus, the identification of immunogens that may be incorporated into prime-boost vaccines to elicit the production of broadly neutralizing antibodies such as VRC01 are exciting prospects for the development of more effective preventative human HIV-1 vaccines in the future.

Interestingly, individuals who remain resistant to natural HIV-1 infections despite being exposed to this virus have stronger CD8+ T cell immunity than individuals who are more susceptible to HIV-1 infections (Kaul et al. 2000). Following prime-boost immunisation robust CD8+ T cell immune responses have been observed in animal models, but unfortunately these outcomes have not translated effectively into human clinical trials. The main reasons for these failures could to be: (a) The route of vaccine delivery – most human prime-boost vaccine clinical trials have used systemic routes (i.m.), which can compromise the avidity of CD8+ T cell immunity as discussed previously. Interestingly, SIV and SHIV challenge studies in non-human primates have demonstrated that the presence of CD8+ T cell responses at mucosae can effectively control virus infection especially when vaccination is conducted via mucosal routes; (b) Not evaluating mucosal immunity – CD8+ T cell immunity measured in these clinical trials have only measured systemic immunity. Therefore, identifying and evaluating methods (i.e. identifying novel mucosal biomarkers) to measure mucosal CD8+ T cell responses and to safely deliver vaccine vectors via mucosal routes may help develop better HIV-1 prime-boost l vaccines in the future.

The presence of non-vaccine sources of pre-existing immunity against vectors used for immune priming or boosting have been shown to dampen immunity against HIV-1. This was shown in the STEP vaccine trial where pre-existing immunity against Ad5 (vector used for vaccination in this trial) was shown to correlate with the lack of efficacy of the vaccine used in this trial (Buchbinder et al. 2008). This may also be a concern if some poxvirus vectors are used in human clinical trials given that significant proportion of the human population prior to 1980 have been immunised against smallpox. Thus, if vectors were first encountered systemically one way to circumvent pre-existing immunity would be to deliver these vaccines via a mucosal route of pre-existing immunity delivery (Belyakov et al. 1999).

Summary

Heterologous prime-boost immunisation have emerged as a strategy for improved vaccination against highly pathogenic intracellular pathogens, which has been clearly shown to yield more robust immunity compared to homologous prime-boost

Table 9.3 Key points to consider when optimising future prime-boost vaccination strategies

Parameter	Consideration	References
Vaccine delivery route	Mucosal routes provide most robust and best quality mucosal immunity	Belyakov and Ahlers (2009b), Goonetilleke et al. (2003), Perrone et al. (2009), Ranasinghe et al. (2007)
	Systemic routes provide most robust systemic immunity	
	Routes that mimic natural infection are desirable for achieving optimal protection against mucosal pathogens	
Choice of vectors	rDNA vectors provide low-level yet persistent immunity	Pal et al. (2006), Ramsay et al. (1999), Ranasinghe et al. (2006), Rerks-Ngarm et al. (2009), Williams et al. (2005)
	Recombinant live viral vectors usually express high levels of encoded antigens and are ideal for immune priming or boosting.	
	Protein formulations of antigens may also be used for multiple boosting strategies if anti-vector immunity is deemed to be a problem	
Vaccine dose	Higher doses of rDNA or viral vectors provide most robust immunity compared to lower doses of the same vectors when used for vaccination	De Rose et al. (2006), Lane et al. (1969), Ranasinghe et al. (2006), Rollman et al. (2005)
	Depending on the viral vectors used, higher doses may also be lethal for vaccines such as immunodeficient individuals or individuals with immunological disorders.	
Choice of vaccine antigens	Antigens that are immunogenic and that do not mutate in the course of a natural infection with a pathogen are ideal for use in a vaccine	Dormitzer et al. (2008), Dzutsev et al. (2007)
	Immunodominant epitopes may be incorporated into vaccine vectors to augment the development of high avidity CTLs	
Molecular adjuvants	Molecular adjuvants can be used to enhance immunity and also bias the Th1 and Th2 immunity	Boyer et al. (2005), Harrison et al. (2006), Ranasinghe et al. (2006), Spellberg and Edwards (2001), Kolibab et al. (2010), Seppala and Makela (1984), Gupta (1998)
	Adjuvants such as unmethylated CpG, IL-12, IL-15 and CCL5 can be used to enhance Th1 1 immune responses	
	Adjuvants such as lipopolysaccharide (LPS) and alum can be used to enhance Th2 immune responses	
Cytokine milieu	Strategies that can block cytokines such as IL-4 and IL-13 can be used to enhance avidity of CD8+ T cells	Ranasinghe and Ramshaw (2009b), Ranasinghe et al. (2007)

vaccination and stand alone rDNA or live viral vector vaccination strategies. Induction of robust and high quality (i.e. avidity and poly-functional) T cell mediated immunity especially at mucosal surfaces where majority of pathogens are initially encountered is crucial for achieving better protective outcomes against intracellular pathogens. Achieving such immunity is not a simple task and we discussed this using the drawbacks of prime-boost vaccination against HIV-1 in human clinical trials. This example also highlights the importance of acquiring sufficient knowledge regarding fundamental protective immune responses against pathogens, which

9 Prime Boost Regimens for Enhancing Immunity

most likely will facilitate the development of better prime-boost vaccine strategies that will yield high avidity T and B cell immunity with enhanced protection. Unfortunately, to date there is no clear immune correlate of protection against HIV-1. Numerous studies have established range of parameters that need to be optimised when designing more effective prime-boost vaccines. These include the route of vaccine delivery, vaccine vector combinations, the dose and choice of vaccine vectors for the prime versus the boost, choice of appropriate immunodominant epitopes (if peptide based vaccines), cytokine milieu and incorporation of effective systemic and/or mucosal molecular adjuvants that generate high magnitude as well as high avidity CMI (Table 9.3).

Financial Disclosure/Acknowledgements   This work and CR was supported by The Australian National Health and Medical Research Council project grant award 525431 (CR)

Conflict of interest: The authors declare no financial or commercial conflict of interest.

References

Ahmed N, Gottschalk S (2009) How to design effective vaccines: lessons from an old success story. Expert Rev Vaccines 8(5):543–546

Alexander-Miller MA (2005) High-avidity CD8+ T cells: optimal soldiers in the war against viruses and tumors. Immunol Res 31(1):13–24

Almeida JR, Price DA, Papagno L, Arkoub ZA, Sauce D, Bornstein E, Asher TE, Samri A, Schnuriger A, Theodorou I, Costagliola D, Rouzioux C, Agut H, Marcelin AG, Douek D, Autran B, Appay V (2007) Superior control of HIV-1 replication by CD8+ T cells is reflected by their avidity, polyfunctionality, and clonal turnover. J Exp Med 204(10):2473–2485

Amara RR, Villinger F, Altman JD, Lydy SL, O'Neil SP, Staprans SI, Montefiori DC, Xu Y, Herndon JG, Wyatt LS, Candido MA, Kozyr NL, Earl PL, Smith JM, Ma HL, Grimm BD, Hulsey ML, Miller J, McClure HM, McNicholl JM, Moss B, Robinson HL (2001) Control of a mucosal challenge and prevention of AIDS by a multiprotein DNA/MVA vaccine. Science 292(5514):69–74

Anderson RJ, Hannan CM, Gilbert SC, Laidlaw SM, Sheu EG, Korten S, Sinden R, Butcher GA, Skinner MA, Hill AV, Dunachie SJ (2004) Enhanced CD8+ T cell immune responses and protection elicited against *Plasmodium berghei* malaria by prime boost immunization regimens using a novel attenuated fowlpox virus prime-boost strategies for malaria vaccine development. J Immunol 172(5):3094–3100

Barouch DH, Kunstman J, Kuroda MJ, Schmitz JE, Santra S, Peyerl FW, Krivulka GR, Beaudry K, Lifton MA, Gorgone DA, Montefiori DC, Lewis MG, Wolinsky SM, Letvin NL (2002) Eventual AIDS vaccine failure in a rhesus monkey by viral escape from cytotoxic T lymphocytes. Nature 415(6869):335–339

Barre-Sinoussi F, Chermann JC, Rey F, Nugeyre MT, Chamaret S, Gruest J, Dauguet C, Axler-Blin C, Vezinet-Brun F, Rouzioux C, Rozenbaum W, Montagnier L (1983) Isolation of a T-lymphotropic retrovirus from a patient at risk for acquired immune deficiency syndrome (AIDS). Science 220(4599):868–871

Belyakov IM, Ahlers JD (2009a) Comment on "trafficking of antigen-specific CD8+ T lymphocytes to mucosal surfaces following intramuscular vaccination". J Immunol 182(4):1779; author reply 1779–1780

Belyakov IM, Ahlers JD (2009b) What role does the route of immunization play in the generation of protective immunity against mucosal pathogens? J Immunol 183(11):6883–6892

Belyakov IM, Moss B, Strober W, Berzofsky JA (1999) Mucosal vaccination overcomes the barrier to recombinant vaccinia immunization caused by preexisting poxvirus immunity. Proc Natl Acad Sci USA 96(8):4512–4517

Belyakov IM, Hel Z, Kelsall B, Kuznetsov VA, Ahlers JD, Nacsa J, Watkins DI, Allen TM, Sette A, Altman J, Woodward R, Markham PD, Clements JD, Genoveffa F, Srober W, Berzofsky JA (2001) Mucosal AIDS vaccine reduces disease and viral load in gut reservoir and blood after mucosal infection of macaques. Nat Med 7(12):1320–1326

Belyakov IM, Kuznetsov VA, Kelsall B, Klinman D, Moniuszko M, Lemon M, Markham PD, Pal R, Clements JD, Lewis MG, Strober W, Franchini G, Berzofsky JA (2006) Impact of vaccine-induced mucosal high-avidity CD8+ CTLs in delay of AIDS viral dissemination from mucosa. Blood 107(8):3258–3264

Bihl F, Frahm N, Di Giammarino L, Sidney J, John M, Yusim K, Woodberry T, Sango K, Hewitt HS, Henry L, Linde CH, Chisholm JV 3rd, Zaman TM, Pae E, Mallal S, Walker BD, Sette A, Korber BT, Heckerman D, Brander C (2006) Impact of HLA-B alleles, epitope binding affinity, functional avidity, and viral coinfection on the immunodominance of virus-specific CTL responses. J Immunol 176(7):4094–4101

Bowman EP, Kuklin NA, Youngman KR, Lazarus NH, Kunkel EJ, Pan J, Greenberg HB, Butcher EC (2002) The intestinal chemokine thymus-expressed chemokine (CCL25) attracts IgA antibody-secreting cells. J Exp Med 195(2):269–275

Boyer JD, Ugen KE, Wang B, Agadjanyan M, Gilbert L, Bagarazzi ML, Chattergoon M, Frost P, Javadian A, Williams WV, Refaeli Y, Ciccarelli RB, McCallus D, Coney L, Weiner DB (1997) Protection of chimpanzees from high-dose heterologous HIV-1 challenge by DNA vaccination. Nat Med 3(5):526

Boyer JD, Kim J, Ugen K, Cohen AD, Ahn L, Schumann K, Lacy K, Bagarazzi ML, Javadian A, Ciccarelli RB, Ginsberg RS, MacGregor RR, Weiner DB, Kim JJ, Nottingham LK, Sin JI, Tsai A, Morrison L, Oh J, Dang K, Hu Y, Kazahaya K, Bennett M, Dentchev T, Wilson DM, Chalian AA, Agadjanyan MG (1999) HIV-1 DNA vaccines and chemokines. Vaccine 17(Suppl 2):S53–S64

Boyer JD, Robinson TM, Kutzler MA, Parkinson R, Calarota SA, Sidhu MK, Muthumani K, Lewis M, Pavlakis G, Felber B, Weiner D (2005) SIV DNA vaccine co-administered with IL-12 expression plasmid enhances CD8 SIV cellular immune responses in cynomolgus macaques. J Med Primatol 34(5–6):262–270

Brave A, Nystrom S, Roos AK, Applequist SE (2010) Plasmid DNA vaccination using skin electroporation promotes poly-functional CD4 T-cell responses. Immunol Cell Biol 89:492–496

Broder S, Gallo RC (1984) A pathogenic retrovirus (HTLV-III) linked to AIDS. N Engl J Med 311(20):1292–1297

Buchan S, Gronevik E, Mathiesen I, King CA, Stevenson FK, Rice J (2005) Electroporation as a "prime/boost" strategy for naked DNA vaccination against a tumor antigen. J Immunol 174(10):6292–6298

Buchbinder SP, Mehrotra DV, Duerr A, Fitzgerald DW, Mogg R, Li D, Gilbert PB, Lama JR, Marmor M, Del Rio C, McElrath MJ, Casimiro DR, Gottesdiener KM, Chodakewitz JA, Corey L, Robertson MN (2008) Efficacy assessment of a cell-mediated immunity HIV-1 vaccine (the step study): a double-blind, randomised, placebo-controlled, test-of-concept trial. Lancet 372(9653):1881–1893

Cai H, Yu DH, Hu XD, Li SX, Zhu YX (2006) A combined DNA vaccine-prime, BCG-boost strategy results in better protection against *Mycobacterium bovis* challenge. DNA Cell Biol 25(8):438–447

Chakrabarti BK, Ling X, Yang ZY, Montefiori DC, Panet A, Kong WP, Welcher B, Louder MK, Mascola JR, Nabel GJ (2005) Expanded breadth of virus neutralization after immunization with a multiclade envelope HIV vaccine candidate. Vaccine 23(26):3434–3445

Chen X, Prow TW, Crichton ML, Jenkins DW, Roberts MS, Frazer IH, Fernando GJ, Kendall MA (2009) Dry-coated microprojection array patches for targeted delivery of immunotherapeutics to the skin. J Control Release 139(3):212–220, Epub 2009 Jul 2003

Corbett M, Bogers WM, Heeney JL, Gerber S, Genin C, Didierlaurent A, Oostermeijer H, Dubbes R, Braskamp G, Lerondel S, Gomez CE, Esteban M, Wagner R, Kondova I, Mooij P, Balla-Jhagjhoorsingh S, Beenhakker N, Koopman G, van der Burg S, Kraehenbuhl JP, Le Pape A

(2008) Aerosol immunization with NYVAC and MVA vectored vaccines is safe, simple, and immunogenic. Proc Natl Acad Sci USA 105(6):2046–2051, Epub 2008 Feb 2011

Coupar BEH, Purcell DFJ, Thomson SA, Ramshaw IA, Kent SJ, Boyle DB (2006) Fowlpox virus vaccines for HIV and SIV clinical and pre-clinical trials. Vaccine 24(9):1378–1388

Cox E, Verdonck F, Vanrompay D, Goddeeris B (2006) Adjuvants modulating mucosal immune responses or directing systemic responses towards the mucosa. Vet Res 37(3):511–539, Epub 2006 Apr 2014

Darrah PA, Patel DT, De Luca PM, Lindsay RW, Davey DF, Flynn BJ, Hoff ST, Andersen P, Reed SG, Morris SL, Roederer M, Seder RA (2007) Multifunctional TH1 cells define a correlate of vaccine-mediated protection against *Leishmania major*. Nat Med 13(7):843–850, Epub 2007 Jun 2010

Day SL, Ramshaw IA, Ramsay AJ, Ranasinghe C (2008) Differential effects of the type I interferons alpha4, beta, and epsilon on antiviral activity and vaccine efficacy. J Immunol 180(11):7158–7166

De Rose R, Sullivan MT, Dale CJ, Kelleher AD, Emery S, Cooper DA, Ramshaw IA, Boyle DB, Kent SJ (2006) Dose-response relationship of DNA and recombinant fowlpox virus primeboost HIV vaccines: implications for future trials. Hum Vaccines 2(3):134–136

Demberg T, Boyer JD, Malkevich N, Patterson LJ, Venzon D, Summers EL, Kalisz I, Kalyanaraman VS, Lee EM, Weiner DB, Robert-Guroff M (2008) Sequential priming with simian immunodeficiency virus (SIV) DNA vaccines, with or without encoded cytokines, and a replicating adenovirus-SIV recombinant followed by protein boosting does not control a pathogenic SIVmac251 mucosal challenge. J Virol 82(21):10911–10921, Epub 12008 Aug 10927

Derby M, Alexander-Miller M, Tse R, Berzofsky J (2001) High-avidity CTL exploit two complementary mechanisms to provide better protection against viral infection than low-avidity CTL. J Immunol 166(3):1690–1697

Dormitzer PR, Ulmer JB, Rappuoli R (2008) Structure-based antigen design: a strategy for next generation vaccines. Trends Biotechnol 26(12):659–667

Duvall MG, Jaye A, Dong T, Brenchley JM, Alabi AS, Jeffries DJ, van der Sande M, Togun TO, McConkey SJ, Douek DC, McMichael AJ, Whittle HC, Koup RA, Rowland-Jones SL (2006) Maintenance of HIV-specific CD4+ T cell help distinguishes HIV-2 from HIV-1 infection. J Immunol 176(11):6973–6981

Dzutsev AH, Belyakov IM, Isakov DV, Margulies DH, Berzofsky JA (2007) Avidity of CD8 T cells sharpens immunodominance. Int Immunol 19(4):497–507

Epstein JE, Charoenvit Y, Kester KE, Wang R, Newcomer R, Fitzpatrick S, Richie TL, Tornieporth N, Heppner DG, Ockenhouse C, Majam V, Holland C, Abot E, Ganeshan H, Berzins M, Jones T, Freydberg CN, Ng J, Norman J, Carucci DJ, Cohen J, Hoffman SL (2004) Safety, tolerability, and antibody responses in humans after sequential immunization with a PfCSP DNA vaccine followed by the recombinant protein vaccine RTS, S/AS02A. Vaccine 22(13–14):1592–1603

Estcourt MJ, Ramsay AJ, Brooks A, Thomson SA, Medveckzy CJ, Ramshaw IA (2002) Primeboost immunization generates a high frequency, high-avidity CD8(+) cytotoxic T lymphocyte population. Int Immunol 14(1):31–37

Ferre AL, Hunt PW, Critchfield JW, Young DH, Morris MM, Garcia JC, Pollard RB, Yee HF Jr, Martin JN, Deeks SG, Shacklett BL (2009) Mucosal immune responses to HIV-1 in elite controllers: a potential correlate of immune control. Blood 113(17):3978–3989, Epub 2008 Dec 3923

Flynn NM, Forthal DN, Harro CD, Judson FN, Mayer KH, Para MF (2005) Placebo-controlled phase 3 trial of a recombinant glycoprotein 120 vaccine to prevent HIV-1 infection. J Infect Dis 191(5):654–665

Fuller DH, Haynes JR (1994) A qualitative progression in HIV type 1 glycoprotein 120-specific cytotoxic cellular and humoral immune responses in mice receiving a DNA-based glycoprotein 120 vaccine. AIDS Res Hum Retrovirus 10(11):1433–1441

Garcia-Hernandez Mde L, Gray A, Hubby B, Kast WM (2007) In vivo effects of vaccination with six-transmembrane epithelial antigen of the prostate: a candidate antigen for treating prostate cancer. Cancer Res 67(3):1344–1351

Gherardi MM, Ramirez JC, Esteban M (2000) Interleukin-12 (IL-12) enhancement of the cellular immune response against human immunodeficiency virus type 1 env antigen in a DNA prime/ vaccinia virus boost vaccine regimen is time and dose dependent: suppressive effects of IL-12 boost are mediated by nitric oxide. J Virol 74(14):6278–6286

Gherardi MM, Najera JL, Perez-Jimenez E, Guerra S, Garcia-Sastre A, Esteban M (2003) Prime-boost immunisation schedules based on influenza virus and vaccinia virus vectors potentiate cellulare immune responses against human immunodeficiency virus Env proteins systemically and in genitorectal draining lymph nodes. J Virol 77(12):7048–7057

Goonetilleke NP, McShane H, Hannan CM, Anderson RJ, Brookes RH, Hill AV (2003) Enhanced immunogenicity and protective efficacy against *Mycobacterium tuberculosis* of bacille Calmette-Guerin vaccine using mucosal administration and boosting with a recombinant modified vaccinia virus Ankara. J Immunol 171(3):1602–1609

Gupta RK (1998) Aluminum compounds as vaccine adjuvants. Adv Drug Deliv Rev 32(3): 155–172

Gurunathan S, Stobie L, Prussin C, Sacks DL, Glaichenhaus N, Fowell DJ, Locksley RM, Chang JT, Wu C-Y, Seder RA (2000) Requirements for the maintenance of Th1 immunity in vivo following DNA vaccination: a potential immunoregulatory role for CD8+ T cells. J Immunol 165:915–924

Hagiwara Y, Kawamura YI, Kataoka K, Rahima B, Jackson RJ, Komase K, Dohi T, Boyaka PN, Takeda Y, Kiyono H, McGhee JR, Fujihashi K (2006) A second generation of double mutant cholera toxin adjuvants: enhanced immunity without intracellular trafficking. J Immunol 177(5):3045–3054

Hansen SG, Vieville C, Whizin N, Coyne-Johnson L, Siess DC, Drummond DD, Legasse AW, Axthelm MK, Oswald K, Trubey CM, Piatak M Jr, Lifson JD, Nelson JA, Jarvis MA, Picker LJ (2009) Effector memory T cell responses are associated with protection of rhesus monkeys from mucosal simian immunodeficiency virus challenge. Nat Med 15(3):293–299

Harding CV, Song R (1994) Phagocytic processing of exogenous particulate antigens by macrophages for presentation by class I MHC molecules. J Immunol 153(11):4925–4933

Harrison JM, Bertram EM, Boyle DB, Coupar BE, Ranasinghe C, Ramshaw IA (2006) 4-1BBL coexpression enhances HIV-specific CD8 T cell memory in a poxvirus prime-boost vaccine. Vaccine 24(47–48):6867–6874

Hill AV, Reece W, Gothard P, Moorthy V, Roberts M, Flanagan K, Plebanski M, Hannan C, Hu JT, Anderson R, Degano P, Schneider J, Prieur E, Sheu E, Gilbert SC (2000) DNA-based vaccines for malaria: a heterologous prime-boost immunisation strategy. Dev Biol (Basel) 104:171–179

Hutchings CL, Gilbert SC, Hill AV, Moore AC (2005) Novel protein and poxvirus-based vaccine combinations for simultaneous induction of humoral and cell-mediated immunity. J Immunol 175(1):599–606

Imrie A, Meeks J, Gurary A, Sukhbataar M, Kitsutani P, Effler P, Zhao Z (2007) Differential functional avidity of dengue virus-specific T-cell clones for variant peptides representing heterologous and previously encountered serotypes. J Virol 81(18):10081–10091

Kallenius G, Pawlowski A, Brandtzaeg P, Svenson S (2007) Should a new tuberculosis vaccine be administered intranasally? Tuberculosis (Edinb) 87(4):257–266, Epub 2007 Feb 2026

Kantele A, Hakkinen M, Moldoveanu Z, Lu A, Savilahti E, Alvarez RD, Michalek S, Mestecky J (1998) Differences in immune responses induced by oral and rectal immunizations with *Salmonella typhi* Ty21a: evidence for compartmentalization within the common mucosal immune system in humans. Infect Immun 66(12):5630–5635

Kaufman DR, Liu J, Carville A, Mansfield KG, Havenga MJ, Goudsmit J, Barouch DH (2008) Trafficking of antigen-specific CD8+ T lymphocytes to mucosal surfaces following intramuscular vaccination. J Immunol 181(6):4188–4198

Kaul R, Plummer FA, Kimani J, Dong T, Kiama P, Rostron T, Njagi E, MacDonald KS, Bwayo JJ, McMichael AJ, Rowland-Jones SL (2000) HIV-1-specific mucosal CD8+ lymphocyte responses in the cervix of HIV-1-resistant prostitutes in Nairobi. J Immunol 164:1602–1611

Kelleher AD, Puls RL, Bebbington M, Boyle D, Ffrench R, Kent SJ, Kippax S, Purcell DFJ, Thomson S, Wand H, Cooper DA, Emery S (2006) A randomised, placebo-controlled phase I trial of DNA prime, recombinant fowlpox virus boost prophylactic vaccine for HIV-1. AIDS 20(2):294–297

Kelso A, Groves P (1997) A single peripheral CD8+ T cell can give rise to progeny expressing type 1 and/or type 2 cytokine genes and can retain its multipotentiality through many cell divisions. Proc Natl Acad Sci USA 94(15):8070–8075

Kent SJ, Zhao A, Best SJ, Chandler JD, Boyle DB, Ramshaw IA (1998) Enhanced T-cell immunogenicity and protective efficacy of a human immunodeficiency virus type 1 vaccine regimen consisting of consecutive priming with DNA and boosting with recombinant fowlpox virus. J Virol 72(12):10180–10188

Kent SJ, Dale CJ, Ranasinghe C, Stratov I, De Rose R, Chea S, Montefiori DC, Thomson S, Ramshaw IA, Coupar BE, Boyle DB, Law M, Wilson KM, Ramsay AJ (2005) Mucosally-administered human-simian immunodeficiency virus DNA and fowlpox virus-based recombinant vaccines reduce acute phase viral replication in macaques following vaginal challenge with CCR5-tropic SHIV(SF162P3). Vaccine 23:5009–5021

Kienzle N, Baz A, Kelso A (2004) Profiling the CD8low phenotype, an alternative career choice for CD8 T cells during primary differentiation. Immunol Cell Biol 82(1):75–83

Kiyono H, Fukuyama S (2004) NALT- versus Peyer's-patch mediated mucosal immunity. Nat Immunol 4:699–710

Klavinskis LS, Barnfield C, Gao L, Parker S (1999) Intranasal immunization with plasmid DNA-lipid complexes elicits mucosal immunity in the female genital and rectal tracts. J Immunol 162(1):254–262

Kolibab K, Yang A, Derrick SC, Waldmann TA, Perera LP, Morris SL (2010) Highly persistent and effective prime/boost regimens against tuberculosis that use a multivalent modified vaccine virus Ankara-based tuberculosis vaccine with interleukin-15 as a molecular adjuvant. Clin Vaccine Immunol 17(5):793–801

Kozlowski PA, Neutra MR (2003) The role of mucosal immunity in prevention of HIV transmission. Curr Mol Med 3(3):217–228

Kutzler MA, Robinson TM, Chattergoon MA, Choo DK, Choo AY, Choe PY, Ramanathan MP, Parkinson R, Kudchodkar S, Tamura Y, Sidhu M, Roopchand V, Kim JJ, Pavlakis GN, Felber BK, Waldmann TA, Boyer JD, Weiner DB (2005) Coimmunization with an optimized IL-15 plasmid results in enhanced function and longevity of CD8 T cells that are partially independent of CD4 T cell help. J Immunol 175(1):112–123

Kwong PD, Wyatt R, Robinson J, Sweet RW, Sodroski J, Hendrickson WA (1998) Structure of an HIV gp120 envelope glycoprotein in complex with the CD4 receptor and a neutralizing human antibody. Nature 393(6686):648–659

La Gruta NL, Turner SJ, Doherty PC (2004) Hierarchies in cytokine expression profiles for acute and resolving influenza virus-specific CD8+ T cell responses: correlation of cytokine profile and TCR avidity. J Immunol 172(9):5553–5560

Lane JM, Ruben FL, Neff JM, Millar JD (1969) Complications of smallpox vaccination. N Engl J Med 281(22):1201–1208

Leong KH, Ramsay AJ, Boyle DB, Ramshaw IA (1994) Selective induction of immune responses by cytokines coexpressed in recombinant fowlpox virus. J Virol 68(12):8125–8130

Leong KH, Ramsay AJ, Morin MJ, Robinson HL, Boyle DB, Ramshaw IA (1995) Molecular approaches to the control of infectious diseases. In: Brown F, Chanock H, Norrby E (eds) Vaccine 95. Cold Spring Harbor Laboratory, New York, pp 327–331

Lillard JW Jr, Boyaka PN, Taub DD, McGhee JR (2001) RANTES potentiates antigen-specific mucosal immune responses. J Immunol 166(1):162–169

Liu J, Yu Q, Stone GW, Yue FY, Ngai N, Jones RB, Kornbluth RS, Ostrowski MA (2008) CD40L expressed from the canarypox vector, ALVAC, can boost immunogenicity of HIV-1 canarypox vaccine in mice and enhance the in vitro expansion of viral specific CD8+ T cell memory responses from HIV-1-infected and HIV-1-uninfected individuals. Vaccine 26(32):4062–4072, Epub 2008 Jun 4062

Mascola JR, Montefiori DC (2010) The role of antibodies in HIV vaccines. Annu Rev Immunol 28:413–444

McConkey SJ, Reece WH, Moorthy VS, Webster D, Dunachie S, Butcher G, Vuola JM, Blanchard TJ, Gothard P, Watkins K, Hannan CM, Everaere S, Brown K, Kester KE, Cummings J, Williams J, Heppner DG, Pathan A, Flanagan K, Arulanantham N, Roberts MT, Roy M, Smith

GL, Schneider J, Peto T, Sinden RE, Gilbert SC, Hill AV (2003) Enhanced T-cell immunogenicity of plasmid DNA vaccines boosted by recombinant modified vaccinia virus Ankara in humans. Nat Med 9(6):729–735

McCormack S, Stohr W, Barber T, Bart PA, Harari A, Moog C, Ciuffreda D, Cellerai C, Cowen M, Gamboni R, Burnet S, Legg K, Brodnicki E, Wolf H, Wagner R, Heeney J, Frachette MJ, Tartaglia J, Babiker A, Pantaleo G, Weber J, Harari A, Bart PA, Stohr W, Tapia G, Garcia M, Medjitna-Rais E, Burnet S, Cellerai C, Erlwein O, Barber T, Moog C, Liljestrom P, Wagner R, Wolf H, Kraehenbuhl JP, Esteban M, Heeney J, Frachette MJ, Tartaglia J, McCormack S, Babiker A, Weber J, Pantaleo G (2008) EV02: a Phase I trial to compare the safety and immunogenicity of HIV DNA-C prime-NYVAC-C boost to NYVAC-C alone. Vaccine 26(25):3162–3174, Epub 2008 May 3166

McMichael AJ, Borrow P, Tomaras GD, Goonetilleke N, Haynes BF (2010) The immune response during acute HIV-1 infection: clues for vaccine development. Nat Rev Immunol 10(1):11–23

Moorthy VS, Imoukhuede EB, Keating S, Pinder M, Webster D, Skinner MA, Gilbert SC, Walraven G, Hill AV (2004) Phase 1 evaluation of 3 highly immunogenic prime-boost regimens, including a 12-month reboosting vaccination, for malaria vaccination in Gambian men. J Infect Dis 189(12):2213–2219, Epub 2004 May 2224

Musey L, Hu Y, Eckert L, Christensen M, Karchmer T, McElrath MJ (1997) HIV-1 induces cytotoxic T lymphocytes in the cervix of infected women. J Exp Med 185(2):293–303

Ogra P (1999) Mucosal immunity, 2nd edn. Academic Press, San Diego, CA

Ogra PL, Faden H, Welliver RC (2001) Vaccination strategies for mucosal immune responses. Clin Microbiol Rev 14(2):430–445

Oh S, Hodge JW, Ahlers JD, Burke DS, Schlom J, Berzofsky JA (2003) Selective induction of high avidity CTL by altering the balance of signals from APC. J Immunol 170(5):2523–2530

Osborn JE (1995) HIV: the more things change, the more they stay the same. Nat Med 1(10):991–993

Pal R, Venzon D, Santra S, Kalyanaraman VS, Montefiori DC, Hocker L, Hudacik L, Rose N, Nacsa J, Edghill-Smith Y, Moniuszko M, Hel Z, Belyakov IM, Berzofsky JA, Parks RW, Markham PD, Letvin NL, Tartaglia J, Franchini G (2006) Systemic immunization with an ALVAC-HIV-1/protein boost vaccine strategy protects rhesus macaques from CD4+ T-cell loss and reduces both systemic and mucosal simian-human immunodeficiency virus SHIVKU2 RNA levels. J Virol 80(8):3732–3742

Perez-Jimenez E, Kochan G, Gherardi MM, Esteban M (2006) MVA-LACK as a safe and efficient vector for vaccination against leishmaniasis. Microbes Infect 8(3):810–822, Epub 2006 Jan 2013

Perrone LA, Ahmad A, Veguilla V, Lu X, Smith G, Katz JM, Pushko P, Tumpey TM (2009) Intranasal vaccination with 1918 influenza virus-like particles protects mice and ferrets from lethal 1918 and H5N1 influenza virus challenge. J Virol 83(11):5726–5734

Pitisuttithum P (2005) HIV-1 prophylactic vaccine trials in Thailand. Curr HIV Res 3(1):17–30

Pitisuttithum P, Gilbert P, Gurwith M, Heyward W, Martin M, van Griensven F, Hu D, Tappero JW, Choopanya K (2006) Randomized, double-blind, placebo-controlled efficacy trial of a bivalent recombinant glycoprotein 120 HIV-1 vaccine among injection drug users in Bangkok, Thailand. J Infect Dis 194(12):1661–1671

Priddy FH, Brown D, Kublin J, Monahan K, Wright DP, Lalezari J, Santiago S, Marmor M, Lally M, Novak RM, Brown SJ, Kulkarni P, Dubey SA, Kierstead LS, Casimiro DR, Mogg R, DiNubile MJ, Shiver JW, Leavitt RY, Robertson MN, Mehrotra DV, Quirk E (2008) Safety and immunogenicity of a replication-incompetent adenovirus type 5 HIV-1 clade B gag/pol/nef vaccine in healthy adults. Clin Infect Dis 46(11):1769–1781

Ramsay AJ, Leong KH, Ramshaw IA (1997) DNA vaccination against virus infection and enhancement of antiviral immunity following consecutive immunization with DNA and viral vectors. Immunol Cell Biol 75(4):382–388

Ramsay AJ, Kent SJ, Strugnell RA, Suhrbier A, Thomson SA, Ramshaw IA (1999) Genetic vaccination strategies for enhanced cellular, humoral and mucosal immunity. Immunol Rev 171:27–44

Ramshaw IA, Ramsay AJ (2000) The prime-boost strategy: exciting prospects for improved vaccination. Immunol Today 21(4):163–165

Ranasinghe C, Ramshaw IA (2009a) Genetic heterologous prime-boost vaccination strategies for improved systemic and mucosal immunity. Expert Rev Vaccines 8(9):1171–1181

Ranasinghe C, Ramshaw IA (2009b) Immunisation route-dependent expression of IL-4/IL-13 can modulate HIV-specific CD8(+) CTL avidity. Eur J Immunol 39(7):1819–1830

Ranasinghe C, Medveczky JC, Woltring D, Gao K, Thomson S, Coupar BE, Boyle DB, Ramsay AJ, Ramshaw IA (2006) Evaluation of fowlpox-vaccinia virus prime-boost vaccine strategies for high-level mucosal and systemic immunity against HIV-1. Vaccine 24(31–32):5881–5895

Ranasinghe C, Turner SJ, McArthur C, Sutherland DB, Kim JH, Doherty PC, Ramshaw IA (2007) Mucosal HIV-1 pox virus prime-boost immunization induces high-avidity CD8+ T cells with regime-dependent cytokine/granzyme B profiles. J Immunol 178(4):2370–2379

Reece JC, Loh L, Alcantara S, Fernandez CS, Stambas J, Sexton A, De Rose R, Petravic J, Davenport MP, Kent SJ (2010) Timing of immune escape linked to success or failure of vaccination. PLoS 5(9), (pii):e12774

Rerks-Ngarm S, Pitisuttithum P, Nitayaphan S, Kaewkungwal J, Chiu J, Paris R, Premsri N, Namwat C, de Souza M, Adams E, Benenson M, Gurunathan S, Tartaglia J, McNeil JG, Francis DP, Stablein D, Birx DL, Chunsuttiwat S, Khamboonruang C, Thongcharoen P, Robb ML, Michael NL, Kunasol P, Kim JH (2009) Vaccination with ALVAC and AIDSVAX to prevent HIV-1 infection in Thailand. N Engl J Med 361(23):2209–2220

Roberts JD, Bebenek K, Kunkel TA (1988) The accuracy of reverse transcriptase from HIV-1. Science 242(4882):1171–1173

Robinson HL, Montefiori DC, Johnson RP, Manson KH, Kalish ML, Lifson JD, Rizvi TA, Lu S, Hu SL, Mazzara GP, Panicali DL, Herndon JG, Glickman R, Candido MA, Lydy SL, Wyand MS, McClure HM (1999) Neutralizing antibody-independent containment of immunodeficiency virus challenges by DNA priming and recombinant pox virus booster immunizations. Nat Med 5(5):526–534

Rollman E, Brave A, Boberg A, Gudmundsdotter L, Engstrom G, Isaguliants M, Ljungberg K, Lundgren B, Blomberg P, Hinkula J, Hejdeman B, Sandstrom E, Liu M, Wahren B (2005) The rationale behind a vaccine based on multiple HIV antigens. Microbes Infect 7(14):1414–1423

Santosuosso M, Zhang X, McCormick S, Wang J, Hitt M, Xing Z (2005) Mechanisms of mucosal and parenteral tuberculosis vaccinations: adenoviral-based mucosal immunization preferentially elicits sustained accumulation of immune protective CD4 and CD8 T cells within the airway lumen. J Immunol 174(12):7986–7994

Seder RA, Darrah PA, Roederer M (2008) T-cell quality in memory and protection: implications for vaccine design. Nat Rev Immunol 8(4):247–258

Sekaly RP (2008) The failed HIV Merck vaccine study: a step back or a launching point for future vaccine development? J Exp Med 205(1):7–12, Epub 2008 Jan 2014

Seppala IJ, Makela O (1984) Adjuvant effect of bacterial LPS and/or alum precipitation in responses to polysaccharide and protein antigens. Immunology 53(4):827–836

Shiver JW, Fu T-M, Chen L, Casimiro DR, Davies M-E, Evans RK, Zhang Z-Q, Simon AJ, Trigona WL, Dubey SA, Huang L, Harris VA, Long RS, Liang X, Handt L, Schlief WA, Zhu L, Freed DC, Persaud NV, Guan L, Punt KS, Tang A, Chen M, Wilson KA, Collins KB, Heidecker GJ, Fernandez VR, Perry HC, Joyce JG, Grimm KM, Cook JC, Keller PM, Kresock DS, Mach H, Troutman RD, Isopi LA, Williams DM, Xu Z, Bohannon KE, Volkin DB, Montefiori DC, Miura A, Krivulka GR, Lifton MA, Kuroda MJ, Schmitz JE, Letvin NL, Caulfield MJ, Bett AJ, Youil R, Kaslow DC, Emini EA (2002) Replication-incompetent adenoviral vaccine vector elicits effective anti-immunodeficiency-virus immunity. Nature 415:331–335

Skinner MA, Buddle BM, Wedlock DN, Keen D, de Lisle GW, Tascon RE, Ferraz JC, Lowrie DB, Cockle PJ, Vordermeier HM, Hewinson RG (2003) A DNA prime-*Mycobacterium bovis* BCG boost vaccination strategy for cattle induces protection against bovine tuberculosis. Infect Immun 71(9):4901–4907

Spellberg B, Edwards JE Jr (2001) Type 1/type 2 immunity in infectious diseases. Clin Infect Dis 32(1):76–102

Staerz UD, Karasuyama H, Garner AM (1987) Cytotoxic T lymphocytes against a soluble protein. Nature 329(6138):449–451

Stambas J, Brown SA, Gutierrez A, Sealy R, Yue W, Jones B, Lockey TD, Zirkel A, Freiden P, Brown B, Surman S, Coleclough C, Slobod KS, Doherty PC, Hurwitz JL (2005) Long lived multi-isotype anti-HIV antibody responses following a prime-double boost immunization strategy. Vaccine 23(19):2454–2464

Tapia E, Perez-Jimenez E, Lopez-Fuertes L, Gonzalo R, Gherardi MM, Esteban M (2003) The combination of DNA vectors expressing IL-12 + IL-18 elicits high protective immune response against cutaneous leishmaniasis after priming with DNA-p36/LACK and the cytokines, followed by a booster with a vaccinia virus recombinant expressing p36/LACK. Microbes Infect 5(2):73–84

Veazey RS, DeMaria M, Chalifoux LV, Shvetz DE, Pauley DR, Knight HL, Rosenzweig M, Johnson RP, Desrosiers RC, Lackner AA (1998) Gastrointestinal tract as a major site of CD4+ T cell depletion and viral replication in SIV infection. Science 280(5362):427–431

Veazey RS, Gauduin MC, Mansfield KG, Tham IC, Altman JD, Lifson JD, Lackner AA, Johnson RP (2001) Emergence and kinetics of simian immunodeficiency virus-specific CD8(+) T cells in the intestines of macaques during primary infection. J Virol 75(21):10515–10519

Vordermeier HM, Villarreal-Ramos B, Cockle PJ, McAulay M, Rhodes SG, Thacker T, Gilbert SC, McShane H, Hill AV, Xing Z, Hewinson RG (2009) Viral booster vaccines improve *Mycobacterium bovis* BCG-induced protection against bovine tuberculosis. Infect Immun 77(8):3364–3373, Epub 2009 Jun 3361

Wagner N, Lohler J, Kunkel EJ, Ley K, Leung E, Krissansen G, Rajewsky K, Muller W (1996) Critical role for beta7 integrins in formation of the gut-associated lymphoid tissue. Nature 382(6589):366–370

Wallace M, Evans B, Woods S, Mogg R, Zhang L, Finnefrock AC, Rabussay D, Fons M, Mallee J, Mehrotra D, Schodel F, Musey L (2009) Tolerability of two sequential electroporation treatments using MedPulser DNA delivery system (DDS) in healthy adults. Mol Ther 17(5):922–928, Epub 2009 Mar 2010

Williams A, Hatch GJ, Clark SO, Gooch KE, Hatch KA, Hall GA, Huygen K, Ottenhoff TH, Franken KL, Andersen P, Doherty TM, Kaufmann SH, Grode L, Seiler P, Martin C, Gicquel B, Cole ST, Brodin P, Pym AS, Dalemans W, Cohen J, Lobet Y, Goonetilleke N, McShane H, Hill A, Parish T, Smith D, Stoker NG, Lowrie DB, Kallenius G, Svenson S, Pawlowski A, Blake K, Marsh PD (2005) Evaluation of vaccines in the EU TB vaccine cluster using a guinea pig aerosol infection model of tuberculosis. Tuberculosis (Edinb) 85(1–2):29–38, Epub 2005 Jan 2020

Wolff JA, Malone RW, Williams P, Chong W, Acsadi G, Jani A, Felgner PL (1990) Direct gene transfer into mouse muscle in vivo. Science 247(4949 Pt 1):1465–1468

Wright PF, Mestecky J, McElrath MJ, Keefer MC, Gorse GJ, Goepfert PA, Moldoveanu Z, Schwartz D, Spearman PW, El Habib R, Spring MD, Zhu Y, Smith C, Flores J, Weinhold KJ (2004) Comparison of systemic and mucosal delivery of 2 canarypox virus vaccines expressing either HIV-1 genes or the gene for rabies virus G protein. J Infect Dis 189(7):1221–1231, Epub 2004 Mar 1215

Xiang ZQ, Pasquini S, Ertl HCJ (1999) Induction of genital immunity by DNA priming and intranasal booster immunisation with a replication-defective adenoviral recombinant. J Immunol 162:6716–6723

Yang K, Whalen BJ, Tirabassi RS, Selin LK, Levchenko TS, Torchilin VP, Kislauskis EH, Guberski DL (2008) A DNA vaccine prime followed by a liposome-encapsulated protein boost confers enhanced mucosal immune responses and protection. J Immunol 180(9):6159–6167

Zhong L, Granelli-Piperno A, Choi Y, Steinman RM (1999) Recombinant adenovirus is an efficient and non-perturbing genetic vector for human dendritic cells. Eur J Immunol 29(3):964–972

Zhou T, Georgiev I, Wu X, Yang ZY, Dai K, Finzi A, Do Kwon Y, Scheid JF, Shi W, Xu L, Yang Y, Zhu J, Nussenzweig MC, Sodroski J, Shapiro L, Nabel GJ, Mascola JR, Kwong PD (2010) Structural basis for broad and potent neutralization of HIV-1 by antibody VRC01. Science 329(5993):811–817

Intralymphatic Vaccination

10

Thomas M. Kündig, Adrian Bot, and Gabriela Senti

The immune response is initiated by dendritic cells and other antigen-presenting cells. These cells are present in nearly all organs and tissues of the body, so that theoretically any organ or tissue could serve as a route for vaccine administration. The choice of route is therefore mainly based on practical aspects. Using conventional needle and syringe the subcutaneous or intramuscular route are standard. The dermis and especially the epidermis are technically more difficult to target, but are likely to gain more interest due to the recent development of micro-needle patches and needle free injection devices. Vaccine administration via mucosal surfaces such as nasal or oral vaccination represents another option for needle free vaccine administration.

While all the above mentioned routes of administration have been proven to work and protect against childhood diseases, influenza and many other infectious agents, the discussion and comparison of these different routes usually focuses on patient convenience, reduction of pain and distress for children, cost and on the possibility for mass vaccination. In this review, however, we would like to focus on how the route of administration can enhance the efficacy of vaccination, in clinical indications that are benefiting to a much lesser extent from conventional vaccination.

Especially in therapeutic vaccination, i.e., in a smaller patient number that already suffers from a disease, vaccination efficiency rather than convenience is the main issue. This is particularly the case in therapeutic cancer vaccines and in allergen specific immunotherapy. Intralymphatic vaccination is a strategy to maximize immunogenicity and therefore vaccine efficacy. The main part of this review will discuss this long known vaccination route and its clinical applicability in therapeutic vaccination, with a special focus on gene vaccines.

T.M. Kündig (✉)
Department of Dermatology, University Hospital of Zurich,
Zurich, Switzerland
e-mail: thomas.kuendig@usz.ch

J. Thalhamer et al. (eds.), *Gene Vaccines*,
DOI 10.1007/978-3-7091-0439-2_10, © Springer-Verlag/Wien, 2012

General Considerations on the Routes of Vaccine Administration

The wide spread introduction of vaccines approximately one century ago likely represents the most significant success in medicine, which together with hygiene and antibiotics have essentially alleviated the modern world from morbidity and mortality caused by infectious diseases. Despite this success, a medical need for improving vaccination remains. For mass vaccination campaigns it would be desirable to increase ease and speed of vaccination. For developing countries the main goal is reduction of cost and elimination of the cold chain. In children, reduction or absence of pain is an important aim. Such improvement of speed, convenience, and cost are the main issues when trying to improve vaccines which already work well, which are generally prophylactic vaccines against infectious agents. For another group of vaccines, e.g. for therapeutic vaccines to treat cancer or allergies, the main goal is to improve their efficacy. Most cancer vaccines so far produced disappointing clinical results (Rosenberg et al. 2004). Allergen specific immunotherapy, also called desensitization or allergy shots, has been proven to work, but only after dozens of vaccine doses and years of treatment (Bousquet et al. 1998). Hence, both in cancer and allergies, a marked improvement of vaccination efficacy is urgently needed. This review will focus on how intralymphatic vaccine administration can enhance the immune response, with a special focus on gene vaccines.

Function of Lymph Nodes

In a series of elegant skin flap experiments Frey and Wenk proved in 1957 (Frey and Wenk 1957) that antigen, in order to induce a T-cell response, needs to reach lymph nodes via afferent lymph vessels. More recent experiments in alymphoplastic (aly/aly) and spleenless (Hox11-/-) mutant mice confirm the importance of secondary lymphoid organs, or neo-lymphoid aggregates (Greter et al. 2009) in generating immune responses (Karrer et al. 1997).

T and B cell receptors have been randomly rearranged early in lymphocyte development generating T and B cells carrying a diverse repertoire of receptors. While this ensures that all possible antigens can be specifically recognized, it also requires that antigens must be presented to approximately 10^7 T and B cells in order to elicit an immune response. Therefore, only antigens that are drained into secondary lymphatic organs, where they can be presented to high numbers of T and B cells will therefore induce an immune response, whereas antigens staying outside of secondary lymphoid organs have little chance to meet with specific T or B cells and are largely ignored, a phenomenon termed the "geographic concept of immunogenicity" (Kundig et al. 1995; Zinkernagel et al. 1997, 2000). In light of the current understanding of immune regulation by dendritic cells (DCs) and T cells, this concept may sound rather simplistic, but it remains valid nevertheless. Today's complexity of immune regulation should not make us forget that the key trigger and regulator of the immune response still is the antigen.

10 Intralymphatic Vaccination

Table 10.1 Intralymphatic vaccination strongly enhances unstable vaccines

Type of vaccine	Dose required s.c./ intralymphatic	Stability in vivo and drainage into lymph node
Naked RNA[a]	$>10^6$	–
Oligopeptide (Johansen et al. 2005)	10^6	+
Naked DNA (Maloy et al. 2001)	10^3–10^4	++
Protein (Martinez-Gomez et al. 2009a)	10^3–10^4	+++
Live virus[b]	1	++++

[a]Kündig TM, unpublished; Kreiter et al. (2010)
[b]Kündig TM, unpublished

Lymphatic Drainage

Lymph vessels have evolved to drain pathogens into lymph nodes so that the immune system can generate an immune response as early as possible. Therefore, small particles sized 20–200 nm, i.e., the size of viruses, drain from peripheral injection sites into lymph nodes quite efficiently and in a free form, but even in this case usually only a few percent of the injected particles drain into the lymph nodes (Manolova et al. 2008). Larger particles sized 500–2000 nm are mostly transported into lymph nodes by DCs (Manolova et al. 2008). Drainage from periphery to lymph nodes of non-particulate antigens, however, can be much less efficient and only very small fractions – between 10^{-3} and 10^{-6} – of the injected doses reach lymph nodes, as summarized in Table 10.1. As many of today's vaccines and immunotherapeutic agents are non-particulate, their direct administration into a lymph node may therefore enhance antigen presentation in the lymph node and therefore the immune response.

Intralymphatic Vaccination Technique

In slack skin animals such as dogs, horses or cattle, subcutaneous lymph nodes are readily palpable and can readily be injected even without ultrasound. Also in humans, many subcutaneous lymph nodes are palpable, especially those in the groin area (Fig. 10.1).

Fine needle punctures of lymph nodes are a routine procedure that many physicians perform even without ultrasound. However, for puncture and injection of lymph nodes in a clinical study setting we recommend ultrasound guidance. Lymph nodes are readily visible by ultrasound, as their paracortical area is hypoechoic (Fig. 10.2). Injection of a superficial lymph node in the groin area can be performed within minutes, even by doctors that have little experience in ultrasound. Especially the lymph nodes in the upper outer quadrant of the groin area are very close to the skin surface, even in overweight patients. On average in this quadrant we find one lymph node that is approx. 1.5 cm long and has a diameter of approx. 5 mm. The pain of intralymphatic injection arises solely from penetrating the skin, whereas lymph nodes are poorly innervated. The pain of an intralymphatic injection is

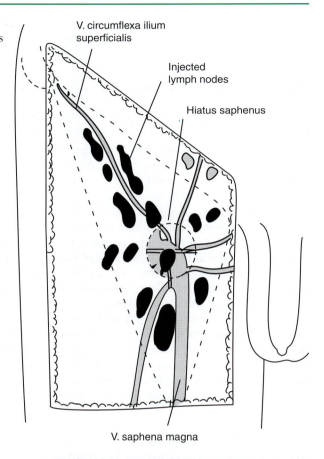

Fig. 10.1 Lymph nodes of the groin area: Lymph vessels and lymph nodes follow the vains of the groin area. Through the hiatus saphenus the superficial venous and lymphatic system of the leg and lower abdomen drain into the deep venous (*V. femoralis*) and lymphatic system. The lymph nodes in the upper outer quadrant of the groin area follow the *V. circumflexa ilium* superficialis. In the latter quadrant, one or two lymph nodes with a length of approx. 1.5 cm and a diameter of approx. 5 mm can be found, which is no more than 5 mm under the skin surface

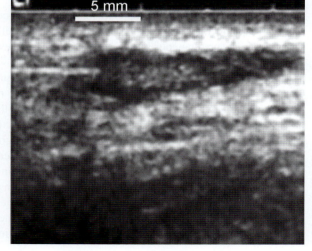

Fig. 10.2 Intralymphatic injection: A sand blasted needle, being inserted into the lymph node from the right was used for better reflection and therefore visibility in the ultrasound. The dark, hypoechoic area represents the paracortex of the lymph node, which is approx. 15 mm long and 5 mm under the skin surface

comparable to the subcutaneous injections. In fact, patients rated intralymphatic injection less painful than venous puncture (Senti et al. 2008).

Biodistribution After Intralymphatic Delivery

Biodistribution studies in mice revealed that 100-fold higher antigen doses reached the lymph nodes after direct lymph-node injection than after subcutaneous injection in the proximity of a draining lymph node (Martinez-Gomez et al. 2009a). Similar results had previously been obtained in dogs where the distribution of intact radiolabelled cells was followed in vivo by whole body gamma scanning. After subcutaneous or intradermal administration most of the label remained at the site of injection and only little drained to lymph nodes and was detectable for a few days only, whereas after infusion into the distal lymph vessels radioactivity was found to concentrate exclusively in the draining lymph node and was retained there for 4 weeks (Juillard et al. 1979).

In humans similar results were obtained when proteins were radiotraced after intralymphatic and subcutaneous injection (Senti et al. 2009). On the right abdominal side, a ^{99m}Tc-labeled protein was injected directly into a superficial inguinal lymph node. On the left side, the same dose was injected subcutaneously, but 10 cm above the inguinal lymph nodes. As shown in Fig. 10.3, only a small fraction of the subcutaneously administered protein reached the lymph nodes after 4 h and this fraction did not increase after 25 h. In contrast, intralymphatic injection caused the protein to drain into the deep subcutaneous lymph nodes and further into one pelvic lymph node already within 20 min. Thus, intralymphatic injection efficiently pulsed five lymph nodes with the full amount of the protein.

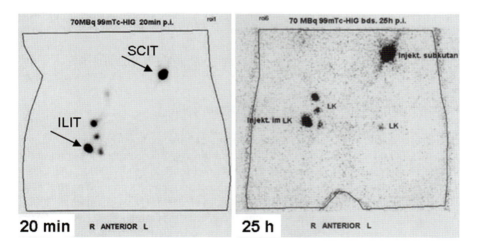

Fig. 10.3 Biodistribution after intralymphatic administration: Biodistribution of ^{99m}Tc-labeled human IgG after intralymphatic (*left abdominal side*) and subcutaneous (*right abdominal side*) injections. Radio tracing was made by gamma-imaging 20 min (*left panel*) and 25 h (*right panel*) after injection. *Arrows* indicate the site of injection (SCIT, subcutaneous, ILIT, intralymphatic)

Intralymphatic Vaccination with Other Types of Vaccines

The first review on intralymphatic vaccination was already written in 1977 (Juillard and Boyer 1977). In the early 1970s Julliard and others aimed at enhancing tumor cell based cancer vaccines in dogs using this method. Ten years later, when researchers wanted to produce antibodies against proteins of which they had been able to purify only very small amounts, they were looking for the most efficient route of immunization. It was already reported in the 1980s that nanogram quantities of protein can elicit immune responses when injected into lymph nodes (Nilsson et al. 1987; Sigel et al. 1983). Thereafter intralymphatic vaccination was performed in various fields where conventional routes of administration produced insufficient results, or where the goal was to maximize the immune response, such as in cancer vaccines or allergen specific immunotherapy. In the following we will list the types of vaccines that are reported to have been used via the intralymphatic route.

Intralymphatic Vaccination with DCs

After subcutaneous or intradermal injection, the main fraction of DCs remains at the injection site (Barratt-Boyes et al. 2000; Morse et al. 1999; De Vries et al. 2003; Lesimple et al. 2003; Quillien et al. 2005; Thomas et al. 1999; Barratt-Boyes et al. 1997). Therefore, intralymphatic and intranodal delivery of DC-based vaccines have been attempted (Lesimple et al. 2006; Mackensen et al. 1999; Grover et al. 2006) in order to enhance the immune response. Antigen-pulsed DCs injected into the lymph node localize to the paracortex (Brown et al. 2003; de Vries et al. 2005; De Vries et al. 2003), and clinical trials suggested that intralymphatic administration of DC vaccines enhanced the immune responses (Lesimple et al. 2003). However, in other clinical trials, no advantage of intranodal delivery over intradermal delivery of DCs was found (Brown et al. 2003; Fong et al. 2001).

Intralymphatic Vaccination with Tumor Cells

Non-professional APC, such as a fibrosarcoma cell line efficiently induced antigen specific CD8+ T-cell responses when injected directly into lymph nodes, but not if injected subcutaneously (Kundig et al. 1995; Ochsenbein et al. 2001). The CD8+ T-cell response was found to be induced via direct antigen presentation on the MHC class I molecule of the fibrosarcoma (Kundig et al. 1995; Ochsenbein et al. 2001). As DCs and T cells are present at very high densities in lymph nodes, costimulatory signals for T and B cell induction may be provided as a bystander effect. Intralymphatic immunization using tumor cells has been tried in both human cancer patients and dogs with indication of success (Juillard and Boyer 1977; Juillard et al. 1976, 1977, 1978, 1979; Boyer et al. 1976).

Intralymphatic Vaccination with MHC Class I Binding Peptides

Aiming at enhancing CD8+ T-cell mediated cancer immunotherapy direct administration of MHC class I-binding peptide vaccines into lymph nodes or spleen was tried and found to dramatically enhance CD8+ T-cell responses in mice (Johansen et al. 2005). Intralymphatic priming with a naked DNA vaccine followed by a peptide boost produced the strongest CD8+ T-cell responses that can be observed in mice, the frequencies of peptide specific CD8+ T cells being as high as 80% (Smith et al. 2009).

Intralymphatic Vaccination with Immunostimulating Complexes (ISCOMS)

The intranasal route was compared to targeted lymph node immunization using HIV formulated in PR8-Flu ISCOM adjuvant in rhesus macaques. Targeting the vaccine to lymph nodes generated significantly stronger T-and B-cell responses (Koopman et al. 2007).

Targeted Lymph-Node Immunization Against Immunodeficiency Viruses

This form of intralymphatic vaccination is extensively documented to be the most efficient means to immunize macaques against SIV. Vaccination using envelope gp120 and core p27 by targeted lymph node immunization was compared to the intradermal, nasal, or intramuscular route. Only targeted lymph node immunization induced protection against the SIV challenge, whereas none of the other routes induced a protective immune response (Lehner et al. 1996). Similar results were obtained in macaques vaccinated with p27 alone (Kawabata et al. 1998), with HSP70 linked either to SIVgp120 or p27 (Lehner et al. 2000), with HSP70 conjugated to HIV gp120, SIV p27 and CCR5 peptides (Bogers et al. 2004a, b), a particulate SIVp27 protein vaccine (Klavinskis et al. 1996), or SIVp27 virus like particles (Lehner et al. 1994).

Targeted lymph-node immunization also proved to be the most efficient route to immunize cats against feline immunodeficiency virus using a protein based vaccine (Finerty et al. 2001). The superior efficacy of lymph node targeting was also confirmed for protein vaccines in cows (Guidry et al. 1994).

Intralymphatic Vaccination with BCG

Julliard et al. report a comparison of intralymphatic versus intradermal vaccination with BCG. It was found that the tuberculin test became positive at an earlier time point (11–23 days) after intralymphatic than after intradermal vaccination (45 days) (Juillard and Boyer 1977).

Intralymphatic Vaccination with Vaccinia Virus

Intranodal immunization with a vaccinia virus encoding multiple antigenic epitopes and costimulatory molecules in patients with metastatic stage III and IV melanoma proved safe and immunogenic in the majority of patients, but did not prove obviously more immunogenic that intradermal administration, although this conclusion was drawn from historical data and not from a direct comparison (Adamina et al. 2010).

Intralymphatic Administration of Adjuvants

Lymph node targeting can also be used to enhance the efficacy of adjuvants. Intralymphatic administration of CpG required 100 times lower doses than subcutaneous administration, thus avoiding unwanted systemic adverse effects of the adjuvant (von Beust et al. 2005). This is in line with reports of better safety profiles and enhanced efficacy of CpG when targeted to lymph nodes using particles (Bourquin et al. 2008; Storni et al. 2004).

Intralymphatic Immunotherapy with Allergens

IgE-mediated allergies, such as allergic rhino-conjunctivitis and asthma today affect up to 35% of the population in westernized countries (Arbes et al. 2005; Verlato et al. 2003; The International Study of Asthma and Allergies in Childhood (ISAAC) Steering Committee 1998; Wuthrich et al. 1996). The gold standard treatment is subcutaneous allergen-specific immunotherapy (SIT), the administration of gradually increasing quantities of an allergen (Bousquet et al. 1998; Lockey 2001; Varney et al. 1991). Immunotherapy confers long term benefit (Durham et al. 1999; Golden et al. 1996; Moller et al. 2002; Pajno et al. 2001), but requires 30–80 doctor visits over 3–5 years,which is compromising patient compliance. SIT is also associated with frequent allergic side effects including a risk of anaphylaxis and even death (Lockey et al. 1987, 1990; Stewart and Lockey 1992).

Allergen immunotherapy shifts the T-cell response from a Th2 towards a Th1 phenotype (Till et al. 2004; Norman 2004), and it also stimulates the production of allergen-specific T-regulatory cells (Vissers et al. 2004; Norman 2004; Till et al. 2004). In the serum, titers of allergen-specific IgG antibodies, especially IgG4, increase (Pierson-Mullany et al. 2000). Which of these immunological mediators is ultimately responsible for ameliorating the allergy symptoms is a matter of debate.

In mice, intralymphatic administration of allergens was shown to significantly enhance the efficiency of immunization, inducing allergen-specific IgG2a antibody responses which were 10–20 times higher with only 0.1% of the allergen dose (Martinez-Gomez et al. 2009a). Also, intralymphatic injection of allergens enhanced IL-2, IFN-γ, IL-4 and IL-10 secretion when compared to subcutaneous injection, suggesting that intralymphatic vaccination does not polarize the response to the allergen, but generated overall stronger Th1, Th2, and T-regulatory responses (Martinez-Gomez et al. 2009a).

Meanwhile, the feasibility, safety and efficacy of intralymphatic allergen immunotherapy has been demonstrated in four separate clinical trials. In a first trial, eight bee-venom allergic patients, who would normally receive 70 subcutaneous injections of bee venom, were given only three low-dose injections of bee venom directly into their inguinal lymph nodes. In this proof of concept trial seven out of the eight treated patients were protected against a subsequent bee sting challenge (Senti et al., manuscript in preparation). Similar results were obtained in a larger multi-center clinical trial with 66 bee venom-allergic patients (Senti et al., manuscript in preparation). In a randomized controlled trial, 165 patients with grass pollen-induced hay fever received either 54 high dose subcutaneous injections with pollen extract over 3 years or three low-dose intralymphatic injections over 2 months. The three low-dose intralymphatic allergen administrations enhanced safety and efficacy of immunotherapy and reduced treatment time from 3 years to 8 weeks (Senti et al. 2008). These data have meanwhile been confirmed in a similar double-blind placebo-controlled trial using intralymphatic vaccination with a modified recombinant cat hair allergen in allergic patients (Imvision Therapeutics 2009).

Targeting Intralymphatic Vaccines to the MHC Class II Pathway

As intralymphatic vaccination brings the antigen directly to the DCs of the lymph node, intracellular translocation sequences and sequences further targeting the antigen to the MHC class II pathway may enhance the CD4+ T cell response. By fusing allergens to a tat-translocation peptide derived from HIV and to a part of the invariant chain, such allergy vaccines can be targeted to MHC class II molecules located in the endoplasmatic reticulum. In several experimental studies, it has been shown that such targeting circumvents the inefficient pinocytosis process as well as enzymatic degradation in phagolysosomes, and that by such means the immunogenicity could be significantly enhanced (Crameri et al. 2007; Martinez-Gomez et al. 2009a, b; Rhyner et al. 2007). This concept has meanwhile also been proven in a first clinical trial (Imvision Therapeutics 2009).

Intralymphatic Vaccination with Naked DNA Vaccines

Intralymphatic injection is shown to also markedly enhance naked DNA vaccines in mice (Maloy et al. 2001; Heinzerling et al. 2006). These murine studies demonstrated that when using three injections the minimal dose of a naked DNA vaccine required to induce ex vivo measurable cytotoxic CD8+ T cell responses was 200 µg if the vaccine was administered via the intradermal and intramuscular route, but could be lowered to 2 µg if administered directly into the spleen and further down to even 0.2 µg when injected directly into a subcutaneous lymph node of the groin.

Thus, direct delivery to the spleen was around 100-fold more potent and administration to a lymph node was around 1,000-times more potent. We found the approx. 10-fold enhanced efficacy of intranodal vs. intrasplenic delivery to be reproducible and consistent, also for other vaccines (TMK unpublished). Because injection into the spleen which in the mouse has a volume of around 100 μl generates lower vaccine concentrations than injection into a subcutaneous lymph node with an estimated volume of around 1 μl, it appears that generating a higher vaccine concentration is more important than pulsing a higher number of professional APCs. This assumption is in line with findings that a few hundred adequately pulsed or transfected APCs are sufficient for generating a biologically relevant immune response (Bot et al. 2000).

While intralymphatic administration of a naked DNA vaccine allows to lower the vaccine doses by three orders of magnitude, we have also demonstrated that, conversely, using the same vaccine dose, intralymphatic injection generates a stronger CD8+ T cell response than intramuscular or intradermal injection. In our hands, only intralymphatic DNA vaccination was able to generate a CD8+ T cell response that protected mice against a tumor challenge (Maloy et al. 2001; Heinzerling et al. 2006).

While plasmid priming induces a high quality immune response, the frequency of specific T cells is relatively low (Smith et al. 2009). In contrast, sequential intralymphatic vaccination with naked DNA followed by a peptide boost, resulted in a considerable higher frequency of antigen-specific CD8+ T cells, i.e. around 5–50% of the total CD8+ T cell population. Boosting with a peptide induced a stepwise functional conversion. First, a rapid loss of CD26L expression, next, initiation of proliferation and expression of CD107a, and finally production of pro-inflammatory cytokines and chemokines. Such induced T cells dominated the T cell repertoire and were able to recognize and clear tumor cells effectively, not only from lymphatic organs, but also from the lung. The significant expansion capability of T cells was mirrored by low PD-1 expression, an important down regulator of T cell immunity. This was in strong contrast to intralymphatic peptide immunization alone which induced high PD-1 expression (Smith et al. 2009). We have found this down regulation of PD-1 to be mediated by TLR-9 signaling, as intralymphatic peptide vaccination adjuvanted with escalating doses of CpG ODN yielded higher numbers of CD8+ T cells with progressively lower PD-1 expression (Wong et al. 2009). By the use of transcriptome microarray analysis and flow cytometry the profile of T cell immunity after intralymphatic vaccination with naked DNA vaccines was extensively analyzed (Smith et al. 2011). In line with the above, repeated intralymphatic administration of naked DNA plasmid induced a markedly different gene signature than vaccination with peptide alone, with transcripts and protein levels of PD-1 being significantly lower in plasmid primed than peptide primed T cells (Smith et al. 2011).

So far, we have performed two clinical trials on intralymphatic administration of naked DNA vaccines. In an attempt to improve on the in vivo generation and amplification of TAA-specific T cells, we clinically evaluated the intra-lymph node administration of two individual plasmids encoding either MART-1/Melan-A or tyrosinase antigen fragments in stage-III and IV melanoma patients with measurable disease (Tagawa et al. 2003; Weber et al. 2008). Despite a correlation between immunity and clinical outcome measured by time to progression, by RECIST criteria there were no objective clinical responses. In hindsight, when looking at the above mentioned mouse studies demonstrating that a peptide boost is necessary to enhance the frequency and to functionally convert the CD8+ T cells response, this outcome is no longer surprising. Clinical trials which are exploiting an intralymphatic naked DNA prime, peptide boost strategy have now been initiated in various forms of cancer and objective tumor regressions are observed (Ribas et al. 2011).

Just recently, intralymphatic vaccination has also been successfully introduced to the veterinary arena. In a pilot study low dose DNA vaccination into the submandibular lymph nodes of ponies using a plasmid expressing the equine influenza virus haemagglutinin successfully led to seroconversion with IgG antibody titers comparable to current commercial protein based equine influenza HA vaccines (Landolt et al. 2010). While T cell responses were not measured, generation of IgG suggests that this procedure also induced CD4+ T cell responses.

Intralymphatic Vaccination with RNA Vaccines

While the feasibility and safety of intradermal vaccination with RNA have been proven in preclinical (Carralot et al. 2004; Scheel et al. 2006) and clinical studies (Weide et al. 2008), induction of CD8+ T cell responses was modest (Weide et al. 2009). A recent study by the group of Ugur Sahin demonstrated that the immunogenicity of mRNA vaccines could be strongly enhanced by administration into the lymph node (Kreiter et al. 2010). This preclinical work demonstrated that intra lymph node administration of a mRNA vaccine generated around 10-fold higher frequencies of specific T cells when compared to subcutaneous, intradermal injection, and also when compared to injection near to the lymph node. Bioluminescence imaging after injection of luciferase encoding RNA via the intranodal, subcutaneous or intradermal route revealed that this enhanced immunogenicity could be attributed to enhanced bioavailability of the encoded antigen in the lymph node. The authors found selective uptake and enrichment of naked RNA by lymph node resident DCs, in particular CD11c+, CD11b+, and CD11c+ CD8+ dendritic cell subpopulations, known to be efficient stimulators of T cells (Banchereau et al. 2000). There was evidence that the mechanism of mRNA uptake was macropinocytosis (Kreiter et al. 2010). Flow cytometric phenotyping of CD11c+ DCs harvested form RNA injected lymph nodes revealed upregulation of maturation markers including CD86, MHC class II, and CD40 within 24 h. Injected lymph nodes also showed higher cellularity and these changes were dependent on TLR3 and TLR7 activation. Also, the same authors observed profound upregulation of the proinflammatory cytokines IL-6, IL-1b, IL-1a and chemokine ligands IP-10, CXCL9, CCL4, and CCL3, as well as IL-12p40, whereas inhibitory molecules IL-10 and TGF-β remained unchanged. All together RNA injection into lymph nodes generated a Th1-type environment. Such immunized T cell responses were robust and completely protected mice against tumor challenge.

Conclusion

Which vaccines profit the most from intralymphatic administration? Those vaccines which are the least stable and do not efficiently drain into lymph nodes after subcutaneous or intramuscular injection, appear to profit the most from direct intralymphatic administration (Table 10.1). Even naked mRNA, despite the presence of RNAses in every tissue, can be used as a vaccine and induces robust and biologically relevant CD8+ T cell responses when administered via the intralymphatic route. On the other end of the spectrum, injection of a stable and particulate vaccine, such as lymphocytic choriomeningitis virus (LCMV) does not become more immunogenic when administered into a lymph node (Senti et al. 2009). Obviously, the virus particles find their way into secondary lymphatic organs efficiently. In line with this, the only report in the literature which does not confirm that the intralymphatic route is superior to other routes, was using a recombinant vaccinia virus (Adamina et al. 2010).

It should also be noted, that intralymphatic delivery should not be regarded as a strategy to replace the adjuvant, but is also a strategy to enhance the effect of the adjuvant, as we have demonstrated for CpG ODN (von Beust et al. 2005) and other biological response modifiers (TMK and AB, unpublished).

Overall, vaccines that work only poorly by subcutaneous or intramuscular administration, or those that need maximization of the immune response such as therapeutic vaccines, profit the most from intralymphatic delivery. Conversely, those vaccines which already induce strong immune responses after subcutaneous or intramuscular administration may not be further enhanced by intralymphatic administration.

References

Adamina M, Rosenthal R, Weber WP, Frey DM, Viehl CT, Bolli M, Huegli RW, Jacob AL, Heberer M, Oertli D, Marti W, Spagnoli GC, Zajac P (2010) Intranodal immunization with a vaccinia virus encoding multiple antigenic epitopes and costimulatory molecules in metastatic melanoma. Mol Ther 18(3):651–659

Arbes SJ Jr, Gergen PJ, Elliott L, Zeldin DC (2005) Prevalences of positive skin test responses to 10 common allergens in the US population: results from the third National Health and Nutrition Examination Survey. J Allergy Clin Immunol 116(2):377–383

Banchereau J, Briere F, Caux C, Davoust J, Lebecque S, Liu YJ, Pulendran B, Palucka K (2000) Immunobiology of dendritic cells. Annu Rev Immunol 18:767–811

Barratt-Boyes SM, Watkins SC, Finn OJ (1997) Migration of cultured chimpanzee dendritic cells following intravenous and subcutaneous injection. Adv Exp Med Biol 417:71–75

Barratt-Boyes SM, Zimmer MI, Harshyne LA, Meyer EM, Watkins SC, Capuano S III, Murphey-Corb M, Falo LD Jr, Donnenberg AD (2000) Maturation and trafficking of monocyte-derived dendritic cells in monkeys: implications for dendritic cell-based vaccines. J Immunol 164(5):2487–2495

Bogers WM, Bergmeier LA, Ma J, Oostermeijer H, Wang Y, Kelly CG, Ten Haaft P, Singh M, Heeney JL, Lehner T (2004a) A novel HIV-CCR5 receptor vaccine strategy in the control of mucosal SIV/HIV infection. AIDS 18(1):25–36

Bogers WM, Bergmeier LA, Oostermeijer H, ten Haaft P, Wang Y, Kelly CG, Singh M, Heeney JL, Lehner T (2004b) CCR5 targeted SIV vaccination strategy preventing or inhibiting SIV infection. Vaccine 22(23–24):2974–2984

Bot A, Stan AC, Inaba K, Steinman R, Bona C (2000) Dendritic cells at a DNA vaccination site express the encoded influenza nucleoprotein and prime MHC class I-restricted cytolytic lymphocytes upon adoptive transfer. Int Immunol 12(6):825–832

Bourquin C, Anz D, Zwiorek K, Lanz AL, Fuchs S, Weigel S, Wurzenberger C, von der Borch P, Golic M, Moder S, Winter G, Coester C, Endres S (2008) Targeting CpG oligonucleotides to the lymph node by nanoparticles elicits efficient antitumoral immunity. J Immunol 181(5):2990–2998

Bousquet J, Lockey R, Malling HJ (1998) Allergen immunotherapy: therapeutic vaccines for allergic diseases. A WHO position paper. J Allergy Clin Immunol 102(4 Pt 1):558–562

Boyer P, Juillard G, Yamashiro C, McCarthy T (1976) Characterization of immune responses to tumor cells following intralymphatic immunization. Proc Am Assoc Cancer Res 17:69

Brown K, Gao W, Alber S, Trichel A, Murphey-Corb M, Watkins SC, Gambotto A, Barratt-Boyes SM (2003) Adenovirus-transduced dendritic cells injected into skin or lymph node prime potent simian immunodeficiency virus-specific T cell immunity in monkeys. J Immunol 171(12): 6875–6882

Carralot JP, Probst J, Hoerr I, Scheel B, Teufel R, Jung G, Rammensee HG, Pascolo S (2004) Polarization of immunity induced by direct injection of naked sequence-stabilized mRNA vaccines. Cell Mol Life Sci 61(18):2418–2424

Crameri R, Fluckiger S, Daigle I, Kundig T, Rhyner C (2007) Design, engineering and in vitro evaluation of MHC class-II targeting allergy vaccines. Allergy 62(2):197–206

De Vries IJ, Krooshoop DJ, Scharenborg NM, Lesterhuis WJ, Diepstra JH, Van Muijen GN, Strijk SP, Ruers TJ, Boerman OC, Oyen WJ, Adema GJ, Punt CJ, Figdor CG (2003) Effective migration of antigen-pulsed dendritic cells to lymph nodes in melanoma patients is determined by their maturation state. Cancer Res 63(1):12–17

de Vries IJ, Lesterhuis WJ, Barentsz JO, Verdijk P, van Krieken JH, Boerman OC, Oyen WJ, Bonenkamp JJ, Boezeman JB, Adema GJ, Bulte JW, Scheenen TW, Punt CJ, Heerschap A, Figdor CG (2005) Magnetic resonance tracking of dendritic cells in melanoma patients for monitoring of cellular therapy. Nat Biotechnol 23(11):1407–1413

Durham SR, Walker SM, Varga EM, Jacobson MR, O'Brien F, Noble W, Till SJ, Hamid QA, Nouri-Aria KT (1999) Long-term clinical efficacy of grass-pollen immunotherapy. N Engl J Med 341(7):468–475

Finerty S, Stokes CR, Gruffydd-Jones TJ, Hillman TJ, Barr FJ, Harbour DA (2001) Targeted lymph node immunization can protect cats from a mucosal challenge with feline immunodeficiency virus. Vaccine 20(1–2):49–58

Fong L, Brockstedt D, Benike C, Wu L, Engleman EG (2001) Dendritic cells injected via different routes induce immunity in cancer patients. J Immunol 166(6):4254–4259

Frey JR, Wenk P (1957) Experimental studies on the pathogenesis of contact eczema in the guinea-pig. Int Arch Allergy Appl Immunol 11(1–2):81–100

Golden DB, Kwiterovich KA, Kagey-Sobotka A, Valentine MD, Lichtenstein LM (1996) Discontinuing venom immunotherapy: outcome after five years. J Allergy Clin Immunol 97(2):579–587

Greter M, Hofmann J, Becher B (2009) Neo-lymphoid aggregates in the adult liver can initiate potent cell-mediated immunity. PLoS Biol 7(5):e1000109

Grover A, Kim GJ, Lizee G, Tschoi M, Wang G, Wunderlich JR, Rosenberg SA, Hwang ST, Hwu P (2006) Intralymphatic dendritic cell vaccination induces tumor antigen-specific, skin-homing T lymphocytes. Clin Cancer Res 12(19):5801–5808

Guidry AJ, O'Brian CN, Oliver SP, Dowlen HH, Douglass LW (1994) Effect of whole *Staphylococcus aureus* and mode of immunization on bovine opsonizing antibodies to capsule. J Dairy Sci 77:2965–2974

Heinzerling L, Basch V, Maloy K, Johansen P, Senti G, Wuthrich B, Storni T, Kundig TM (2006) Critical role for DNA vaccination frequency in induction of antigen-specific cytotoxic responses. Vaccine 24(9):1389–1394

Imvision Therapeutics (2009) Positive phase I clinical results for treatment of cat dander allergy. http://www.imvision-therapeutics.com

Johansen P, Haffner AC, Koch F, Zepter K, Erdmann I, Maloy K, Simard JJ, Storni T, Senti G, Bot A, Wuthrich B, Kundig TM (2005) Direct intralymphatic injection of peptide vaccines enhances immunogenicity. Eur J Immunol 35(2):568–574

Juillard GJ, Boyer PJ (1977) Intralymphatic immunization: current status. Eur J Cancer 13(4–5):439–440

Juillard GJ, Boyer PJ, Snow HD (1976) Intralymphatic infusion of autochthonous tumor cells in canine lymphoma. Int J Radiat Oncol Biol Phys 1(5–6):497–503

Juillard GJ, Boyer PJ, Yamashiro CH, Snow HD, Weisenburger TH, McCarthy T, Miller RJ (1977) Regional intralymphatic infusion (ILI) of irradiated tumor cells with evidence of distant effects. Cancer 39(1):126–130

Juillard GJ, Boyer PJ, Yamashiro CH (1978) A phase I study of active specific intralymphatic immunotherapy (ASILI). Cancer 41(6):2215–2225

Juillard GJ, Boyer PJ, Niewisch H, Hom M (1979) Distribution and consequences of cell suspensions following intralymphatic infusion. Bull Cancer 66(3):217–228

Karrer U, Althage A, Odermatt B, Roberts CW, Korsmeyer SJ, Miyawaki S, Hengartner H, Zinkernagel RM (1997) On the key role of secondary lymphoid organs in antiviral immune responses studied in alymphoplastic (aly/aly) and spleenless (Hox11(–)/–) mutant mice. J Exp Med 185(12):2157–2170

Kawabata S, Miller CJ, Lehner T, Fujihashi K, Kubota M, McGhee JR, Imaoka K, Hioi T, Kiyono H (1998) Induction of Th2 cytokine expression for p27-specific IgA B-cell responses after targeted lymph node immunization with simian immunodeficiency virus in rhesus macaques. J Infect Dis 177:26–33

Klavinskis LS, Bergmeier LA, Gao L, Mitchell E, Ward RG, Layton G, Brookes R, Meyers NJ, Lehner T (1996) Mucosal or targeted lymph node immunization of macaques with a particulate SIVp27 protein elicits virus-specific CTL in the genito-rectal mucosa and draining lymph nodes. J Immunol 157(6):2521–2527

Koopman G, Bogers WM, van Gils M, Koornstra W, Barnett S, Morein B, Lehner T, Heeney JL (2007) Comparison of intranasal with targeted lymph node immunization using PR8-Flu ISCOM adjuvanted HIV antigens in macaques. J Med Virol 79(5):474–482

Kreiter S, Selmi A, Diken M, Koslowski M, Britten CM, Huber C, Tureci O, Sahin U (2010) Intranodal vaccination with naked antigen-encoding RNA elicits potent prophylactic and therapeutic antitumoral immunity. Cancer Res 70(22):9031–9040

Kundig TM, Bachmann MF, DiPaolo C, Simard JJ, Battegay M, Lother H, Gessner A, Kuhlcke K, Ohashi PS, Hengartner H et al (1995) Fibroblasts as efficient antigen-presenting cells in lymphoid organs. Science 268(5215):1343–1347

Landolt GA, Hussey SB, Kreutzer K, Quintana A, Lunn DP (2010) Low-dose DNA vaccination into the submandibular lymph nodes in ponies. Vet Rec 167(8):302–303

Lehner T, Bergmeier LA, Tao L, Panagiotidi C, Klavinskis LS, Hussain L, Ward RG, Meyers N, Adams SE, Gearing AJ et al (1994) Targeted lymph node immunization with simian immunodeficiency virus p27 antigen to elicit genital, rectal, and urinary immune responses in nonhuman primates. J Immunol 153(4):1858–1868

Lehner T, Wang Y, Cranage M, Bergmeier LA, Mitchell E, Tao L, Hall G, Dennis M, Cook N, Brookes R, Klavinskis L, Jones I, Doyle C, Ward R (1996) Protective mucosal immunity elicited by targeted iliac lymph node immunization with a subunit SIV envelope and core vaccine in macaques. Nat Med 2(7):767–775

Lehner T, Mitchell E, Bergmeier L, Singh M, Spallek R, Cranage M, Hall G, Dennis M, Villinger F, Wang Y (2000) The role of gammadelta T cells in generating antiviral factors and beta-chemokines in protection against mucosal simian immunodeficiency virus infection. Eur J Immunol 30(8):2245–2256

Lesimple T, Moisan A, Carsin A, Ollivier I, Mousseau M, Meunier B, Leberre C, Collet B, Quillien V, Drenou B, Lefeuvre-Plesse C, Chevrant-Breton J, Toujas L (2003) Injection by various routes of melanoma antigen-associated macrophages: biodistribution and clinical effects. Cancer Immunol Immunother 52(7):438–444

Lesimple T, Neidhard EM, Vignard V, Lefeuvre C, Adamski H, Labarriere N, Carsin A, Monnier D, Collet B, Clapisson G, Birebent B, Philip I, Toujas L, Chokri M, Quillien V (2006) Immunologic and clinical effects of injecting mature peptide-loaded dendritic cells by intra-lymphatic and intranodal routes in metastatic melanoma patients. Clin Cancer Res 12(24):7380–7388

Lockey RF (2001) "ARIA": global guidelines and new forms of allergen immunotherapy. J Allergy Clin Immunol 108(4):497–499

Lockey RF, Benedict LM, Turkeltaub PC, Bukantz SC (1987) Fatalities from immunotherapy (IT) and skin testing (ST). J Allergy Clin Immunol 79(4):660–677

Lockey RF, Turkeltaub PC, Olive ES, Hubbard JM, Baird-Warren IA, Bukantz SC (1990) The hymenoptera venom study. III: safety of venom immunotherapy. J Allergy Clin Immunol 86(5):775–780

Mackensen A, Krause T, Blum U, Uhrmeister P, Mertelsmann R, Lindemann A (1999) Homing of intravenously and intralymphatically injected human dendritic cells generated in vitro from CD34+ hematopoietic progenitor cells. Cancer Immunol Immunother 48(2–3):118–122

Maloy KJ, Erdmann I, Basch V, Sierro S, Kramps TA, Zinkernagel RM, Oehen S, Kundig TM (2001) Intralymphatic immunization enhances DNA vaccination. Proc Natl Acad Sci USA 98(6):3299–3303

Manolova V, Flace A, Bauer M, Schwarz K, Saudan P, Bachmann MF (2008) Nanoparticles target distinct dendritic cell populations according to their size. Eur J Immunol 38(5):1404–1413

Martinez-Gomez JM, Johansen P, Erdmann I, Senti G, Crameri R, Kundig TM (2009a) Intralymphatic injections as a new administration route for allergen-specific immunotherapy. Int Arch Allergy Immunol 150(1):59–65

Martinez-Gomez JM, Johansen P, Rose H, Steiner M, Senti G, Rhyner C, Crameri R, Kundig TM (2009b) Targeting the MHC class II pathway of antigen presentation enhances immunogenicity and safety of allergen immunotherapy. Allergy 64(1):172–178

Moller C, Dreborg S, Ferdousi HA, Halken S, Host A, Jacobsen L, Koivikko A, Koller DY, Niggemann B, Norberg LA, Urbanek R, Valovirta E, Wahn U (2002) Pollen immunotherapy reduces the development of asthma in children with seasonal rhinoconjunctivitis (the PAT-study). J Allergy Clin Immunol 109(2):251–256

Morse MA, Coleman RE, Akabani G, Niehaus N, Coleman D, Lyerly HK (1999) Migration of human dendritic cells after injection in patients with metastatic malignancies. Cancer Res 59(1):56–58

Nilsson BO, Svalander PC, Larsson A (1987) Immunization of mice and rabbits by intrasplenic deposition of nanogram quantities of protein attached to Sepharose beads or nitrocellulose paper strips. J Immunol Methods 99(1):67–75

Norman PS (2004) Immunotherapy: 1999–2004. J Allergy Clin Immunol 113(6):1013–1023; quiz 1024

Ochsenbein AF, Sierro S, Odermatt B, Pericin M, Karrer U, Hermans J, Hemmi S, Hengartner H, Zinkernagel RM (2001) Roles of tumour localization, second signals and cross priming in cytotoxic T-cell induction. Nature 411(6841):1058–1064

Pajno GB, Barberio G, De Luca F, Morabito L, Parmiani S (2001) Prevention of new sensitizations in asthmatic children monosensitized to house dust mite by specific immunotherapy. A six-year follow-up study. Clin Exp Allergy 31(9):1392–1397

Pierson-Mullany LK, Jackola D, Blumenthal M, Rosenberg A (2000) Altered allergen binding capacities of Amb a 1-specific IgE and IgG4 from ragweed-sensitive patients receiving immunotherapy. Ann Allergy Asthma Immunol 84(2):241–243

Quillien V, Moisan A, Carsin A, Lesimple T, Lefeuvre C, Adamski H, Bertho N, Devillers A, Leberre C, Toujas L (2005) Biodistribution of radiolabelled human dendritic cells injected by various routes. Eur J Nucl Med Mol Imag 32(7):731–741

Ribas A, Weber JS, Chmielowski B, Comin-Anduix B, Lu D, Douek M, Ragavendra N, Raman S, Seja E, Rosario D, Miles S, Diamond DC, Qiu Z, Obrocea M, Bot A (2011). Intra-lymph node prime-boost vaccination against Melan A and tyrosinase for the treatment of metastatic melanoma: results of a phase 1 clinical trial. Clin Cancer Res 17(9):2987-2996

Rhyner C, Kundig T, Akdis CA, Crameri R (2007) Targeting the MHC II presentation pathway in allergy vaccine development. Biochem Soc Trans 35(Pt 4):833–834

Rosenberg SA, Yang JC, Restifo NP (2004) Cancer immunotherapy: moving beyond current vaccines. Nat Med 10(9):909–915

Scheel B, Aulwurm S, Probst J, Stitz L, Hoerr I, Rammensee HG, Weller M, Pascolo S (2006) Therapeutic anti-tumor immunity triggered by injections of immunostimulating single-stranded RNA. Eur J Immunol 36(10):2807–2816

Senti G, Prinz Vavricka BM, Erdmann I, Diaz MI, Markus R, McCormack SJ, Simard JJ, Wuthrich B, Crameri R, Graf N, Johansen P, Kundig TM (2008) Intralymphatic allergen administration renders specific immunotherapy faster and safer: a randomized controlled trial. Proc Natl Acad Sci USA 105(46):17908–17912

Senti G, Johansen P, Kundig TM (2009) Intralymphatic immunotherapy. Curr Opin Allergy Clin Immunol 9(6):537–543

Sigel MB, Sinha YN, VanderLaan WP (1983) Production of antibodies by inoculation into lymph nodes. Methods Enzymol 93:3–12

Smith KA, Tam VL, Wong RM, Pagarigan RR, Meisenburg BL, Joea DK, Liu X, Sanders C, Diamond D, Kundig TM, Qiu Z, Bot A (2009) Enhancing DNA vaccination by sequential injection of lymph nodes with plasmid vectors and peptides. Vaccine 27(19):2603–2615

Smith KA, Qiu Z, Wong R, Tam VL, Tam BL, Joea DK, Quach A, Liu X, Pold M, Malyankar UM, Bot A (2011) Multivalent immunity targeting tumor-associated antigens by intra-lymph node DNA-prime, peptide-boost vaccination. Cancer Gene Ther 18(1):63–76

Stewart GE II, Lockey RF (1992) Systemic reactions from allergen immunotherapy. J Allergy Clin Immunol 90(4 Pt 1):567–578

Storni T, Ruedl C, Schwarz K, Schwendener RA, Renner WA, Bachmann MF (2004) Nonmethylated CG motifs packaged into virus-like particles induce protective cytotoxic T cell responses in the absence of systemic side effects. J Immunol 172(3):1777–1785

Tagawa ST, Lee P, Snively J, Boswell W, Ounpraseuth S, Lee S, Hickingbottom B, Smith J, Johnson D, Weber JS (2003) Phase I study of intranodal delivery of a plasmid DNA vaccine for patients with stage IV melanoma. Cancer 98(1):144–154

The International Study of Asthma and Allergies in Childhood (ISAAC) Steering Committee (1998) Worldwide variation in prevalence of symptoms of asthma, allergic rhinoconjunctivitis, and atopic eczema: ISAAC. Lancet 351(9111):1225–1232

Thomas R, Chambers M, Boytar R, Barker K, Cavanagh LL, MacFadyen S, Smithers M, Jenkins M, Andersen J (1999) Immature human monocyte-derived dendritic cells migrate rapidly to draining lymph nodes after intradermal injection for melanoma immunotherapy. Melanoma Res 9(5):474–481

Till SJ, Francis JN, Nouri-Aria K, Durham SR (2004) Mechanisms of immunotherapy. J Allergy Clin Immunol 113(6):1025–1034, quiz 1035

Varney VA, Gaga M, Frew AJ, Aber VR, Kay AB, Durham SR (1991) Usefulness of immunotherapy in patients with severe summer hay fever uncontrolled by antiallergic drugs. BMJ 302(6771):265–269

Verlato G, Corsico A, Villani S, Cerveri I, Migliore E, Accordini S, Carolei A, Piccioni P, Bugiani M, Lo Cascio V, Marinoni A, Poli A, de Marco R (2003) Is the prevalence of adult asthma and allergic rhinitis still increasing? results of an Italian study. J Allergy Clin Immunol 111(6):1232–1238

Vissers JL, van Esch BC, Hofman GA, Kapsenberg ML, Weller FR, van Oosterhout AJ (2004) Allergen immunotherapy induces a suppressive memory response mediated by IL-10 in a mouse asthma model. J Allergy Clin Immunol 113(6):1204–1210

von Beust BR, Johansen P, Smith KA, Bot A, Storni T, Kundig TM (2005) Improving the therapeutic index of CpG oligodeoxynucleotides by intralymphatic administration. Eur J Immunol 35(6):1869–1876

Weber J, Boswell W, Smith J, Hersh E, Snively J, Diaz M, Miles S, Liu X, Obrocea M, Qiu Z, Bot A (2008) Phase 1 trial of intranodal injection of a Melan-A/MART-1 DNA plasmid vaccine in patients with stage IV melanoma. J Immunother 31(2):215–223

Weide B, Carralot JP, Reese A, Scheel B, Eigentler TK, Hoerr I, Rammensee HG, Garbe C, Pascolo S (2008) Results of the first phase I/II clinical vaccination trial with direct injection of mRNA. J Immunother 31(2):180–188

Weide B, Pascolo S, Scheel B, Derhovanessian E, Pflugfelder A, Eigentler TK, Pawelec G, Hoerr I, Rammensee HG, Garbe C (2009) Direct injection of protamine-protected mRNA: results of a phase 1/2 vaccination trial in metastatic melanoma patients. J Immunother 32(5):498–507

Wong RM, Smith KA, Tam VL, Pagarigan RR, Meisenburg BL, Quach AM, Carrillo MA, Qiu Z, Bot AI (2009) TLR-9 signaling and TCR stimulation co-regulate CD8(+) T cell-associated PD-1 expression. Immunol Lett 127(1):60–67

Wuthrich B, Schindler C, Medici TC, Zellweger JP, Leuenberger P (1996) IgE levels, atopy markers and hay fever in relation to age, sex and smoking status in a normal adult Swiss population. SAPALDIA (Swiss study on air pollution and lung diseases in adults) team. Int Arch Allergy Immunol 111(4):396–402

Zinkernagel RM (2000) Localization dose and time of antigens determine immune reactivity. Semin Immunol 12(3):163–171; discussion 257–344

Zinkernagel RM, Ehl S, Aichele P, Oehen S, Kundig T, Hengartner H (1997) Antigen localisation regulates immune responses in a dose-and time-dependent fashion: a geographical view of immune reactivity. Immunol Rev 156:199–209

Messenger RNA Vaccines

11

Jochen Probst, Mariola Fotin-Mleczek, Thomas Schlake, Andreas Thess, Thomas Kramps, and Karl-Josef Kallen

Twenty years after the seminal observation of Wolff et al. that injection of naked RNA and DNA vectors results in protein expression in vivo, messenger RNA (mRNA) vaccines have found entry into clinical development. Through improved vector design, formulation, and delivery, mRNA, initially perceived as unstable and difficult to manipulate, has been developed into a convenient, efficacious, and flexible vaccine platform. Importantly, the same production process can be used to produce a variety of different vaccines, independent of the specifics of particular constructs, which ultimately decreases costs and development time.

mRNA represents an inherently safe and universally applicable vector that eliminates the risks of genomic integration and uncontrolled expression. In contrast to DNA, mRNA only requires delivery to the cytoplasm to achieve antigen expression. It also has intriguing self-adjuvanting activity, i.e. it directly stimulates immunological pattern recognition receptors to galvanize the host response against the mRNA-encoded antigen. There is now ample evidence from nonclinical and clinical studies that mRNA-based vaccines can induce balanced immune responses comprising the activation of persistent, antigen-specific CD8+ and CD4+ T cells as well as B cells, not just in mice.

In summary, mRNA offers an effective, flexible, and safe vaccine vector. This leads us to believe that mRNA-based vaccines are highly attractive not just for cancer immunotherapy, but also for prophylactic – and maybe even therapeutic – vaccination against infectious diseases. A clinically effective mRNA-based approach to vaccination will represent a game-changing "disruptive technology".

J. Probst(✉)
CureVac GmbH, Tübingen, Germany
e-mail: jochen.probst@curevac.com

J. Thalhamer et al. (eds.), *Gene Vaccines*,
DOI 10.1007/978-3-7091-0439-2_11, © Springer-Verlag/Wien, 2012

The Promises of mRNA Vaccines

A viable vaccine product must be efficacious and safe, i.e. the benefits of using it have to outweigh associated risks. It also must be cost effective, which requires that costs for production, distribution, and use outweigh the human and economic costs associated with disease (Levine 2009).

While messenger RNA (mRNA) vaccines are a budding technology that has to prove its value in the clinic and the market, we posit that, conceptually, they constitute an ideal vaccine platform (Hilleman 1994) fulfilling the above prerequisites. We argue that, if these conceptual strengths are tapped to their full potential, mRNA vaccines could become a "disruptive innovation" (as defined by Christensen (1997), Kaslow (2004)) for the benefit of society.

Unique Strengths

Messenger RNA vaccines exhibit safety advantages that set them apart from other vaccine vectors (Pascolo 2006):

mRNA is a natural and ubiquitous intermediate of protein synthesis that can be employed as the minimal, antigen-encoding vector. As such, it contains neither promoter sequences nor gene cassettes for selective markers (antibiotic resistance, etc.). Hence, mRNA lacks the risk of unintended genetic interactions or immunogenicity (and concurrent adverse effects) potentially associated with such elements.

Furthermore, mRNA cannot integrate into the host genome. This is important as, particularly for prophylactic vaccines, which may be administered to many millions of young and healthy individuals over time, genomic integration would likely undermine acceptance due to perceived risk of, e.g., tumour induction upon disruption or misregulation of genomic loci. For DNA vaccines (Schleef 2005), for instance, the risk of stable genomic integration – albeit very low (FDA Guidance for Industry 2006) – is vividly demonstrated by plasmid DNA (pDNA)-mediated generation of stable transfectants. Throughout clinical use of DNA vaccines genomic integration will, therefore, almost certainly occur and has in fact been demonstrated in nonclinical studies in mice (Wang et al. 2004).

Irrespective of genomic integration, mRNA cannot induce persistent genetic transformation. As the genetic vector is only transiently active and metabolically decays within a few days (Probst et al. 2007), antigen-expression and immunological stimulation remain defined and tightly controlled (we like the descriptive term "immunize and disappear" put forward by Roesler et al. (2009)). Although single-stranded RNA molecules might undergo recombination with each other (Jäschke and Helm 2003; Chetverin 2004), any resulting changes would not be perpetual (as the vector could not replicate) or penetrant (as an affected mRNA would produce relatively little protein). Under any circumstance, they would be exceedingly rare and undirected (virtually eliminating chances of a productive outcome).

Strengths Shared with Other Genetic Vaccines

mRNA vaccines combine immunological characteristics of live attenuated vaccines (e.g. endogenous antigen expression, induction of T cells) with those of killed or subunit vaccines (safety, defined composition, etc.) (Hilleman 1994; Liu 2010). At the same time, they overcome insufficient immunogenicity observed for protein subunit vaccines due to a class-specific adjuvant effect.

As other vaccine vectors and approaches detailed in this book, mRNA-based vaccines can principally encode any protein of interest, including artificial, specifically designed sequences or non-pathogen-associated antigens. They may be used to target antigens in, e.g., infectious diseases, cancer, or allergic disorders. Importantly, encoded antigens are not limited to soluble proteins or protein fragments that are comparatively easy to produce, but may be difficult entities such as transmembrane proteins or complex protein assemblies for which production of a defined subunit vaccine would be otherwise difficult or impossible. mRNA-mediated expression allows for the faithful reproduction of relevant posttranslational modifications and native protein folding.

The production of mRNA-based vaccines, a fully synthetic format, requires only the relevant gene sequence, i.e. a corresponding string of nucleotides on a computer, to initiate production. Thus, the same production process and facility can be used to produce vaccines against very different antigens, adding flexibility and lowering cost. In principle, the process is scalable and can be geared to supply ready-to-use vaccines very quickly, i.e. within a few weeks after receipt of the antigen sequence. In addition, the production process is simple (by standards of other biotechnological products) and can be run with relatively generic equipment, akin to production of plasmid DNA. This flexibility could facilitate rapid and decentralized production of large vaccine quantities and would be particularly important in case of a rapidly emerging pandemic threatening the global human population (Forde 2005; Hoare et al. 2005; Ulmer et al. 2006).

Finally, with the flexibility of a synthetic, nucleotide-based format, individualized (patient-specific) therapeutic approaches, e.g. by targeting a cocktail of patient-specific tumor mutations, become technically feasible.

RNA is chemically quite stable and, therefore, development of lyophilized formulations may obviate the requirement of a cold-chain, facilitating storage and distribution even with limiting infrastructure.

Technological Basis

Despite these attractive conceptual strengths, few systematic efforts and comparatively limited funds have been devoted to realizing the potential of mRNA vaccines. We think this is mainly due to the fact that mRNA is widely considered unstable and difficult to handle. Indeed, for mRNA to become a well accepted and widely used platform technology that is, ultimately, competitive in the demanding and price-sensitive prophylactic vaccine market, central issues remain to be addressed.

In this section, we will delineate the design of mRNA-based vaccines. We will consider the molecular processes acting on mRNA, the understanding of which is key to the development of an effective mRNA-based vaccine: First, mRNA production is briefly outlined (section "Vector Synthesis"). Second, we discuss vaccine delivery, including factors influencing extracellular stability and adjuvanticity (section "Vaccine Delivery"). Third, we present mRNA vector design and factors impacting intracellular stability and efficient translation (section "Considerations Guiding Vector Design"). Finally, we summarize current thought on the vaccine mode-of-action (section "Mode-of-Action").

Vector Synthesis

Eukaryotic mRNA molecules contain discrete elements that are required for efficient translation (Fig. 11.1a): a typical molecule starts with a 5′ Cap structure that is a 7-methyl-guanosine residue joined to the remaining mRNA molecule via a 5′–5′ triphosphate linkage (Banerjee 1980). In vivo, the Cap structure is added enzymatically and may be further modified by 2′-O-methylation of the first or the first and second transcribed nucleotides. Downstream of the Cap structure, the protein-encoding open reading frame (ORF) is typically flanked by untranslated regions (UTRs), the 5′- and 3′-UTR. Finally, mRNA molecules are terminated by a tail of adenosine residues (poly(A) tail) added enzymatically after transcription (Wickens 1990).

The production of pharmaceutical grade mRNA is performed in vitro in a reaction termed run-off transcription (Fig. 11.1b) (Pascolo 2006): Template plasmid DNA (pDNA) containing a RNA polymerase promoter and all structural mRNA elements (except the 5′ Cap and, in some protocols, the 3′ poly(A) tail) is propagated in bacteria. Purified pDNA is linearized by sequence-specific cleavage with a restriction enzyme to ensure defined termination of transcription and is then used as a template for in vitro transcription. Besides linearized pDNA, the in vitro transcription reaction mixture contains reaction buffer, recombinant RNA polymerase, nucleotides (chemically modified nucleotides can be included, but may adversely affect yield) and, in some protocols, Cap analogue. Alternative protocols include a separate enzymatic capping reaction after transcription. Transcription stops as the RNA polymerase reaches the end of the DNA template releasing both the template DNA and the newly synthesized mRNA. Polyadenylation of the mRNA molecule is either performed by including a poly(T) sequence of about 50 nucleotides in the template DNA or by adding the tail enzymatically in a subsequent reaction. Finally, different protocols are employed to purify the mRNA, all of which include a step of nuclease digestion for subsequent removal of template DNA. We have shown that a Good Manufacturing Practice (GMP)-compliant chromatographic method increases the activity of the mRNA molecules up to about fivefold (in terms of protein expression in vivo) (Probst et al. 2007). Importantly, the complete mRNA production process as described above can be adapted to a GMP process at reasonable cost of goods.

Fig. 11.1 Vector structure and synthesis. (**a**) Schematic representation of eukaryotic mRNA elements. (**b**) mRNA production. For details see main text. *P*, promoter; *R*, restriction site for linearization

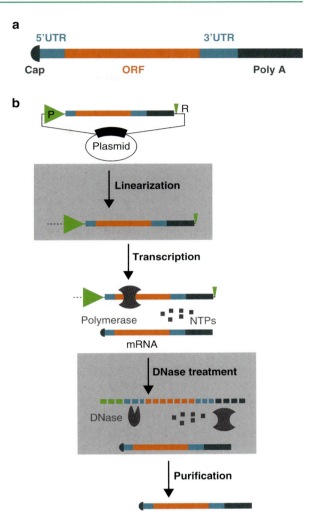

Vaccine Delivery

Extracellular RNA Stability

Most people with a life science background are (by training or painful experience) aware that RNA molecules extracted from natural samples like cell or tissue extracts are prone to degradation. This instability of the molecule is not due to its chemical nature but, rather, the virtual omnipresence of ribonucleases (RNases) within and outside of cells (Sorrentino 1998).

Due to their ubiquity, digestion by extracellular ribonucleases is one of the critical steps affecting the efficacy of mRNA based vaccines in vivo. For example, exposure of naked RNA to simple skin wash preparations, i.e. mixtures of water-soluble molecules washed off the skin surface, destroys mRNA within seconds (Probst et al. 2006). Besides extracellular RNases (and cytosolic mRNA decay machinery, see section "Intracellular RNA Stability"), administered mRNA may have to bypass endosomal degradation, if uptake via the endocytic route is of relevance. Here, chemical degradation via depurination under acidic conditions (in mature lysosomes) may play the dominant role (Sederoff et al. 1975). Therefore, ensuring quick uptake of the mRNA by target cells and/or protection of the mRNA by formulation is critical for clinical efficacy and/or vaccine dose-sparing. Appropriate formulation of mRNA vaccines should protect the cargo from (extracellular) degradation and improve the uptake into (particular) target cells. Due to the complexity and extension of the field of mRNA delivery, we direct the reader to separate reviews (Friedmann 2007; Yamamoto et al. 2009). In the section on applications (see section "Applications to Vaccine Development") we mostly discuss approaches using direct injection by needle and syringe.

Adjuvanticity

In addition to a suitable target antigen, an efficient vaccine should also contain a powerful adjuvant to provide a danger signal for initiating and supporting the adaptive immune response (Pulendran and Ahmed 2006). We now know that ribonucleic acid (RNA)-sensing receptors are particularly diverse and powerful adjuvant targets that probably evolved to detect and counter viral infections by orchestrating innate and adaptive immune responses (Sadler and Williams 2008; McCartney and Colonna 2009).

The immunostimulatory potential of RNA was first recognized in the 1960s by Alick Isaacs and coworkers. They discovered that exposure to "foreign" RNA (i.e. extracted from virus or chemically altered extracts from vertebrate cells) was necessary and sufficient for interferon induction in exposed cells (Isaacs et al. 1963). These observations were extended to the production of double-stranded RNA as synthetic inducers of interferon by Maurice Hilleman and coworkers (Field et al. 1967), but toxic side effects of these early formulations soon limited clinical use (Absher and Stinebring 1969). Throughout the last decade, a spate of studies described the immunostimulatory activity of in vitro transcribed RNA and underlying molecular mechanism in great detail (Karikó et al. 2004; Kim et al. 2004; Scheel et al. 2004, 2005):

At the molecular level, we now know that single-stranded RNA (ssRNA) and double-stranded (dsRNA) are recognized in the endosome by toll-like receptor (TLR) 7/8 (Heil et al. 2004; Diebold et al. 2004) and TLR3 (Alexopoulou et al. 2001), respectively. For ssRNA, optimal sequence motifs were identified (Hornung et al. 2008; Diebold et al. 2006; Saito et al. 2008; Uzri and Gehrke 2009). More recently, recognition of uncapped RNA molecules that bear a 5' triphosphate moiety by the cytosolic helicase RIG-I was shown (Hornung et al. 2006; Pichlmair et al. 2006; Rehwinkel et al. 2010). Still other pattern recognition receptors (PRRs) may in certain situations contribute to the immunostimulatory activity of mRNA vaccines, including PKR, 2'–5' oligo (A) synthetase, and MDA5 (Wilkins and Gale 2010; Nallagatla et al. 2007; Hovanessian 2007; Kato et al. 2006). Intriguingly, the

11 Messenger RNA Vaccines

immunostimulatory potential of in vitro transcribed mRNA can be further tuned by nucleotide modifications, generally ablating immunostimulary capacity, with possible applications in genetic substitution therapy (Karikó et al. 2005; Karikó and Weissman 2007; Karikó et al. 2008; Uzri and Gehrke 2009).

PRR-mediated recognition of nucleic acids has been shown to require additional "sentinel" proteins as well, including HMGB (Yanai et al. 2009), scavenger receptors (Amiel et al. 2009), and antimicrobial peptides (Lande et al. 2007). The apparent role of at least some of these factors in cytosolic nucleic acid uptake is striking (see section "Mode-of-Action"). As a consequence, formulation certainly modulates the immunostimulatory activity of the mRNA vaccine, possibly by influencing mRNA stability (Scheel et al. 2004), but also the route of uptake which could affect exposure to distinct PRRs. Hence, formulation is not only critical for mRNA stability (see section "Intracellular RNA Stability"), but also for adjuvanticity, and offers an important layer for rational vaccine design (Bachmann and Jennings 2010).

In conclusion, relevant immunostimulatory structures of mRNA-based vaccines likely include single-stranded, and double-stranded regions, as well as 5′-triphosphorylated side products. However, this hypothesis and the identity of relevant receptors remain to be addressed experimentally.

Special Delivery Methods

In contrast to DNA vaccines, RNA vaccines only have to cross one membrane barrier. This might lower the requirements for successful transfection in vivo (Yamamoto et al. 2009), but the point remains to be proven. In fact, passive transfection of different (even non-dividing) mammalian cells with mRNA invariably results in expression of protein, which is not true for passive transfection with pDNA (our unpublished data). Appropriate application devices may deliver an mRNA vaccine to more relevant target cells compared to conventional injection and, thereby, further improve immunogenicity or enable vaccine dose-sparing.

Following this idea, gene gun bombardment was successfully used to vaccinate mice against human alpha 1 antitrypsin (Qiu et al. 1996) or the melanoma-associated antigen TRP2 (Steitz et al. 2006). Some optimization of relevant parameters was also reported (Sohn et al. 2001).

More recently, electroporation has emerged as a way to dramatically improve the activity of pDNA vaccines (see Chaps. 7 and 8 of this book for details). However, it remains to be seen, if mRNA vaccines profit from such an approach likewise. Initial reports suggest that this may not hold true, possibly due to the simpler mode of entry for mRNA compared to pDNA (J. Thalhamer, personal communication).

Though not the focus of this chapter, ex vivo mRNA transfection of professional antigen presenting cells (pAPCs) is the most frequently used application of mRNA in the clinic today. Originally described by Boczkowski et al. (1996), this approach has been studied in several clinical trials (Nair et al. 1998; Heiser et al. 2001; Su et al. 2005). While in vitro transfection allows for direct manipulation of dendritic cells with mRNA, the procedure is very time consuming, laborious and requires patient-specific (autologous) cell preparations. Bearing these tremendous logistical challenges in mind, feasibility may remain limited to highly specialized laboratories or clinical centers. It is difficult to see how this approach could be made available on a broad scale. However, the future success of companies pioneering autologous therapeutic modalities in the marketplace (Kantoff et al. 2010) will likely shape the fate of this field.

A conceptually simple, albeit technically challenging approach aimed at targeting pAPCs in vivo is intranodal injection as described in Chap. 10 of this book. A recent report suggests that certain mRNA vaccine formats may require intranodal injection (see section "Nonclinical Studies").

Looking ahead, we think that low cost of goods and convenient administration are prerequisites for the general success of new application methods.

Considerations Guiding Vector Design

Intracellular RNA Stability

Inside the cell, mRNA is subject to complex machinery that finely tunes RNA decay. In eukaryotic cells, cytosolic mRNA decay is catalyzed predominantly by exonucleases (Parker and Song 2004). At the same time, the ends of eukaryotic mRNAs are protected by specific terminal structures and their associated proteins: the Cap at the 5' end and the poly(A) tail at the 3' end (see Fig. 11.1a). Thus, the "default state" of an mRNA in an eukaryotic cell is one of relative stability (Meyer et al. 2004). In the decay of such stable mRNAs, the first and rate limiting step is usually removal of the poly(A) tail (deadenylation) (Yamashita et al. 2005).

Decay of individual mRNAs may be accelerated by specific *cis*-acting elements, i.e. RNA segments on the same molecule as the ORF. Still, these pathways use the same enzymes responsible for general mRNA decay, involving mechanisms for targeting of specific mRNAs to deadenylation. Of note, diverse control mechanisms of mRNA degradation such as decay mediated by destabilizing elements in protein coding regions (Chang et al. 2004; Grosset et al. 2000), decay triggered by AU-rich elements in the 3'-UTR (Chen et al. 1995), decay directed by micro RNAs (Wu et al. 2006), or decay due to premature termination codons known as nonsense mediated decay (Chen and Shyu 2003) all converge on deadenylation as the first step of mRNA degradation in mammalian cells.

Mammalian deadenylation is mediated by the concerted action of two different poly(A) nuclease complexes. Poly(A) tails, initially between 200 and 250 nucleotides in length, are first shortened to about 110 nucleotides by Pan2 in association with Pan3 (Uchida et al. 2004). In the second phase of deadenylation, a complex composed of Ccr4 and Caf1 catalyzes further shortening of the poly(A) tail to oligo(A) (Yamashita et al. 2005).

In the decay of normal mRNA, activation of both deadenylation complexes is coupled to translation termination. When eRF3, part of the termination complex, is released from poly(A) binding protein (PABP), in turn the deadenylase complexes bind to PABP, leading to their activation (Funakoshi et al. 2007). eRF3 family members have also been shown to play key roles in other pathways of mRNA decay.

During and/or after the second phase of deadenylation, decapping by the decapping enzyme Dcp1 may occur (Yamashita et al. 2005). Recently, a further mammalian decapping enzyme, Nudt16, ubiquitously expressed in mouse tissue, has been identified (Song et al. 2010). Deadenylation appears to be linked to subsequent decapping by a protein interacting with both, deadenylation and decapping enzyme; in humans, Pat1b serves as such a scaffold protein (Ozgur et al. 2010). Once decapped, the mRNA body is then progressively degraded by the 5′ exonuclease Xrn1.

Alternatively, after deadenylation, the mRNA body may be degraded by a complex of 3′ exonucleases termed exosome. The remaining Cap structure is then hydrolyzed by the scavenger mRNA-decapping enzyme DcpS (Liu and Kiledjian 2006).

As already mentioned, specific *cis*-acting elements of many kinds can accelerate mRNA decay. However, mRNA may also be stabilized by such elements. For example, it has been shown that the 3′-UTR of alpha-globin mRNA assembles the so called alpha-complex which, by interacting with PABP, functions to reduce deadenylation (Wang et al. 1999).

Efficient Translation

Within the cytosol, the vaccine mRNA needs to be efficiently translated to produce protein antigen. Translation takes place in three phases: initiation (usually the rate-limiting step), elongation, and termination.

Cap and poly(A) tail are not only essential for mRNA stability, both are also required for efficient translation. In fact, Cap and poly(A) tail synergize to regulate mRNA translation efficiency (Gallie 1991). The synergistic effect of Cap and poly(A) appears to be mediated by the interaction of Cap and PABP: The poly(A) tail's stimulation of translation is mediated by PABP (Tarun and Sachs 1995; Blobel 1973) which interacts with eukaryotic initiation factor 4G (eIF4G) (Imataka et al. 1998; Tarun and Sachs 1996). eIF4G in turn is part of the Cap binding eIF4F complex. This interaction between PABP and eIF4G is required for the cooperative action of Cap and poly(A) (Michel et al. 2000). Remarkably, PABP and initiation factors mutually increase their affinity for poly(A) and the Cap, respectively (Wei et al. 1998; Le et al. 1997).

Apart from Cap and poly(A), UTRs also affect the efficiency of translation. In addition to specific *cis* elements such as binding motifs for regulatory molecules, the secondary structure of the 5′ UTR close to the Cap is of critical importance for efficient translation (Babendure et al. 2006).

Codon usage is also considered as a factor affecting the efficiency of translation in many species. However, in humans codon usage bias does not correlate with tRNA levels and gene expression (Duret 2002; Kanaya et al. 2001). In conclusion, codon optimization cannot be expected to (generally) improve mRNA translation in humans, particularly if the ORF is already of human (or even mammalian) origin.

One possible hurdle for effective mRNA vaccines might actually be the stress induced by the RNA itself due to its adjuvant nature. Activation of protein kinase R (PKR) leads to phosphorylation of eIF2α which in turn inhibits Cap-dependent

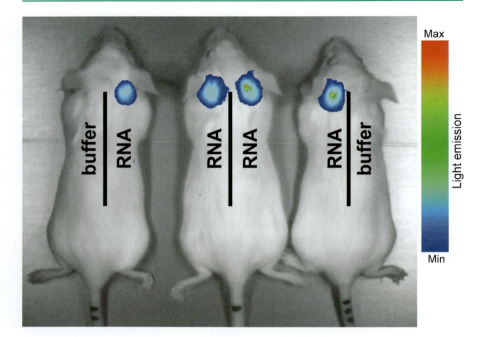

Fig. 11.2 Expression of mRNA in vivo. BALB/c mice were injected intradermally into the ear pinna with either 20 μg of *Photinus pyralis* luciferase (*Pp*luc) encoding mRNA or with injection buffer. 17 h post injection, luciferase expression was visualized in living animals by optical imaging

translation (Anderson et al. 2010). Incorporation of modified nucleotides like pseudouridine may largely counteract these effects (Karikó et al. 2008), however at the expense of the immune stimulatory capacity of the RNA molecule (Karikó et al. 2005).

Mode-of-Action

At the molecular level, many aspects of mRNA vaccines' mode-of-action remain relatively poorly understood.

Naked mRNA injected into mice clearly (and unexpectedly considering its size, charge and the ubiquitous presence of RNases) translocates across the cell membrane barrier into the cytosol for translation to take place (Probst et al. 2007; Wolff et al. 1990) (Fig. 11.2). Similarly, it was observed that receptor-mediated virus entry was not required for viral mRNA to be expressed (Freigang et al. 2003; Mandl et al. 1998). In vitro, cells appear to be generally capable of transferring mRNA molecules from the environment into the cytosol (all primary cells and cell lines we have tested in vitro take up and express naked mRNA; Lorenz et al. 2011. We also found that uncomplexed mRNA predominantly enters mammalian cells via an endocytic route involving scavenger receptor(s). Intriguingly, as discussed in section "Adjuvanticity", scavenger receptors also appear to be required as co-receptors for TLR-dependent signaling and may, therefore, play a role in facilitating not only mRNA expression, but also adjuvanticity. How mRNA subsequently escapes the endocytic pathway to reach the cytosol is a subject of ongoing research. For local injection methods hydrodynamic pressure possibly contributes to the efficacy of target cell transfection (Herweijer and Wolff 2007). Moreover, cellular mRNA uptake can be modulated by appropriate formulation and route of administration.

It is still a matter of debate whether locally administered mRNA is preferentially taken up by restricted cell types and to what extent different cell types may contribute to mRNA vaccine immunogenicity. For example, mRNA may get directly internalized by pAPCs, but other cells may equally well (or even more efficiently) take up and express the mRNA. At least for intradermal injection we have shown that pAPCs do not exclusively take up and express mRNA (Probst et al. 2007).

Depending on the predominant target cell population in vivo, the immune response that is typically observed after local administration of antigen-encoding mRNA may be induced by one of at least two (mutually not exclusive) mechanisms: Either the mRNA directly enters pAPCs, enabling these cells to express, process, and present the antigen directly and to prime an immune response in the draining lymph node after pAPC maturation and migration. Or the mRNA enters primarily non-antigen presenting cells that, by expressing the exogenous RNA, provide antigen (either by release of the antigen or by death of the transfected cell) for the subsequent processing and presentation by pAPCs (a process termed cross priming). Irrespective of the relative contribution of either mechanism, we believe that the intrinsic capability of the mRNA molecule to serve as an adjuvant (Scheel et al. 2004) (see section "Adjuvanticity") plays a pivotal role in the immunogenicity of mRNA-based vaccines. Indeed, we and others have shown that activation of TLR7 and possibly TLR3 are critical for an mRNA vaccine to prime immune responses (Fotin-Mleczek et al. 2011; Kreiter et al. 2010). Other pattern recognition receptors like TLR8 (in humans), RIG-I, or MDA-5 may be of similar importance for the functionality of mRNA based vaccines.

Applications to Vaccine Development

A handful (literally) of seminal studies in the 1990s established that mRNA can be used to induce significant adaptive immune responses in animals (Wolff et al. 1990; Martinon et al. 1993; Conry et al. 1995; Hoerr et al. 2000; Granstein et al. 2000). These pioneering works have been recently extended and led to first clinical trials of mRNA-based cancer immunotherapeutics.

Infectious Disease

Direct injection of mRNA requires optimization to ensure immunogenicity at reasonable vaccine doses. To improve efficacy, the first report on successful vaccination with mRNA used cholesterol/phosphatidylcholine/phosphatidylserine liposomes for enhanced delivery. Vaccine directed against influenza A virus nucleoprotein was injected intraperitoneally or subcutaneously in different mouse strains and resulted in the induction of antigen-specific B and T cell responses (Martinon et al. 1993). Despite this success, the authors, unfortunately, did not address protection against virus challenge that was shown by independent groups working with plasmid DNA (Ulmer et al. 1993).

With no systematic studies on the use of mRNA vaccines against infectious pathogens published, the efficacy of mRNA-based vaccination against infectious diseases remains unproven. Recently, we have initiated a nonclinical program to address this question with encouraging results against a variety of disparate antigens from different pathogens (Petsch et al., manuscript in preparation).

Cancer Vaccines

With regard to potential clinical application, mRNA vaccines have been most frequently and extensively used in the context of cancer immunotherapy.

Nonclinical Studies

The use of mRNA as a new generation tumor vaccine was initiated 15 years ago by Conry et al. (Conry et al. 1995). Inspired by their own results obtained with human carcinoembryonic antigen (CEA, an oncogenic protein)-encoding DNA vaccines, they reasoned that the safety of their genetic vaccine could be improved by using a short-lived mRNA vector for vaccination. This would avoid inadvertent malignant transformation by stable expression, e.g. from persistently integrated DNA vector. Their work also constitutes the first publication on the use of naked mRNA for vaccination and demonstrated an antigen-specific antibody response in a heterologous prime-boost schedule (repeated RNA vaccination, challenge with tumor cell line). Their construct was stabilized by the human β-globin 5′ and 3′ UTRs, but, taking into account the shorter (compared to DNA) duration of antigen expression from mRNA, they adapted the vaccination schedule: mice were injected intramuscularly twice a week for 5 weeks and then challenged with syngenic tumor cells overexpressing human CEA. Antigen-specific antibodies could be detected in five of seven vaccinated mice, yet, unfortunately, none of these animals was protected against tumor challenge. Thus, this paper demonstrated the general feasibility of using an mRNA vaccine to elicit an immune response, but also revealed the necessity to further optimize the vaccine format. Thus, the pursuit of more potent mRNA tumor vaccines had been initiated.

Some groups concentrated on alternative delivery strategies and RNA molecules formulated with different components. Zhou et al. designed a Hemagglutinating virus of Japan (HVJ)–liposome delivery to introduce mRNA encoding melanoma antigen gp100 into mice. Despite the use of this elaborate delivery technology, anti-tumor activity was only elicited when the vaccine was injected directly into the spleen (Zhou et al. 1999).

Two publications in 2000 advanced the field further by describing skin as a suitable injection site for mRNA vaccination and for the induction of antigen-specific immune responses: First, Hoerr et al. showed that intradermally injected naked mRNA induced both, antigen-specific antibodies and T cells with lytic activity against β-galactosidase, a model antigen (Hoerr et al. 2000). Then, Granstein et al. demonstrated that either Langerhans cells, professional antigen presenting cells of the epidermis, pulsed with mRNA and used as a vaccine, or direct intradermal injection of tumor-derived mRNA could induce effective anti-tumoral responses (Granstein et al. 2000). These studies demonstrated that RNA could be easily administered in vivo to induce significant therapeutic effects.

More recently, systemic injection of MART1 mRNA encapsulated in histidylated lipopolyplexes was reported to prevent B16 melanoma from progression and from metastasis (Mockey et al. 2007).

The inclusion of adjuvants to further improve the mRNA vaccine's potency was variously addressed. To this end, different strategies have been devised, mostly based on the addition of a heterologous (non RNA-based) adjuvant, e.g. granulocyte macrophage colony-stimulating factor (GM-CSF) (Carralot et al. 2004) or GM-CSF and Interleukin-2 (IL-2) (Hess et al. 2006) or on the coexpression of costimulatory molecules such as CD80 (Hess et al. 2006). For such combinations, defining suitable, i.e. effective and practical, treatment regimens remains challenging.

We recently described an alternative, simplified approach, by combining naked mRNA with protamine formulated mRNA that results in two distinct, simultaneously applied vaccine components with complementary functions (Fotin-Mleczek et al. 2011). Both components contained the same mRNA but differed in their particle size (Fig. 11.3a). Component 1 with an average size of 50 nm was naked mRNA, component 2 consisted of mRNA:protamine complexes with a diameter of 250–350 nm. Once formed, mRNA:protamine complexes were very stable as revealed by fluorescence correlation spectroscopy (FCS, our unpublished data): In a solution containing differently labeled components 1 and 2, both components remained separate over time, i.e., there was no detectable mRNA exchange between the components. Moreover, a confocal microscopy study showed that both components were taken up by cells via distinct endocytic pathways as no co-localization between the two components could be detected (Fig. 11.3b). These two distinct components apparently fulfilled different functions within the vaccine – free mRNA supported optimal antigen expression (Fig. 11.3c), whereas protamine-complexed mRNA exhibited stronger immunostimulatory properties by TLR7 (Fig. 11.3d). Further, we showed that such formulations (a) induced CD4[+] T helper cells that supported the generation of CD8[+] effector and memory T cells and (b) exerted better anti-tumoral effects in mice than adjusted doses of either component alone (Fig. 11.3e).

The simultaneous activation of both adaptive and innate immunity is crucial for effective vaccination. Two-component mRNA vaccines fulfill this requirement displaying antigenic and adjuvant activity simultaneously to the same target cell population.

Recently, Sahin and coworkers developed a novel mRNA vector platform by introducing different features: First, the use of a duplicated 3′ globin UTR and a particularly long poly A-tail (Holtkamp et al. 2006) probably enhancing the

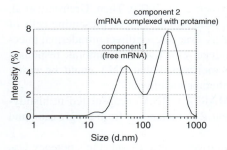

a Two-component complexation of Luc-mRNA size distribution by intensity

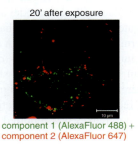

b Uptake of two-component vaccine by human dendritic cells

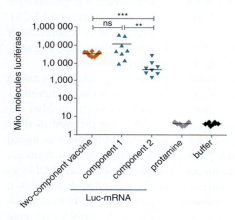

c Expression of *Photinus pyralis* luciferase in vivo

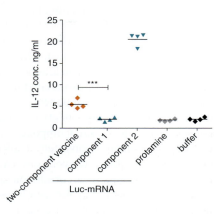

d Interleukin-12 secretion in mice

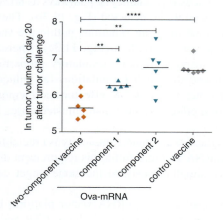

e Inhibition of E.G7-OVA tumor growth upon different treatments

Fig. 11.3 **Two-component mRNA vaccine.** (**a**) mRNA encoding *Pp*luc was produced using the RNActive® technology. The size of particles composing the vaccine solution was analyzed by dynamic light scattering using a Nano ZS Zetasizer (Malvern Instruments). (**b**) mRNA fluorescently labeled with AlexaFluor 488 (component 1) was mixed (at the mass ratio 1:1) with mRNA fluorescently labeled with AlexaFluor 647 and complexed with protamine at the mass ratio of 2:1 (component 2). 10 µg of RNA mixture was added to human dendritic cells and the cellular uptake was monitored by confocal laser scanning microscopy. (**c**) BALB/c mice were treated intradermally with 10 µg of mRNA coding for *Pp*luc administered either as two-component vaccine, free (component 1), or complexed with protamine at a mass ratio of mRNA:protamine of 2:1 (component 2). Luciferase expression was analyzed in eight independent samples. (**d**) mRNA coding for *Pp*luc was administered intravenously either as two-component vaccine, component 1 or component 2. Serum levels of IL-12 in BALB/c mice 4 h after injection were analyzed using standard ELISA. (**e**) C57BL/6 mice (n=6) were vaccinated intradermally on days 1 and 15 with 64 µg of either two-component OVA vaccine or single components of OVA vaccine. Control two-component vaccine or injection buffer were used as controls. Mice were challenged subcutaneously with 1×10E6 syngenic E.G7-OVA tumor cells on day 23 (Reproduced with permission in part from Fotin-Mleczek et al. (2011))

---

interaction between 5′- and 3′-end of the mRNA, thereby supporting translation. Second, modified Cap structures (Kuhn et al. 2010) were introduced to stabilize the mRNA. Third, protein design was used to target the mRNA-encoded antigen into the MHC class I antigen loading compartment (Kreiter et al. 2008). Using such mRNA vectors, Kreiter et al. (2010) compared intradermal, subcutaneous, perinodal and intranodal injections for the delivery of naked (non-complexed) mRNA vaccines and could demonstrate good immunogenicity against influenza A virus hemagglutinin and chicken ovalbumin upon repeated, frequent injections into the lymph node. As the authors point out, no such immune responses could be raised by intradermal (or perinodal) injections. This apparent discrepancy vis-à-vis older, independent results obtained with naked mRNA (Hoerr et al. 2000; Granstein et al. 2000; Carralot et al. 2004) and, much more recently, with formulated mRNA (Fotin-Mleczek et al. 2011) remains a mystery.

Clinical Studies

Very few clinical studies with mRNA-based vaccines have been published so far. The first clinical trial on mRNA vaccination in humans made use of autologous mRNA libraries prepared from melanoma lesions (Weide et al. 2009a; Carralot et al. 2005): 15 melanoma patients (six with stage III, nine with stage IV disease) were treated intradermally with 200 µg of autologous mRNA libraries prepared from tumor biopsies. 24 h later, GM-CSF was injected subcutaneously at the same sites as the mRNA. The first four vaccinations were given every 2 weeks followed by six once-monthly injections. Four patients received further injections as compassionate treatment. The treatment was safe and well tolerated, the most frequent side effects being injection site reactions of grade I and few of grade II according to WHO criteria. Five out of 13 immunologically evaluable patients showed a transient enhancement of CD4[+] and CD8[+] T cell frequencies upon restimulation with cRNA library-transfeced autologous peripheral blood mononuclear cells (PBMCs). The humoral response was assessed by measuring binding of IgG antibodies to three different allogeneic melanoma cell lines (SK-Mel 37, SK-Mel 28, MeWo). A reproducible, significantly increased binding to all cell lines was detected in four patients. An objective response was not observed in the 6 stage IV patients with measurable disease, but favorable clinical courses (stable disease for more than 18 months) were reported in two patients. Two more patients showed a mixed response and regressing metastases during chemotherapy combined with the mRNA vaccine.

In a subsequent study by the same investigators a cocktail of protamine-complexed mRNAs encoding melan-A, tyrosinase, gp100, Mage-A1, Mage-A3, and survivin was administered intradermally in an intensified treatment regimen (Weide et al. 2009b): Three vaccinations were given in the first week, followed by six once-monthly vaccinations and three vaccinations every 2 months. 21 patients with metastatic melanoma (14 patients with stage III, seven with stage IV disease) were included into the trial. GM-CSF was administered 1 day after mRNA injection, in addition ten patients received keyhole limpet hemocyanin (KLH). Again, the most frequent side effects were injection site reactions of WHO grade I or II, that were stronger in the KLH+ arm. The next most common side effects, generally mild, were fatigue, and flu-like symptoms. Probably owing to the addition of protamine, the injection site reactions were more pronounced than in the first trial, but still judged as transient and mild. Two of four immunologically assessable patients showed an increase of vaccine directed T cell frequencies. Six of seven patients with measurable disease had rapid disease progression. However, a seventh patient in the KLH- arm with lung metastases showed a partial response after 12 vaccinations and developed a complete response at month 13, having received additional vaccinations as compassionate treatment. A histopathologically confirmed bone metastasis was detected and surgically removed. Five months later the complete remission was established. The treatment was continued nonetheless and the patient remained disease free thereafter (44 months at the time of manuscript preparation). Three years after start of vaccination, 5 of the 14 patients with stage III disease had no evidence of disease.

In a third trial (Rittig et al. 2011), 30 patients with renal cell carcinoma stage IV were vaccinated with a naked mRNA cocktail encoding MUC1, CEA, Her-2/neu, telomerase, survivin and MAGE-A1 together with GM-CSF administered 24 h after vaccination. Arm A (14 patients) received vaccinations on days 0, 14, 28 and 42. Arm B (16 patients) received an intensified schedule with vaccinations on days 0–3, 7–10, 28 and 42. In both arms, vaccinations were continued on a monthly basis until progression. Severe side effects were not reported and the treatment was considered to be well-tolerated. Clinical benefits consisted of six stable diseases and one partial remission in arm A (median survival 24 months) and nine stable diseases in arm B (median survival 29 months). Induction of antigen specific T cell responses against several of the antigens administered was demonstrated by IFNγ-ELISPOT and chromium release assays.

11 Messenger RNA Vaccines

At CureVac, we have initiated clinical studies in two different indications, castrate resistant prostate carcinoma patients with rising PSA and existing metastasis and patients with NSCLC stage IV (http://www.curevac.de/development_pipeline.php). In both indications, cocktails of optimized versions of protamine-complexed mRNA-based vaccines, which we termed RNActive® (Fotin-Mleczek et al. 2011), are employed. The prostate carcinoma cocktail CV9103 encodes PSA, PSMA, PSCA and STEAP-1. A total of five vaccinations were administered intradermally over a period of 23 weeks in a phase I/IIa trial. The prostate carcinoma trial, conducted at sites in Italy and Germany, is advanced furthest and has yielded first, preliminary data. The most common side effects consisted of injection site reactions similar to the academic studies cited above. The first immunological read-outs obtained indicate a surprisingly high immunogenicity. At least 70% of patients showed a T cell response to at least one of the antigens encoded. Immune responses were detected to each of the antigens contained in the cocktail and the majority of immunological responders (65%) reacted to more than one antigen. While it is too early to make any statements on the clinical course of the patients vaccinated at the time of writing, these first data obtained with an optimized, protamine-complexed mRNA-based vaccine suggest safety and biological activity of the optimized RNActive® vaccines.

Taken together, the clinical data summarized above indicate that mRNA is a suitable polynucleotide format to elicit immune responses against diverse full-length antigens in humans. However, schedule and design of the mRNA-based vaccine may have a major impact on the strength and robustness of the immune response. Identifying these pitfalls is easy, but it remains a formidable challenge to optimize these parameters under clinical conditions, given the regulatory confinements to even small variations in clinical trials and our technically still very demanding approaches to immunomonitoring. Polynucoletide-based formats encoding full-length antigens inherently avoid biased selection of target epitopes when compared to peptide vaccines. However, this functional advantage comes at the price of more difficult immunomonitoring, since the best epitopes for restimulation are often also unknown. This does not even consider an assessment of the correlation of immune responses with clinical benefits. Despite these challenges, the first clinical trials with mRNA-based tumor vaccines underline our view that mRNA-based vaccination is a workable principle in humans. Biological activity in terms of immunogenicity has been observed in all trials and moreover, clear signs of clinical benefit have been reported for some patients. It would appear that the task is now no longer to establish, whether the principle of mRNA-mediated immunization is applicable to humans, but to make it stronger and robust and to establish clinical activity beyond reasonable doubt.

Allergy

As discussed in detail in Chap. 12 of this book, mRNA vaccines might be ideally suited for the development of the first prophylactic vaccine against allergies as well (Weiss et al. 2010). Of note, besides using RNA replicons, Roesler et al. also succeeded in inducing immune responses against different allergens by using mRNA constructs containing a 5'-β-globin UTR and an A30 segment flanking the ORF (Roesler et al. 2009).

Conclusions

A growing body of immunological data provides strong evidence that mRNA-vaccines hold great clinical promise. It has now been firmly demonstrated that mRNA vaccines, particularly if formulated properly, induce broad immune responses, including the activation of antigen-specific $CD8^+$ and $CD4^+$ T cells and B cells. Moreover, immune responses are long-lived and functional as shown by anti tumor activity. Intriguingly, mRNA vaccines are self-adjuvanting, thus making the addition of separate adjuvants dispensable. The efficacy of mRNA vaccines is complemented by an excellent safety profile. Like other genetic vaccines described in this book, mRNA vaccines profit from the flexibility offered by modern molecular cloning techniques as well as the transferability of the production process to different constructs. Further clinical trials in humans are now required to validate these findings and to pave the way towards new and highly innovative therapeutics for unmet medical needs.

Taken together, we believe that mRNA vaccines hold promise in becoming a game-changing vaccine technology platform.

References

Absher M, Stinebring WR (1969) Toxic properties of a synthetic double-stranded RNA. Endotoxin-like properties of poly I. poly C, an interferon stimulator. Nature 223(5207):715–717

Alexopoulou L, Holt AC, Medzhitov R, Flavell RA (2001) Recognition of double-stranded RNA and activation of NF-kappaB by Toll-like receptor 3. Nature 413(6857):732–738

Amiel E, Alonso A, Uematsu S, Akira S, Poynter ME, Berwin B (2009) Pivotal advance: toll-like receptor regulation of scavenger receptor-A-mediated phagocytosis. J Leukoc Biol 85(4):595–605

Anderson BR, Muramatsu H, Nallagatla SR, Bevilacqua PC, Sansing LH, Weissman D, Karikó K (2010) Incorporation of pseudouridine into mRNA enhances translation by diminishing PKR activation. Nucleic Acids Res 38(17):5884–5892

Babendure JR, Babendure JL, Ding JH, Tsien RY (2006) Control of mammalian translation by mRNA structure near caps. RNA (New York) 12(5):851–861

Bachmann MF, Jennings GT (2010) Vaccine delivery: a matter of size, geometry, kinetics and molecular patterns. Nat Rev Immunol 10(11):787–796

Banerjee AK (1980) 5'-terminal cap structure in eucaryotic messenger ribonucleic acids. Microbiol Rev 44(2):175–205

Blobel G (1973) A protein of molecular weight 78,000 bound to the polyadenylate region of eukaryotic messenger RNAs. Proc Natl Acad Sci USA 70(3):924–928

Boczkowski D, Nair SK, Snyder D, Gilboa E (1996) Dendritic cells pulsed with RNA are potent antigen-presenting cells in vitro and in vivo. J Exp Med 184(2):465–472

Carralot JP, Probst J, Hoerr I, Scheel B, Teufel R, Jung G, Rammensee HG, Pascolo S (2004) Polarization of immunity induced by direct injection of naked sequence-stabilized mRNA vaccines. Cell Mol Life Sci 61(18):2418–2424

Carralot J-P, Weide B, Schoor O, Probst J, Scheel B, Teufel R, Hoerr I, Garbe C, Rammensee H-G, Pascolo S (2005) Production and characterization of amplified tumor-derived cRNA libraries to be used as vaccines against metastatic melanomas. Genet Vaccin Ther 3:6–6

Chang T-C, Yamashita A, Chen C-YA, Yamashita Y, Zhu W, Durdan S, Kahvejian A, Sonenberg N, Shyu A-B (2004) UNR, a new partner of poly(A)-binding protein, plays a key role in translationally coupled mRNA turnover mediated by the c-fos major coding-region determinant. Genes Dev 18(16):2010–2023

Chen C-YA, Shyu A-B (2003) Rapid deadenylation triggered by a nonsense codon precedes decay of the RNA body in a mammalian cytoplasmic nonsense-mediated decay pathway. Mol Cell Biol 23(14):4805–4813

Chen CY, Xu N, Shyu AB (1995) mRNA decay mediated by two distinct AU-rich elements from c-fos and granulocyte-macrophage colony-stimulating factor transcripts: different deadenylation kinetics and uncoupling from translation. Mol Cell Biol 15(10):5777–5788

Chetverin AB (2004) Replicable and recombinogenic RNAs. FEBS Lett 567(1):35–41

Christensen C (1997) The innovator's dilemma: when new technologies cause great firms to fail. Harvard Business School Press, Boston Mass

Conry RM, LoBuglio AF, Wright M, Sumerel L, Pike MJ, Johanning F, Benjamin R, Lu D, Curiel DT (1995) Characterization of a messenger RNA polynucleotide vaccine vector. Cancer Res 55(7):1397–1400

Diebold SS, Kaisho T, Hemmi H, Akira S, Reise Sousa (2004) Innate antiviral responses by means of TLR7-mediated recognition of single-stranded RNA. Science (New York) 303(5663): 1529–1531

Diebold SS, Massacrier C, Akira S, Paturel C, Morel Y, Reis e Sousa C (2006) Nucleic acid agonists for Toll-like receptor 7 are defined by the presence of uridine ribonucleotides. Eur J Immunol 36(12):3256–3267

Duret L (2002) Evolution of synonymous codon usage in metazoans. Curr Opin Genet Dev 12(6):640–649

FDA Guidance for Industry (2006) Gene therapy clinical trials; observing subjects for delayed adverse events. http://www.fda.gov/downloads/BiologicsBloodVaccines/GuidanceComplianceRegulatoryInformation/Guidances/CellularandGeneTherapy/ucm078719.pdf. Accessed 12 july 2011

Field AK, Tytell AA, Lampson GP, Hilleman MR (1967) Inducers of interferon and host resistance. II. Multistranded synthetic polynucleotide complexes. Proc Natl Acad Sci USA 58(3):1004–1010

Forde GM (2005) Rapid-response vaccines – does DNA offer a solution? Nat Biotechnol 23(9): 1059–1062

Fotin-Mleczek M, Duchardt KM, Lorenz C, Pfeiffer R, Ojkić-Zrna S, Probst J, Kallen K-J (2011) Messenger RNA-based vaccines with dual activity induce balanced TLR-7 dependent adaptive immune responses and provide antitumor activity. J Immunother (Hagerstown, MD: 1997) 34(1):1–15

Freigang S, Egger D, Bienz K, Hengartner H, Zinkernagel RM (2003) Endogenous neosynthesis vs. cross-presentation of viral antigens for cytotoxic T cell priming. Proc Natl Acad Sci USA 100(23):13477–13482

Friedmann T (2007) Gene transfer: delivery and expression of DNA and RNA: a laboratory manual. Cold Spring Harbor Laboratory Press, Cold Spring Harbor, New York

Funakoshi Y, Doi Y, Hosoda N, Uchida N, Osawa M, Shimada I, Tsujimoto M, Suzuki T, Katada T, Hoshino S-i (2007) Mechanism of mRNA deadenylation: evidence for a molecular interplay between translation termination factor eRF3 and mRNA deadenylases. Genes Dev 21(23): 3135–3148

Gallie DR (1991) The cap and poly(A) tail function synergistically to regulate mRNA translational efficiency. Genes Dev 5(11):2108–2116

Granstein RD, Ding W, Ozawa H (2000) Induction of anti-tumor immunity with epidermal cells pulsed with tumor-derived RNA or intradermal administration of RNA. J Investig Dermatol 114(4):632–636

Grosset C, Chen CY, Xu N, Sonenberg N, Jacquemin-Sablon H, Shyu AB (2000) A mechanism for translationally coupled mRNA turnover: interaction between the poly(A) tail and a c-fos RNA coding determinant via a protein complex. Cell 103(1):29–40

Heil F, Hemmi H, Hochrein H, Ampenberger F, Kirschning C, Akira S, Lipford G, Wagner H, Bauer S (2004) Species-specific recognition of single-stranded RNA via toll-like receptor 7 and 8. Science (New York) 303(5663):1526–1529

Heiser A, Maurice MA, Yancey DR, Wu NZ, Dahm P, Pruitt SK, Boczkowski D, Nair SK, Ballo MS, Gilboa E, Vieweg J (2001) Induction of polyclonal prostate cancer-specific CTL using dendritic cells transfected with amplified tumor RNA. J Immunol (Baltimore, MD: 1950) 166(5):2953–2960

Herweijer H, Wolff JA (2007) Gene therapy progress and prospects: hydrodynamic gene delivery. Gene Ther 14(2):99–107

Hess PR, Boczkowski D, Nair SK, Snyder D, Gilboa E (2006) Vaccination with mRNAs encoding tumor-associated antigens and granulocyte-macrophage colony-stimulating factor efficiently primes CTL responses, but is insufficient to overcome tolerance to a model tumor/self antigen. Cancer Immunol Immunother 55(6):672–683

Hilleman MR (1994) Recombinant vector vaccines in vaccinology. Dev Biol Stand 82:3–20

Hoare M, Levy MS, Bracewell DG, Doig SD, Kong S, Titchener-Hooker N, Ward JM, Dunnill P (2005) Bioprocess engineering issues that would be faced in producing a DNA vaccine at up to 100 m^3 fermentation scale for an influenza pandemic. Biotechnol Prog 21(6):1577–1592

Hoerr I, Obst R, Rammensee HG, Jung G (2000) In vivo application of RNA leads to induction of specific cytotoxic T lymphocytes and antibodies. Eur J Immunol 30(1):1–7

Holtkamp S, Kreiter S, Selmi A, Simon P, Koslowski M, Huber C, Türeci O, Sahin U (2006) Modification of antigen-encoding RNA increases stability, translational efficacy, and T-cell stimulatory capacity of dendritic cells. Blood 108(13):4009–4017

Hornung V, Ellegast J, Kim S, Brzózka K, Jung A, Kato H, Poeck H, Akira S, Conzelmann K-K, Schlee M, Endres S, Hartmann G (2006) 5′-Triphosphate RNA is the ligand for RIG-I. Science (New York) 314(5801):994–997

Hornung V, Barchet W, Schlee M, Hartmann G (2008) RNA recognition via TLR7 and TLR8. Handb Exp Pharmacol 183:71–86

Hovanessian AG (2007) On the discovery of interferon-inducible, double-stranded RNA activated enzymes: the 2′–5′ oligoadenylate synthetases and the protein kinase PKR. Cytokine Growth Factor Rev 18(5–6):351–361

Imataka H, Gradi A, Sonenberg N (1998) A newly identified N-terminal amino acid sequence of human eIF4G binds poly(A)-binding protein and functions in poly(A)-dependent translation. EMBO J 17(24):7480–7489

Isaacs A, Cox RA, Rotem Z (1963) Foreign nucleic acids as the stimulus to make interferon. Lancet 2(7299):113–116

Jäschke A, Helm M (2003) RNA sex. Chem Biol 10(12):1148–1150

Kanaya S, Yamada Y, Kinouchi M, Kudo Y, Ikemura T (2001) Codon usage and tRNA genes in eukaryotes: correlation of codon usage diversity with translation efficiency and with CG-dinucleotide usage as assessed by multivariate analysis. J Mol Evol 53(4–5):290–298

Kantoff PW, Higano CS, Shore ND, Berger ER, Small EJ, Penson DF, Redfern CH, Ferrari AC, Dreicer R, Sims RB, Xu Y, Frohlich MW, Schellhammer PF (2010) Sipuleucel-T immunotherapy for castration-resistant prostate cancer. N Engl J Med 363(5):411–422

Karikó K, Weissman D (2007) Naturally occurring nucleoside modifications suppress the immunostimulatory activity of RNA: implication for therapeutic RNA development. Curr Opin Drug Discov Dev 10(5):523–532

Karikó K, Ni H, Capodici J, Lamphier M, Weissman D (2004) mRNA is an endogenous ligand for Toll-like receptor 3. J Biol Chem 279(13):12542–12550

Karikó K, Buckstein M, Ni H, Weissman D (2005) Suppression of RNA recognition by Toll-like receptors: the impact of nucleoside modification and the evolutionary origin of RNA. Immunity 23(2):165–175

Karikó K, Muramatsu H, Welsh FA, Ludwig J, Kato H, Akira S, Weissman D (2008) Incorporation of pseudouridine into mRNA yields superior nonimmunogenic vector with increased translational capacity and biological stability. Mol Ther J Am Soc Gene Ther 16(11):1833–1840

Kaslow DC (2004) A potential disruptive technology in vaccine development: gene-based vaccines and their application to infectious diseases. Trans R Soc Trop Med Hyg 98(10):593–601

Kato H, Takeuchi O, Sato S, Yoneyama M, Yamamoto M, Matsui K, Uematsu S, Jung A, Kawai T, Ishii KJ, Yamaguchi O, Otsu K, Tsujimura T, Koh C-S, Reis e Sousa C, Matsuura Y, Fujita T, Akira S (2006) Differential roles of MDA5 and RIG-I helicases in the recognition of RNA viruses. Nature 441(7089):101–105

Kim D-H, Longo M, Han Y, Lundberg P, Cantin E, Rossi JJ (2004) Interferon induction by siRNAs and ssRNAs synthesized by phage polymerase. Nat Biotechnol 22(3):321–325

Kreiter S, Selmi A, Diken M, Sebastian M, Osterloh P, Schild H, Huber C, Türeci O, Sahin U (2008) Increased antigen presentation efficiency by coupling antigens to MHC class I trafficking signals. J Immunol (Baltimore, MD: 1950) 180(1):309–318

Kreiter S, Selmi A, Diken M, Koslowski M, Britten CM, Huber C, Türeci O, Sahin U (2010) Intranodal vaccination with naked antigen-encoding rna elicits potent prophylactic and therapeutic antitumoral immunity. Cancer Res 70:9031–9040

Kuhn AN, Diken M, Kreiter S, Selmi A, Kowalska J, Jemielity J, Darzynkiewicz E, Huber C, Türeci O, Sahin U (2010) Phosphorothioate cap analogs increase stability and translational efficiency of RNA vaccines in immature dendritic cells and induce superior immune responses in vivo. Gene Ther 17(8):961–971

Lande R, Gregorio J, Facchinetti V, Chatterjee B, Wang Y-H, Homey B, Cao W, Wang Y-H, Su B, Nestle FO, Zal T, Mellman I, Schröder J-M, Liu Y-J, Gilliet M (2007) Plasmacytoid dendritic cells sense self-DNA coupled with antimicrobial peptide. Nature 449(7162): 564–569

Le H, Tanguay RL, Balasta ML, Wei CC, Browning KS, Metz AM, Goss DJ, Gallie DR (1997) Translation initiation factors eIF-iso4G and eIF-4B interact with the poly(A)-binding protein and increase its RNA binding activity. J Biol Chem 272(26):16247–16255

Levine M (2009) New generation vaccines. Informa Healthcare, New York

Liu MA (2010) Immunologic basis of vaccine vectors. Immunity 33(4):504–515

Liu H, Kiledjian M (2006) Decapping the message: a beginning or an end. Biochem Soc Trans 34(Pt 1):35–38

Mandl CW, Aberle JH, Aberle SW, Holzmann H, Allison SL, Heinz FX (1998) In vitro-synthesized infectious RNA as an attenuated live vaccine in a flavivirus model. Nat Med 4(12):1438–1440

Martinon F, Krishnan S, Lenzen G, Magné R, Gomard E, Guillet JG, Lévy JP, Meulien P (1993) Induction of virus-specific cytotoxic T lymphocytes in vivo by liposome-entrapped mRNA. Eur J Immunol 23(7):1719–1722

McCartney SA, Colonna M (2009) Viral sensors: diversity in pathogen recognition. Immunol Rev 227(1):87–94

Meyer S, Temme C, Wahle E (2004) Messenger RNA turnover in eukaryotes: pathways and enzymes. Crit Rev Biochem Mol Biol 39(4):197–216

Michel YM, Poncet D, Piron M, Kean KM, Borman AM (2000) Cap-Poly(A) synergy in mammalian cell-free extracts. Investigation of the requirements for poly(A)-mediated stimulation of translation initiation. J Biol Chem 275(41):32268–32276

Mockey M, Bourseau E, Chandrashekhar V, Chaudhuri A, Lafosse S, Le Cam E, Quesniaux VFJ, Ryffel B, Pichon C, Midoux P (2007) mRNA-based cancer vaccine: prevention of B16 melanoma progression and metastasis by systemic injection of MART1 mRNA histidylated lipopolyplexes. Cancer Gene Ther 14(9):802–814

Nair SK, Boczkowski D, Morse M, Cumming RI, Lyerly HK, Gilboa E (1998) Induction of primary carcinoembryonic antigen (CEA)-specific cytotoxic T lymphocytes in vitro using human dendritic cells transfected with RNA. Nat Biotechnol 16(4):364–369

Nallagatla SR, Hwang J, Toroney R, Zheng X, Cameron CE, Bevilacqua PC (2007) 5'-triphosphate-dependent activation of PKR by RNAs with short stem-loops. Science (New York) 318(5855):1455–1458

Ozgur S, Chekulaeva M, Stoecklin G (2010) Human Pat1b connects deadenylation with mRNA decapping and controls the assembly of processing bodies. Mol Cell Biol 30(17):4308–4323

Parker R, Song H (2004) The enzymes and control of eukaryotic mRNA turnover. Nat Struct Mol Biol 11(2):121–127

Pascolo S (2006) Vaccination with messenger RNA. Methods Mol Med 127:23–40

Pichlmair A, Schulz O, Tan CP, Näslund TI, Liljeström P, Weber F, Reise Sousa C (2006) RIG-I-mediated antiviral responses to single-stranded RNA bearing 5′-phosphates. Science (New York) 314(5801):997–1001

Probst J, Brechtel S, Scheel B, Hoerr I, Jung G, Rammensee H-G, Pascolo S (2006) Characterization of the ribonuclease activity on the skin surface. Genet Vaccin Ther 4:4–4

Probst J, Weide B, Scheel B, Pichler BJ, Hoerr I, Rammensee HG, Pascolo S (2007) Spontaneous cellular uptake of exogenous messenger RNA in vivo is nucleic acid-specific, saturable and ion dependent. Gene Ther 14(15):1175–1180

Pulendran B, Ahmed R (2006) Translating innate immunity into immunological memory: implications for vaccine development. Cell 124(4):849–863

Qiu P, Ziegelhoffer P, Sun J, Yang NS (1996) Gene gun delivery of mRNA in situ results in efficient transgene expression and genetic immunization. Gene Ther 3(3):262–268

Rehwinkel J, Tan CP, Goubau D, Schulz O, Pichlmair A, Bier K, Robb N, Vreede F, Barclay W, Fodor E, Reis e Sousa C (2010) RIG-I detects viral genomic RNA during negative-strand RNA virus infection. Cell 140(3):397–408

Rittig SM, Haentschel M, Weimer KJ, Heine A, Muller MR, Brugger W, Horger MS, Maksimovic O, Stenzl A, Hoerr I, Rammensee H-G, Holderried TA, Kanz L, Pascolo S, Brossart P (2011) Intradermal vaccinations with RNA coding for TAA generate CD8(+) and CD4(+) immune responses and induce clinical benefit in vaccinated patients. Mol Ther 19(5):990-999

Roesler E, Weiss R, Weinberger EE, Fruehwirth A, Stoecklinger A, Mostböck S, Ferreira F, Thalhamer J, Scheiblhofer S (2009) Immunize and disappear-safety-optimized mRNA vaccination with a panel of 29 allergens. J Allergy Clin Immunol 124(5):1070–1077, e1071-1011-1070-1077.e1071-1011

Sadler AJ, Williams BRG (2008) Interferon-inducible antiviral effectors. Nat Rev Immunol 8(7):559–568

Saito T, Owen DM, Jiang F, Marcotrigiano J, Gale M (2008) Innate immunity induced by composition-dependent RIG-I recognition of hepatitis C virus RNA. Nature 454(7203):523–527

Scheel B, Braedel S, Probst J, Carralot J-P, Wagner H, Schild H, Jung G, Rammensee H-G, Pascolo S (2004) Immunostimulating capacities of stabilized RNA molecules. Eur J Immunol 34(2):537–547

Scheel B, Teufel R, Probst J, Carralot J-P, Geginat J, Radsak M, Jarrossay D, Wagner H, Jung G, Rammensee H-G, Hoerr I, Pascolo S (2005) Toll-like receptor-dependent activation of several human blood cell types by protamine-condensed mRNA. Eur J Immunol 35(5):1557–1566

Schleef M (2005) DNA pharmaceuticals: formulation and delivery in gene therapy, DNA vaccination and immunotherapy. Wiley-VCH, Weinheim

Sederoff R, Lowenstein L, Mayer A, Stone J, Birnboim HC (1975) Acid treatment of Drosophila deoxyribonucleic acid. J Histochem Cytochem: Off J Histochem Soc 23(7):482–492

Sohn RL, Murray MT, Schwarz K, Nyitray J, Purray P, Franko AP, Palmer KC, Diebel LN, Dulchavsky SA (2001) In-vivo particle mediated delivery of mRNA to mammalian tissues: ballistic and biologic effects. Wound Repair Regen: Off Publ Wound Heal Soc Eur Tissue Repair Soc 9(4):287–296

Song M-G, Li Y, Kiledjian M (2010) Multiple mRNA decapping enzymes in mammalian cells. Mol Cell 40(3):423–432

Sorrentino S (1998) Human extracellular ribonucleases: multiplicity, molecular diversity and catalytic properties of the major RNase types. Cell Mol Life Sci 54(8):785–794

Steitz J, Britten CM, Wölfel T, Tüting T (2006) Effective induction of anti-melanoma immunity following genetic vaccination with synthetic mRNA coding for the fusion protein EGFP.TRP2. Cancer Immunol Immunother 55(3):246–253

Su Z, Dannull J, Yang BK, Dahm P, Coleman D, Yancey D, Sichi S, Niedzwiecki D, Boczkowski D, Gilboa E, Vieweg J (2005) Telomerase mRNA-transfected dendritic cells stimulate antigen-specific CD8+ and CD4+ T cell responses in patients with metastatic prostate cancer. J Immunol (Baltimore, MD: 1950) 174(6):3798–3807

11 Messenger RNA Vaccines

Tarun SZ, Sachs AB (1995) A common function for mRNA 5′ and 3′ ends in translation initiation in yeast. Genes Dev 9(23):2997–3007

Tarun SZ, Sachs AB (1996) Association of the yeast poly(A) tail binding protein with translation initiation factor eIF-4G. EMBO J 15(24):7168–7177

Uchida N, Hoshino S-I, Katada T (2004) Identification of a human cytoplasmic poly(A) nuclease complex stimulated by poly(A)-binding protein. J Biol Chem 279(2):1383–1391

Ulmer JB, Donnelly JJ, Parker SE, Rhodes GH, Felgner PL, Dwarki VJ, Gromkowski SH, Deck RR, DeWitt CM, Friedman A (1993) Heterologous protection against influenza by injection of DNA encoding a viral protein. Science (New York) 259(5102):1745–1749

Ulmer JB, Valley U, Rappuoli R (2006) Vaccine manufacturing: challenges and solutions. Nat Biotechnol 24(11):1377–1383

Uzri D, Gehrke L (2009) Nucleotide sequences and modifications that determine RIG-I/RNA binding and signaling activities. J Virol 83(9):4174–4184

Wang Z, Day N, Trifillis P, Kiledjian M (1999) An mRNA stability complex functions with poly(A)-binding protein to stabilize mRNA in vitro. Mol Cell Biol 19(7):4552–4560

Wang Z, Troilo PJ, Wang X, Griffiths TG, Pacchione SJ, Barnum AB, Harper LB, Pauley CJ, Niu Z, Denisova L, Follmer TT, Rizzuto G, Ciliberto G, Fattori E, Monica NL, Manam S, Ledwith BJ (2004) Detection of integration of plasmid DNA into host genomic DNA following intramuscular injection and electroporation. Gene Ther 11(8):711–721

Wei CC, Balasta ML, Ren J, Goss DJ (1998) Wheat germ poly(A) binding protein enhances the binding affinity of eukaryotic initiation factor 4F and (iso)4F for cap analogues. Biochemistry 37(7):1910–1916

Weide B, Carralot J-P, Reese A, Scheel B, Eigentler TK, Hoerr I, Rammensee H-G, Garbe C, Pascolo S (2009a) Results of the first phase I/II clinical vaccination trial with direct injection of mRNA. J Immunother (Hagerstown, MD: 1997) 31(2):180–188

Weide B, Pascolo S, Scheel B, Derhovanessian E, Pflugfelder A, Eigentler TK, Pawelec G, Hoerr I, Rammensee H-G, Garbe C (2009b) Direct injection of protamine-protected mRNA: results of a phase 1/2 vaccination trial in metastatic melanoma patients. J Immunother (Hagerstown, MD: 1997) 32(5):498–507

Weiss R, Scheiblhofer S, Roesler E, Ferreira F, Thalhamer J (2010) Prophylactic mRNA vaccination against allergy. Curr Opin Allergy Clin Immunol 10(6):567–574

Wickens M (1990) How the messenger got its tail: addition of poly(A) in the nucleus. Trends Biochem Sci 15(7):277–281

Wilkins C, Gale M (2010) Recognition of viruses by cytoplasmic sensors. Curr Opin Immunol 22(1):41–47

Wolff JA, Malone RW, Williams P, Chong W, Acsadi G, Jani A, Felgner PL (1990) Direct gene transfer into mouse muscle in vivo. Science (New York) 247(4949 Pt 1):1465–1468

Wu L, Fan J, Belasco JG (2006) MicroRNAs direct rapid deadenylation of mRNA. Proc Natl Acad Sci USA 103(11):4034–4039

Yamamoto A, Kormann M, Rosenecker J, Rudolph C (2009) Current prospects for mRNA gene delivery. Eur J Pharm Biopharm: Off J Arbeitsgemeinschaft Für Pharm Verfahrenstechnik eV 71(3):484–489

Yamashita A, Chang T-C, Yamashita Y, Zhu W, Zhong Z, Chen C-YA, Shyu A-B (2005) Concerted action of poly(A) nucleases and decapping enzyme in mammalian mRNA turnover. Nat Struct Mol Biol 12(12):1054–1063

Yanai H, Ban T, Wang Z, Choi MK, Kawamura T, Negishi H, Nakasato M, Lu Y, Hangai S, Koshiba R, Savitsky D, Ronfani L, Akira S, Bianchi ME, Honda K, Tamura T, Kodama T, Taniguchi T (2009) HMGB proteins function as universal sentinels for nucleic-acid-mediated innate immune responses. Nature 462(7269):99–103

Zhou WZ, Hoon DS, Huang SK, Fujii S, Hashimoto K, Morishita R, Kaneda Y (1999) RNA melanoma vaccine: induction of antitumor immunity by human glycoprotein 100 mRNA immunization. Hum Gene Ther 10(16):2719–2724

DNA and RNA Vaccines for Prophylactic and Therapeutic Treatment of Type I Allergy

12

Richard Weiss, Sandra Scheiblhofer, Elisabeth Rösler, and Josef Thalhamer

The constant rise in allergies in Western industrialized countries has fueled efforts to develop novel therapies to treat the immunological cause of disease rather than merely ameliorating symptoms. Gene vaccines against allergic diseases may be an attractive alternative to classical specific immunotherapy (SIT) avoiding its pitfalls such as potential side effects as well as low patient compliance. While SIT is commonly believed to rely on the generation of regulatory immune reactions and blocking antibodies, gene based allergy vaccines rather exert immune deviation by balancing allergic TH2 reactions through the generation of allergen specific TH1 cells. In contrast to SIT, gene based allergy vaccines may also have a high potential for prophylactic applications. Already small amounts of translated allergen in the context of DNA/RNA vaccine-inherent danger signals prime a milieu that counteracts the induction of allergic immune responses. Such prophylactic vaccines may very well resemble naturally acquired protection from allergy as it is observed in individuals exposed to microbial compounds during early childhood (hygiene hypothesis). In this chapter, we will discuss different types of DNA vaccines that have been designed to prevent from allergy, and the potential safety hazards associated with their application for prophylactic vaccination of children. Furthermore, we will demonstrate that RNA vaccines are as effective as DNA vaccines, yet with a much higher safety profile, thus making them the most promising candidates for prophylactic vaccination against allergic diseases.

J. Thalhamer (✉)
Department of Molecular Biology, Division of Allergy and Immunology,
University of Salzburg, Salzburg, Austria
e-mail: Josef.Thalhamer@sbg.ac.at

J. Thalhamer et al. (eds.), *Gene Vaccines*,
DOI 10.1007/978-3-7091-0439-2_12, © Springer-Verlag/Wien, 2012

247

Introduction

DNA vaccines have initially been recognized for their potential to induce TH1 driven induction of cytotoxic T cells (CTLs), and to this day, the main focus of gene vaccine-related research is still on anti-viral vaccines and cancer therapy (as discussed in the previous chapters of this book). However, as early as 1996, Raz et al. demonstrated that DNA vaccination can modulate ongoing IgE responses in an antigen-specific manner (Raz et al. 1996). As generation of IgE antibodies represents the hallmark event during induction of type I allergies, this publication initiated a large number of studies dealing with the potential of DNA vaccines to interfere with allergic disease.

In general, type I allergy is characterized by the generation of inappropriate immune responses against otherwise harmless environmental antigens, such as tree, grass, and weed pollen, insect venom, house dust mite and cockroaches, animal dander, latex, certain drugs, moulds, as well as foods. Over the past decades, the prevalence of atopic diseases has considerably increased not only in industrialized countries but also in emerging economies. To date, the only curative approach targeting the immunological defect underlying type I allergy is specific immunotherapy (SIT), which relies on frequent injections of increasing amounts of allergen extracts or purified allergens. However, the efficacy of SIT is still in need of improvement, and moreover, due to frequent side effects, the approach suffers from bad compliance. Therefore, the majority of current therapies are simple symptom relieving, using immunosuppressive and anti-inflammatory agents, such as anti-histamines, corticosteroids, and beta agonists. At present, more than one quarter of the world population is affected with allergic diseases causing an enormous economic burden on public health systems. There is an urgent need not only for more efficient therapeutic approaches, but also for a shift of opinion towards the development of prophylactic strategies against this growing pandemic.

General Mechanisms of Type I Allergy

Type I allergic immune responses are characterized by the synthesis of allergen-specific IgE antibodies and production of the key cytokines IL-4, IL-5, and IL-13. Re-exposure of atopic individuals to the respective allergen leads to the induction of immediate as well as delayed symptoms of atopy. Cross-linking of IgE bound to high affinity FcεR on mast cells or basophils results in the release of inflammatory mediators such as histamine, which cause the immediate symptoms. The subsequent late phase reaction after some hours is mainly dependent on mediators including prostaglandins, leukotrienes, and platelet activating factor released by recruited inflammatory cells. Mast cell mediators and TH2 cytokines induce mucus secretion by goblet cells as well as invasion of eosinophilic granulocytes and TH2 lymphocytes into the lung. During the early stage of type I allergy, reactions are mainly restricted to the mucosa of the upper airways (rhino-conjunctivitis), but progression of the disease leads to the so-called "Etagenwechsel" (allergic-March) to the lower airways. Increased maturation and recruitment of eosinophils via TH2 lymphocyte secreted IL-5/IL-13 triggers damage of the vascular and bronchial epithelium, and ultimately, an asthmatic phenotype. At the final stages of the disease, exacerbation of allergic asthma results in tissue remodeling and fibrosis.

Factors Associated with the Generation of Allergic Diseases

Though we are constantly exposed to a broad range of environmental allergens, only a minority of individuals develops type I allergies. Complex interactions between genetic and environmental factors account for the fact that atopic persons are prone to mount TH2 type immune responses. We are only just beginning to elucidate the genetic polymorphisms associated with the development of atopy. For example, mutations in the filaggrin gene associated with the integrity of the skin barrier, have been shown to facilitate the transition from eczema to asthma and can be used as a predictive asthma marker before the onset of symptoms (Marenholz et al. 2009). Also certain polymorphisms in innate immune receptors, such as toll like receptor (TLR) 4 have been linked to a reduced prevalence of hay fever and atopy (Senthilselvan et al. 2008). This is in line with epidemiological studies, which showed that the immune repertoire shaped through the exposure to environmental pathogens during early childhood is of special importance for the development of allergies.

Naturally Acquired Immune Responses Against Allergens and the Hygiene Hypothesis

Many factors of the Western life-style have been proposed to contribute to the increase of atopic diseases, such as dietary habits and air pollution (ozone, diesel exhaust, sulphur dioxide, particulate matter, and passive smoking), but especially the reduced childhood infections due to increased hygiene standards and vaccinations seem to be dominant risk factors (Floistrup et al. 2006). The so-called "hygiene hypothesis" postulates that a reduced exposure to microbial agents during early childhood leads to a decreased stimulation of the innate immune system and a shift towards TH2-type adaptive immune response against environmental allergens. This postulated shift has also been termed "missing immune deviation" (Romagnani 2004). Braun-Fahrländer et al. first reported in the late 1990s that farmers' children in Switzerland have a significantly reduced risk for allergic sensitization compared to children grown up in the same areas but without close contact to livestock and stables (Braun-Fahrlander et al. 1999). Several studies confirming these findings followed within a short period of time (Braun-Fahrlander et al. 2002; Riedler et al. 2000, 2001; Von Ehrenstein et al. 2000). High concentrations of grass pollen and other plant-derived substances, such as water-soluble polysaccharides arabinogalactans, have been found in cowsheds and also in farm children's mattresses (Peters et al. 2010; Sudre et al. 2009). The key factors associated with a farming lifestyle that contribute to the reduced risk of asthma and allergies in farm children are contact with livestock (cattle, pigs, poultry), contact with animal feed (hay, grain, straw, silage) and the consumption of unprocessed cow's milk (von Mutius and Vercelli 2010). Inhalation and ingestion have been identified as the two main routes of exposure. Strongest protective effects have been observed for exposures occurring in utero and during the first years of life (Ege et al. 2006; Riedler et al. 2001). Components identified by studying immune responses in farm children and experimental animal models are of bacterial and fungal origin. Whereas levels of muramic acid (a component predominantly found in the cell-wall of gram positive bacteria) and extracellular polysaccharides derived from fungal species Penicillium and Aspergillus display strong inverse relationships with asthma and wheeze (Ege et al. 2007; van Strien et al. 2004), lipopolysaccharide (a cell-wall component of gram negative bacteria) was only found to be inversely related with allergic sensitization, but not with childhood asthma and wheeze (Vogel et al. 2008). At school age, peripheral blood cells from farm children express significantly higher levels of CD14, TLR2 and TLR4 mRNA than cells from non-farm children (Ege et al. 2006; Lauener et al. 2002), confirming the hypothesis that the innate immune system senses the signals delivered by the high microbial burden associated with farming and influences the adaptive immune system. In cord blood of infants whose mothers had not been exposed to animal sheds and grass, significantly increased seasonal allergen-specific IgE responses were observed, which were correlated with reduced production of the TH1 cell cytokines IFN-γ and TNF (Pfefferle et al. 2008). Whether a missing immune deviation is the sole mechanism responsible for the constant rise in allergies is still under debate. Alternatively, a lack of immune suppression due to decreased activity of regulatory T cells (Tregs) has been suggested. Experimental evidence and epidemiological findings indicate that both mechanisms might be involved (Romagnani 2004).

Taken together, we can postulate five basic types of immune reactions against environmental allergens:

1. The TH2 type: This immune profile results in atopy and development of allergy.
2. The TH1 type: Priming of allergen specific TH1 memory inhibits the induction of allergic immune responses. TH1 primed individuals remain asymptomatic.
3. The Treg type: The presence of allergen specific regulatory T cells down regulates allergic TH2 responses, thus no allergic symptoms develop. This type of immunosuppression protects bee keepers from allergy, and is predominant after SIT against insect venoms.
4. The modified TH2 type: Atopic individuals with a high allergen specific IgE titer can also remain asymptomatic due to simultaneous presence of high titers of so-called blocking IgG, which competes for the binding of epitopes on allergens. SIT against pollen allergens has been observed to induce this type of response.
5. Immunological ignorance: From a theoretical point of view, individuals might also acquire tolerance against environmental allergens due to clonal deletion or anergy of allergen specific T cell clones. However, it is unclear under which conditions and to which extent this takes place during natural exposure.

Prophylactic Vaccination Versus the Natural Immune Response

Prophylactic vaccination against allergy today is seriously discussed as an alternative to existing therapeutic approaches. Such an approach would require selection of children at an early stage before immune deviation towards the TH2 phenotype takes place. Due to the improvement of risk assessment in infants, sensitization to inhalant allergens can be predicted from family history, the occurrence of food allergies early in life (milk, egg white, wheat), and from genetic polymorphisms (Kulig et al. 1998; Marenholz et al. 2009; Senthilselvan et al. 2008), thus, prophylactic vaccination against allergic diseases has come within reach. The question remains, whether the immune profile induced by prophylactic vaccination would resemble the naturally acquired immune response observed in non-atopic, healthy individuals. We and others have shown that DNA and RNA gene vaccines against allergy are clearly based on TH1 immune deviation rather than induction of regulatory responses. In preliminary experiments we could demonstrate that, whereas peripheral blood mononuclear cells from an allergic individual displayed high proliferation rates and an elevated percentage of IL-4 secreting T cells upon re-stimulation with the respective allergen, cells purified from the blood of non-atopics were either non-responsive or mounted strong allergen-specific proliferation associated almost exclusively with IFN-γ secretion (Fig. 12.1). The latter immunophenotype closely resembles the immune status of rodents immunized with allergen-encoding DNA or RNA vaccines as discussed in detail below. The observation that immune responses against allergens in healthy individuals are rather of a mixed TH1/Treg type than solely Treg dominated has also been made in studies characterizing the cytokine profile and surface markers of individual T helper cells (Bullens et al. 2005; Van Overtvelt et al. 2008). In an ongoing clinical study with a large cohort of non-atopic individuals with or without farming background we are currently investigating the distribution of the immunophenotypes described above in the non-atopic part of the population. This data will provide the immunological foundation for the design of tailored gene vaccines mimicking naturally acquired protection against allergy.

Gene Vaccines Against Allergy

The first study demonstrating the anti-allergic capacity of DNA vaccination was published in 1996 by Raz et al. In this study, the authors injected BALB/c mice with plasmid DNA encoding the model allergen β-galactosidase or with the recombinant protein adjuvanted with aluminium hydroxide. While DNA vaccination induced TH1 biased immune responses characterized by the secretion of IFN-γ by CD4 as well as CD8 T cells, protein immunization triggered IgG1, IgE and IL-4 dominated immune responses. Moreover, DNA immunization prevented from the subsequent induction of TH2 immune responses and could also modulate an ongoing TH2 response. Transfer experiments showed that both, CD4 and CD8 positive T cells from DNA immunized mice contributed to the anti-allergic effects (Raz et al. 1996). In the same year, the first study utilizing a clinically relevant allergen, namely Der

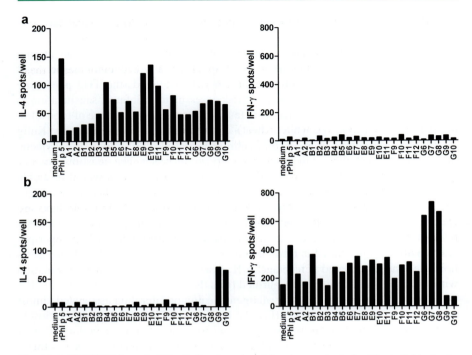

Fig. 12.1 ELISPOT data of a Phl p 5 allergic patient (**a**) and a nonatopic, healthy individual, who was raised and still lives in a farming environment (**b**). Peripheral blood mononuclear cells (PBMCs) were expanded by re-stimulation with rPhl p 5 and after a resting period assayed by ELISPOT without stimulation (medium), or re-stimulation with rPhl p 5, or immunodominant peptides resembling class II epitopes of Phl p 5 (A1–G10) (Reproduced with permission from Weiss et al. (2010))

p 5 from house dust mite, showed that DNA vaccination not only prevents from IgE induction but also from induction of lung inflammation induced upon aerosol challenge with recombinant allergen (Hsu et al. 1996).

Since then, a great number of studies evaluating clinically relevant allergens such as the cow's milk allergen β-lactoglobulin, the house dust mite allergens Der p 1, Der p 2 and Der f 11, pollen allergens from birch, cedar, and grasses as well as peanut allergens have been performed in various rodent models of allergy. For a review of these studies see (Weiss et al. 2006).

Our own lab mainly focused on DNA immunization against the major birch pollen allergen Bet v 1a and the timothy grass pollen allergen Phl p 5. In 1999 Hartl et al. demonstrated that intradermal (i.d.) immunization with plasmids encoding Bet v 1a elicited immune responses characterized by elevated levels of IFN-γ, low levels of IL-4, and a complete absence of IgE (Hartl et al. 1999a). Plasmids encoding the two isoforms Bet v 1a and Bet v 1d induced comparable humoral responses, however, cytokine profiles remarkably differed and only Bet v 1a led to significant allergen specific proliferation (Hartl et al. 1999b). Later, we demonstrated that DNA based immunization with constructs encoding Bet v 1a or derivates thereof could

12 Gene Vaccines for Prophylactic and Therapeutic Treatment of Allergy

prevent from allergic sensitization as indicated by a complete lack of allergen-specific IgE and a shift of the T helper cell profile towards TH1. Additionally, we could also show the suppression of already established TH2 responses in terms of downregulation of IgE, passive cutaneous anaphylaxis, and TH2 cytokines in these studies (Hartl et al. 2004; Hochreiter et al. 2003).

Second Generation DNA Vaccines Against Allergy

After these initial studies demonstrating the principle applicability of DNA vaccination against type I allergy we decided to exploit the vast possibilities of the DNA vaccine technology in terms of antigen modifications to induce tailored immune responses meeting the requirements of anti-allergic vaccines. Ideally, gene vaccines against allergic diseases will have to meet the following requirements:
1. Appropriate expression of the antigen to induce sufficient immunogenicity.
2. Induction of TH1 biased immune reactions.
3. Reduced IgE binding of the translated gene product to avoid therapy-induced side effects.
4. Self-removal of the vaccine from the body after inducing the desired immune response.
5. Highest possible safety profile for prophylactic application in children.

In the following chapters, we will discuss various approaches to address these issues.

Generation of Hypoallergenic DNA Vaccines

One major drawback of SIT is the risk of anaphylactic reaction via cross-linking of pre-existing IgE antibodies bound to mast cells. Additionally, application of high amounts of allergen during SIT can lead to novel, therapy-induced generation of IgE (Ball et al. 1999; Van Ree et al. 1997). To avoid these shortcomings, molecules with a reduced binding capacity to patient-derived allergen-specific IgE, so-called hypoallergens, can be employed. Such molecules are currently in development as recombinant proteins, or chemically modified proteins (allergoids) for SIT (Valenta et al. 2010).

Although the risk associated with wild type allergens may be low in the context of gene vaccines, due to the low concentration of translated protein compared to the high amounts used during SIT, the safety profile of anti-allergic gene vaccines can be further enhanced by various strategies. One approach to generate hypoallergenic derivates of wild type allergens utilizes fragmentation of allergens, which retains the original T cell epitopes while simultaneously changing their folding and thereby reducing IgE reactivity. Hochreiter et al. have demonstrated, that DNA vaccination with the N or C terminal fragments of Bet v 1a induces no Bet v 1a reactive antibodies, but protects from IgE induction in an antigen-specific manner (Hochreiter et al. 2003). The same molecules have recently been used as recombinant proteins in a clinical trial of SIT in birch pollen allergic patients (Purohit et al. 2008). Another possibility is the use of isoforms or mutants of allergen which display reduced IgE binding capacity (Hochreiter et al. 2003; Hartl et al. 1999b).

All of these approaches require a detailed knowledge of the structural features of the molecules and evaluation of the derivatives on an individual basis. Indeed, our own experiments have shown that cutting allergens into fragments has completely different outcomes for different molecules, indicating that creating hypoallergens by fragmentation is not predictable but random (unpublished data). Therefore, we sought for more general methods to generate hypoallergenic derivatives with broad applicability.

One possibility would be the use of peptides, which retain their T cell stimulation capacity but lack the IgE binding propensity of their parental molecules. Such peptide approaches have been intensely studied for cat allergy. DNA vaccination offers an elegant solution for combining the safety and efficacy of peptide vaccines with the simple and cost efficient generation of gene vaccines. We have demonstrated that targeting gene expression of Bet v 1a towards the proteasome by covalently linking ubiquitin to the N-terminus, results in complete degradation of the native allergen as indicated by the lack of antibody induction by this vaccines. However, T cell stimulation and IFN-γ induction is largely unaffected, suggesting that proteasome generated peptides are not solely loaded on MHC class I molecules – the default pathway – but also reach the MHC class II compartment. This phenomenon has been described previously and has been attributed to the autophagy machinery of the cell (Bonifaz et al. 1999; Lich et al. 2000; Mukherjee et al. 2001). Consequently, the ubiquitinated vaccine could protect from allergic sensitization and lung inflammation and also displayed therapeutic efficacy (Bauer et al. 2006). Similar strategies employed by us and others include the targeting of allergens directly into the class II pathway by using the major constituent of the lysosomal membrane, the glycoprotein LAMP (lysosome-associated membrane protein) or LIMP (lysosomal integral membrane protein) (Cheng et al. 2001; Dobano et al. 2007; Kim et al. 2003; Lu et al. 2003; Marques et al. 2003; Rodriguez et al. 2001). However, suppression of antibodies against native epitopes may not be as complete as seen with ubiquitinated allergens (unpublished observations).

Another strategy for systematic generation of hypoallergens recently employed by our group is the in silico mutation approach. This method utilizes the calculation of z-scores, which allows prediction of the consequences of mutations on fold stability. Using z-score calculations we generated novel hypoallergens based on protein destabilization that displayed reduced IgE binding capacity while maintaining T cells stimulation activity. The robustness of the method could be confirmed by calculating z-scores for hypoallergens known from the literature (Thalhamer et al. 2010).

Allergen Recoding and Self-Replicating Vaccines

DNA vaccination efficacy correlates with transgene expression levels, which depend on several parameters including choice of promoter, use of introns, stability and conformation of the encoded RNA, and codon usage of the encoded antigen. The pattern of codon usage differs between genes and organisms, due to a variety of selective evolutionary pressures. The codons of plant allergens are usually suboptimal with respect to expression in mammalian cells. Recoding of antigens has been demonstrated to dramatically improve expression levels and immunogenicity in many cases, however, the predictive validity of codon adaption on expression levels still needs improvement.

As an example, a gene vaccine encoding the major house dust mite allergen precursor ProDer p1 resulted in five to ten times higher protein levels compared to the wild type molecule and resulted in enhanced vaccination efficacy and protection from allergy (Jacquet et al. 2003; Massaer et al. 2001). Similarly, adapting the codon usage of the major mugwort allergen Art v 1a led to about 180-fold increased levels of protein expression and strong TH1 biased immunogenicity whereas the wild type induced no measureable immune response (Bauer et al. 2003). In contrast, other plant-derived allergens with similar codon usage to Art v 1a display excellent immunogenicity without sequence adaptations or display no noticeable change in vaccine efficacy after recoding (unpublished observation). These observations exemplify that the effect of codon adaption is difficult to predict, yet in certain cases, a dramatic increase in protein expression and immunogenicity can be achieved.

Vaccine types, which were originally believed to exert their excellent immunogenicity via the increase of protein expression, are self-replicating RNA and DNA vaccines. However, recent investigations elicited additional mechanisms underlying the potent immunogenicity of self-replicating vaccines. A detailed background about the molecular and immunological mechanisms of self-replicating vaccines is given in Chap. 3 in this book. Briefly, self replicating RNA vaccines encode an alpha virus-derived replicase molecule that drives its own amplification, and subsequently transcription and translation of the antigen if interest (which has been substituted for the genes encoding the viral structural proteins). Self replicating DNA vaccines have been generated by cloning such self replicating RNAs into eukaryotic expression vectors.

We have demonstrated that self replicating DNA vaccines encoding the timothy grass pollen allergen Phl p 5, or the model allergen β-galactosidase, exert their therapeutic and prophylactic efficacy at doses 100-fold lower than those of conventional DNA vaccines. Although their immunostimulatory capacity relies on different sensors of genetic material, i.e. detection of dsRNA intermediates vs. detection of plasmid DNA, we could show that similar to conventional DNA vaccines, the anti-allergic potential of self-replicating DNA constructs strictly depend on IFN-γ and partially on IL-12 (Scheiblhofer et al. 2006; Gabler et al. 2006). These data demonstrate that while the upstream processes of immune stimulation of conventional vs. self-replicating DNA vaccines may be different, the essential anti-allergic pathways addressed by both vaccines result in the generation of IFN-γ secreting TH1 cells. Similarly, we could recently demonstrate that also self-replicating RNA vaccines encoding Phl p 5 effectively prevent from induction of type I allergy, as will be discussed below.

Self-Removal of Gene Vaccines and the Safety Profile of Prophylactic Allergy Vaccines

Beyond the questions, how to increase immunogenicity and decrease allergenicity, a childhood gene vaccine against allergy must address the potential risks associated with the gene vaccine itself, which include the following concerns:

1. Long term expression of the encoded antigen and associated immunological side effects.
2. Long term persistence of the plasmid DNA itself, which might be associated with the generation of anti-DNA antibodies and autoimmunity.
3. Integration into the genome and induction of oncogenic events.

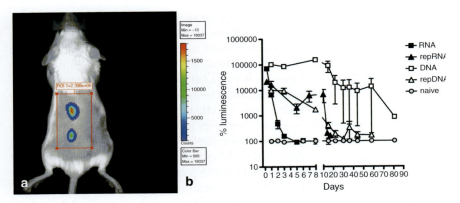

Fig. 12.2 In vivo RNA expression is short lived. In vivo expression of luciferase in mice (n=3) was quantitated on an Ivis Lumina imaging system (**a**) and expressed as a percentage of luminescence compared with that of naive mice injected with luciferin (**b**) (Reproduced from Roesler et al. (2009))

Although most of these concerns appear largely hypothetical today, and are of no relevance for vaccines against life threatening diseases such as HIV and cancer, the situation gets different when a vaccine has to be applied to healthy children, such as a prophylactic allergy vaccine.

Points 1 and 2, i.e. long term expression and long term persistence, can at least partly be addressed by the use of self-replicating vaccines. As described in Chap. 3 of this book, the generation of dsRNA intermediates during replication of the mRNA results in the triggering of apoptotic pathways, thereby removing transfected cells from the body. Indeed, we could demonstrate that protein expression from a self replicating DNA vaccine is essentially restricted to the first 20 days following immunization, while expression from conventional plasmids can last for several months. However, sporadic low level expression was also detectable in the self-replicating DNA group over extended time periods (Fig. 12.2) (Roesler et al. 2009). This is in line with data from Morris-Downes et al. (Morris-Downes et al. 2001), who were able to detect plasmids encoding self-replicating RNA vaccines via sensitive PCR methods over long periods of time, comparable to that of conventional DNA vaccines.

This gave rise to our decision to favour naked mRNA for a prophylactic allergy gene vaccine, which will be described in detail in the following section.

Prophylactic mRNA Vaccines Against Allergy

Like DNA vaccines, mRNA-based vaccines are able to carry exogenous genetic information into cells, and thus trigger an effective humoral and cellular immune reaction against the encoded antigen in vivo (Tavernier et al. 2010). Moreover, RNA based vaccines are an elegant solution to avoid safety risks associated with DNA vaccines. They represent minimal vectors lacking control sequences such as antibiotic resistance genes or promoters/terminators. In its purest form, a mRNA

12 Gene Vaccines for Prophylactic and Therapeutic Treatment of Allergy

vaccine is only composed of the gene of interest, a poly-adenosine (Poly(A)) tail of more than 30 residues at the 3' end and a 7-methyl guanosine cap structure (m7G(5')ppp(5')G) at the 5' end. In addition, 3' and/or 5' untranslated regions (UTRs) might be incorporated to enhance stability and protein levels. Because RNA exerts its function in the cytoplasm, RNA vaccines do not depend on transport mechanisms into and out of the nucleus, and on the cellular transcription machinery. RNA cannot integrate into the host genome, thus being free of any oncogenic risk. Furthermore, the low stability of RNA in the presence of ubiquitous RNAses limits the half life of such this vaccine type, and therefore the persistence in the body. Indeed, we could demonstrate that protein expression driven by a conventional RNA vaccine is completely abrogated within 5 days after intradermal injection, while expression from a self replicating RNA vaccine lasts for about 10 days (Fig. 12.2). Moreover, in contrast to DNA, no anti-RNA antibody reactions in the context of autoimmune diseases are known, suggesting that RNA has a low or no potential to induce autoimmune responses. Taken together, these features attribute a very high safety profile to RNA vaccines. This is also reflected by the fact, that the Food and Drug Administration (FDA) in the USA and the Paul Ehrlich Institute in Germany have classified non-replicative mRNA-based vaccines as non-gene therapy, facilitating access to human clinical trials (Pascolo 2008). RNA vaccines therefore represent the logical alternative to DNA vaccines for prophylactic vaccination against allergy.

Since the first report that injection of naked RNA encoding a reporter molecule induced transfection of muscle cells (Wolff et al. 1990), mRNA was mainly used for induction of anti-tumour immune responses and is currently evaluated in clinical trials of malignant melanoma (see Chap. 11 of this book).

Immune Responses Induced by RNA Vaccination

Initial data from Carralot et al. suggested that mRNA vaccination induced a TH2-polarized immune response type and co-application of GM-CSF was necessary to trigger a predominant TH1 response (Carralot et al. 2004). Recent publications, including our own, indicate that RNA vaccines are equally potent TH1 triggers as DNA vaccines. mRNA vaccines encoding a great variety of antigens proved to prime TH1-biased immune responses without additional adjuvantation. In general, the immunogenicity of RNA vaccines seems to be slightly lower, compared to their DNA counterparts, as we observed upon comparing the immunogenicity of both, conventional as well as self-replicating RNA and DNA vaccines coding for the timothy grass pollen allergen Phl p 5 (Roesler et al. 2009). This seems not to impair the efficacy of RNA vaccines, as data from a mouse model of allergy provided evidence, that even subtle TH1-priming by RNA vaccines gave rise to the recruitment of TH1 cells. Allergen exposure led to expansion of these cells, which retained their specificity and original TH1 polarization, resembling the mechanism of boosting a vaccine-induced memory by naturally occurring infectious agents. Consequently, RNA vaccines also protected mice from induction of IgE (Fig. 12.3). These results indicate that even relatively weak priming may be sufficient for long-term prevention of an allergic phenotype, due to natural

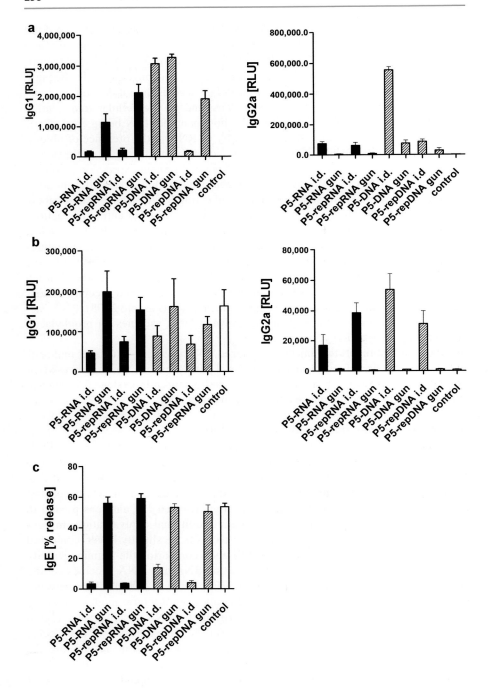

Fig. 12.3 Immune responses after vaccination with RNA (*solid bars*) and DNA (*hatched bars*) vaccines encoding Phl p 5 (P5-RNA, P5-DNA) and their self-replicating counterparts (P5-repRNA, P5-repDNA) were compared. Mice were immunized three times in weekly intervals by intradermal injection or via gene gun (gun). Sensitization controls (control, *open bars*) were naive prior to sensitization. (**a**) Phl p 5-specific IgG1 and IgG2a after the third vaccination. (**b**) IgG1 and IgG2a levels of the corresponding groups after a subsequent challenge using two subcutaneous injections with recombinant allergen in alum (**c**). Allergen-specific IgE after sensitization. Data are shown as means ± SEM (n=4) of relative light units (RLU) of a luminescence-based ELISA assay (**a** and **b**) or mediator release in a basophil release assay (**c**). Serum dilutions were 1:1,000 (**a**), 1:100,000 (**b**), and 1:100 (**c**) (Reproduced with permission from Weiss et al. (2010))

boosting of allergen-specific TH1 immunity, e.g. via allergen exposure during the pollen season.

Induction of a primary TH1-biased immune response is a necessary prerequisite for gene vaccine-mediated protection against allergy. Application of DNA-coated particles with a biolistic device, however, has been shown to trigger a serological TH2 polarization (Scheiblhofer et al. 2007; Weiss et al. 2002). Similarly, this TH2 bias seems to be valid for gene gun immunization with mRNA, as demonstrated by the failure to induce a TH1 milieu and to prevent from an allergic sensitization (Fig. 12.3).

Suppression of Type I Allergy Parameters by RNA Vaccination

Based on these findings, we characterized the anti-allergic potential of conventional and self-replicating Phl p 5 RNA vaccines in a prophylactic dose response study (Roesler et al. 2009) and found that as little as 10 µg of conventional or 1 µg of self-replicating RNA was sufficient to induce complete inhibition of IgE induction and a switch to a TH1 biased memory profile in the spleen. This immune profile was characterized by the induction of IFN-γ-secreting T cells and a suppression of IL-4, IL-5, and IL-13. In agreement with previous studies using DNA based vaccines (Gabler et al. 2006), no induction of IL-10 producing cells could be demonstrated. More importantly, RNA vaccination not only prevented from IgE induction, but also could suppress lung inflammation, as indicated by reduced numbers of total leukocytes, especially eosinophils in bronchoalveloar lavage fluids, and alleviate airway hyperresponsiveness. The latter was assessed by both, non-invasive whole body plethysmography, as well as direct invasive measurement of resistance and dynamic compliance. Finally, by applying this vaccination approach to 28 additional allergens, representing the major groups of tree, grass, weed pollens as well as food allergens, dust mite, animal dander, moulds and latex allergens, we could exemplify the broad applicability of the method (Thalhamer et al. 2009).

Future Perspectives

In summary, gene vaccines are promising candidates for prophylactic vaccination against allergy in children with an elevated risk of atopy. Although self-replicating DNA and RNA vaccines provide an elegant method to induce protective immunity at minimal doses, such vaccines might not pass the high regulatory requirements for clinical application in children. However, we could clearly demonstrate that even a minimal naked RNA vaccine in its purest form, utilizing only a 5′-cap structure, a minimal 5′ UTR, the allergen gene of interest, and a synthetic polyA tail, is sufficient to prevent from allergic sensitization. Consequently, as the RNA is rapidly degraded after initiation of the desired immune response, we termed our approach "immunize and disappear."

In contrast to gene vaccines designed to treat tumors or viral diseases, a prophylactic vaccine against allergy does not have to, yes it even should not, induce potent immune responses, but just set a specific subtle immunological bias. Natural exposure, as in the case of pollen allergens, will then recall and strengthen the initially set type of immune response. Therefore, such a vaccine might not even require booster immunizations but provide life-long protection once the correct immune bias has been triggered. We are currently investigating how this repeated revoking of anti-allergic immune responses via aerosol exposure will affect the observed immune responses in the long run, with respect to memory, stability of polarization, and long-term protection.

These data will insert the last piece parts of the jigsaw puzzle upon preparing the logical step forward, i.e. evaluation of safety and the generation of TH1 memory T cells in a phase I/IIa clinical trial.

Acknowlegement This work was supported by Biomay AG, Vienna, Austria and the Christian Doppler Research Association, Vienna, Austria.

References

Ball T, Sperr WR, Valent P, Lidholm J, Spitzauer S, Ebner C, Kraft D, Valenta R (1999) Induction of antibody responses to new B cell epitopes indicates vaccination character of allergen immunotherapy. Eur J Immunol 29(6):2026–2036

Bauer R, Himly M, Dedic A, Ferreira F, Thalhamer J, Hartl A (2003) Optimization of codon usage is required for effective genetic immunization against Art v 1, the major allergen of mugwort pollen. Allergy 58(10):1003–1010

Bauer R, Scheiblhofer S, Kern K, Gruber C, Stepanoska T, Thalhamer T, Hauser-Kronberger C, Alinger B, Zoegg T, Gabler M, Ferreira F, Hartl A, Thalhamer J, Weiss R (2006) Generation of hypoallergenic DNA vaccines by forced ubiquitination: preventive and therapeutic effects in a mouse model of allergy. J Allergy Clin Immunol 118(1):269–276

Bonifaz LC, Arzate S, Moreno J (1999) Endogenous and exogenous forms of the same antigen are processed from different pools to bind MHC class II molecules in endocytic compartments. Eur J Immunol 29(1):119–131

Braun-Fahrlander C, Gassner M, Grize L, Neu U, Sennhauser FH, Varonier HS, Vuille JC, Wuthrich B (1999) Prevalence of hay fever and allergic sensitization in farmer's children and their peers living in the same rural community. SCARPOL team. Swiss study on childhood allergy and respiratory symptoms with respect to air pollution. Clin Exp Allergy 29(1):28–34

Braun-Fahrlander C, Riedler J, Herz U, Eder W, Waser M, Grize L, Maisch S, Carr D, Gerlach F, Bufe A, Lauener RP, Schierl R, Renz H, Nowak D, von Mutius E (2002) Environmental exposure to endotoxin and its relation to asthma in school-age children. N Engl J Med 347(12):869–877

Bullens DM, De Swerdt A, Dilissen E, Kasran A, Kroczek RA, Cadot P, Casaer P, Ceuppens JL (2005) House dust mite-specific T cells in healthy non-atopic children. Clin Exp Allergy 35(12):1535–1541

Carralot JP, Probst J, Hoerr I, Scheel B, Teufel R, Jung G, Rammensee HG, Pascolo S (2004) Polarization of immunity induced by direct injection of naked sequence-stabilized mRNA vaccines. Cell Mol Life Sci 61(18):2418–2424

Cheng WF, Hung CF, Hsu KF, Chai CY, He L, Ling M, Slater LA, Roden RB, Wu TC (2001) Enhancement of sindbis virus self-replicating RNA vaccine potency by targeting antigen to endosomal/lysosomal compartments. Hum Gene Ther 12(3):235–252

Dobano C, Rogers WO, Gowda K, Doolan DL (2007) Targeting antigen to MHC class I and class II antigen presentation pathways for malaria DNA vaccines. Immunol Lett 111(2):92–102

Ege MJ, Bieli C, Frei R, van Strien RT, Riedler J, Ublagger E, Schram-Bijkerk D, Brunekreef B, van Hage M, Scheynius A, Pershagen G, Benz MR, Lauener R, von Mutius E, Braun-Fahrlander C (2006) Prenatal farm exposure is related to the expression of receptors of the innate immunity and to atopic sensitization in school-age children. J Allergy Clin Immunol 117(4): 817–823

Ege MJ, Frei R, Bieli C, Schram-Bijkerk D, Waser M, Benz MR, Weiss G, Nyberg F, van Hage M, Pershagen G, Brunekreef B, Riedler J, Lauener R, Braun-Fahrlander C, von Mutius E (2007) Not all farming environments protect against the development of asthma and wheeze in children. J Allergy Clin Immunol 119(5):1140–1147

Floistrup H, Swartz J, Bergstrom A, Alm JS, Scheynius A, van Hage M, Waser M, Braun-Fahrlander C, Schram-Bijkerk D, Huber M, Zutavern A, von Mutius E, Ublagger E, Riedler J, Michaels KB, Pershagen G (2006) Allergic disease and sensitization in Steiner school children. J Allergy Clin Immunol 117(1):59–66

Gabler M, Scheiblhofer S, Kern K, Leitner WW, Stoecklinger A, Hauser-Kronberger C, Alinger B, Lechner B, Prinz M, Vrtala S, Valenta R, Thalhamer J, Weiss R (2006) Immunization with a low-dose replicon DNA vaccine encoding Phl p 5 effectively prevents allergic sensitization. J Allergy Clin Immunol 118(3):734–741

Hartl A, Kiesslich J, Weiss R, Bernhaupt A, Mostbock S, Scheiblhofer S, Ebner C, Ferreira F, Thalhamer J (1999a) Immune responses after immunization with plasmid DNA encoding Bet v 1, the major allergen of birch pollen. J Allergy Clin Immunol 103(1 Pt 1):107–113

Hartl A, Kiesslich J, Weiss R, Bernhaupt A, Mostbock S, Scheiblhofer S, Flockner H, Sippl M, Ebner C, Ferreira F, Thalhamer J (1999b) Isoforms of the major allergen of birch pollen induce different immune responses after genetic immunization. Int Arch Allergy Immunol 120(1): 17–29

Hartl A, Hochreiter R, Stepanoska T, Ferreira F, Thalhamer J (2004) Characterization of the protective and therapeutic efficiency of a DNA vaccine encoding the major birch pollen allergen Bet v 1a. Allergy 59(1):65–73

Hochreiter R, Stepanoska T, Ferreira F, Valenta R, Vrtala S, Thalhamer J, Hartl A (2003) Prevention of allergen-specific IgE production and suppression of an established Th2-type response by immunization with DNA encoding hypoallergenic allergen derivatives of Bet v 1, the major birch-pollen allergen. Eur J Immunol 33(6):1667–1676

Hsu CH, Chua KY, Tao MH, Lai YL, Wu HD, Huang SK, Hsieh KH (1996) Immunoprophylaxis of allergen-induced immunoglobulin E synthesis and airway hyperresponsiveness in vivo by genetic immunization. Nat Med 2(5):540–544

Jacquet A, Magi M, Haumont M, Jurado M, Garcia L, Bollen A (2003) Absence of immunoglobulin E synthesis and airway eosinophilia by vaccination with plasmid DNA encoding ProDer p 1. Clin Exp Allergy 33(2):218–225

Kim TW, Hung CF, Boyd D, Juang J, He L, Kim JW, Hardwick JM, Wu TC (2003) Enhancing DNA vaccine potency by combining a strategy to prolong dendritic cell life with intracellular targeting strategies. J Immunol 171(6):2970–2976

Kulig M, Bergmann R, Niggemann B, Burow G, Wahn U (1998) Prediction of sensitization to inhalant allergens in childhood: evaluating family history, atopic dermatitis and sensitization to food allergens. The MAS study group. Multicentre allergy study. Clin Exp Allergy 28(11):1397–1403

Lauener RP, Birchler T, Adamski J, Braun-Fahrlander C, Bufe A, Herz U, von Mutius E, Nowak D, Riedler J, Waser M, Sennhauser FH (2002) Expression of CD14 and toll-like receptor 2 in farmers' and non-farmers' children. Lancet 360(9331):465–466

Lich JD, Elliott JF, Blum JS (2000) Cytoplasmic processing is a prerequisite for presentation of an endogenous antigen by major histocompatibility complex class II proteins. J Exp Med 191(9):1513–1524

Lu Y, Raviprakash K, Leao IC, Chikhlikar PR, Ewing D, Anwar A, Chougnet C, Murphy G, Hayes CG, August TJ, Marques ET Jr (2003) Dengue 2 PreM-E/LAMP chimera targeted to the MHC class II compartment elicits long-lasting neutralizing antibodies. Vaccine 21(17–18): 2178–2189

Marenholz I, Kerscher T, Bauerfeind A, Esparza-Gordillo J, Nickel R, Keil T, Lau S, Rohde K, Wahn U, Lee YA (2009) An interaction between filaggrin mutations and early food sensitization improves the prediction of childhood asthma. J Allergy Clin Immunol 123(4):911–916

Marques ET Jr, Chikhlikar P, de Arruda LB, Leao IC, Lu Y, Wong J, Chen JS, Byrne B, August JT (2003) HIV-1 p55Gag encoded in the lysosome-associated membrane protein-1 as a DNA plasmid vaccine chimera is highly expressed, traffics to the major histocompatibility class II compartment, and elicits enhanced immune responses. J Biol Chem 278(39):37926–37936

Massaer M, Mazzu P, Haumont M, Magi M, Daminet V, Bollen A, Jacquet A (2001) High-level expression in mammalian cells of recombinant house dust mite allergen ProDer p 1 with optimized codon usage. Int Arch Allergy Immunol 125(1):32–43

Morris-Downes MM, Phenix KV, Smyth J, Sheahan BJ, Lileqvist S, Mooney DA, Liljestrom P, Todd D, Atkins GJ (2001) Semliki forest virus-based vaccines: persistence, distribution and pathological analysis in two animal systems. Vaccine 19(15–16):1978–1988

Mukherjee P, Dani A, Bhatia S, Singh N, Rudensky AY, George A, Bal V, Mayor S, Rath S (2001) Efficient presentation of both cytosolic and endogenous transmembrane protein antigens on MHC class II is dependent on cytoplasmic proteolysis. J Immunol 167(5):2632–2641

Pascolo S (2008) Vaccination with messenger RNA (mRNA). Handb Exp Pharmacol 183: 221–235

Peters M, Kauth M, Scherner O, Gehlhar K, Steffen I, Wentker P, von Mutius E, Holst O, Bufe A (2010) Arabinogalactan isolated from cowshed dust extract protects mice from allergic airway inflammation and sensitization. J Allergy Clin Immunol 126(3):648–656, e641-644

Pfefferle PI, Sel S, Ege MJ, Buchele G, Blumer N, Krauss-Etschmann S, Herzum I, Albers CE, Lauener RP, Roponen M, Hirvonen MR, Vuitton DA, Riedler J, Brunekreef B, Dalphin JC, Braun-Fahrlander C, Pekkanen J, von Mutius E, Renz H (2008) Cord blood allergen-specific IgE is associated with reduced IFN-gamma production by cord blood cells: the protection against allergy-study in rural environments (PASTURE) study. J Allergy Clin Immunol 122(4):711–716

Purohit A, Niederberger V, Kronqvist M, Horak F, Gronneberg R, Suck R, Weber B, Fiebig H, van Hage M, Pauli G, Valenta R, Cromwell O (2008) Clinical effects of immunotherapy with genetically modified recombinant birch pollen Bet v 1 derivatives. Clin Exp Allergy 38(9):1514–1525

Raz E, Tighe H, Sato Y, Corr M, Dudler JA, Roman M, Swain SL, Spiegelberg HL, Carson DA (1996) Preferential induction of a Th1 immune response and inhibition of specific IgE antibody formation by plasmid DNA immunization. Proc Natl Acad Sci USA 93(10):5141–5145

Riedler J, Eder W, Oberfeld G, Schreuer M (2000) Austrian children living on a farm have less hay fever, asthma and allergic sensitization. Clin Exp Allergy 30(2):194–200

Riedler J, Braun-Fahrlander C, Eder W, Schreuer M, Waser M, Maisch S, Carr D, Schierl R, Nowak D, von Mutius E (2001) Exposure to farming in early life and development of asthma and allergy: a cross-sectional survey. Lancet 358(9288):1129–1133

Rodriguez F, Harkins S, Redwine JM, de Pereda JM, Whitton JL (2001) CD4(+) T cells induced by a DNA vaccine: immunological consequences of epitope-specific lysosomal targeting. J Virol 75(21):10421–10430

Roesler E, Weiss R, Weinberger EE, Fruehwirth A, Stoecklinger A, Mostbock S, Ferreira F, Thalhamer J, Scheiblhofer S (2009) Immunize and disappear-safety-optimized mRNA vaccination with a panel of 29 allergens. J Allergy Clin Immunol 124(5):1070–1077, e1071-1011

Romagnani S (2004) The increased prevalence of allergy and the hygiene hypothesis: missing immune deviation, reduced immune suppression, or both? Immunology 112(3):352–363

Scheiblhofer S, Gabler M, Leitner WW, Bauer R, Zoegg T, Ferreira F, Thalhamer J, Weiss R (2006) Inhibition of type I allergic responses with nanogram doses of replicon-based DNA vaccines. Allergy 61(7):828–835

Scheiblhofer S, Stoecklinger A, Gruber C, Hauser-Kronberger C, Alinger B, Hammerl P, Thalhamer J, Weiss R (2007) Gene gun immunization with clinically relevant allergens aggravates allergen induced pathology and is contraindicated for allergen immunotherapy. Mol Immunol 44(8):1879–1887

Senthilselvan A, Rennie D, Chenard L, Burch LH, Babiuk L, Schwartz DA, Dosman JA (2008) Association of polymorphisms of toll-like receptor 4 with a reduced prevalence of hay fever and atopy. Ann Allergy Asthma Immunol 100(5):463–468

Sudre B, Vacheyrou M, Braun-Fahrlander C, Normand AC, Waser M, Reboux G, Ruffaldi P, von Mutius E, Piarroux R (2009) High levels of grass pollen inside European dairy farms: a role for the allergy-protective effects of environment? Allergy 64(7):1068–1073

Tavernier G, Andries O, Demeester J, Sanders NN, De Smedt SC, Rejman J (2010) mRNA as gene therapeutic: How to control protein expression. J Control Release 150(3):238–247

Thalhamer J, Weiss R, Roesler E, Scheiblhofer S, Fruehwirth A (2009) RNA vaccines. WO/2009/040443

Thalhamer T, Dobias H, Stepanoska T, Proll M, Stutz H, Dissertori O, Lackner P, Ferreira F, Wallner M, Thalhamer J, Hartl A (2010) Designing hypoallergenic derivatives for allergy treatment by means of in silico mutation and screening. J Allergy Clin Immunol 125(4):926–934, e910

Valenta R, Ferreira F, Focke-Tejkl M, Linhart B, Niederberger V, Swoboda I, Vrtala S (2010) From allergen genes to allergy vaccines. Annu Rev Immunol 28:211–241

Van Overtvelt L, Wambre E, Maillere B, von Hofe E, Louise A, Balazuc AM, Bohle B, Ebo D, Leboulaire C, Garcia G, Moingeon P (2008) Assessment of Bet v 1-specific CD4+ T cell responses in allergic and nonallergic individuals using MHC class II peptide tetramers. J Immunol 180(7):4514–4522

Van Ree R, Van Leeuwen WA, Dieges PH, Van Wijk RG, De Jong N, Brewczyski PZ, Kroon AM, Schilte PP, Tan KY, Simon-Licht IF, Roberts AM, Stapel SO, Aalberse RC (1997) Measurement of IgE antibodies against purified grass pollen allergens (Lol p 1, 2, 3 and 5) during immunotherapy. Clin Exp Allergy 27(1):68–74

van Strien RT, Engel R, Holst O, Bufe A, Eder W, Waser M, Braun-Fahrlander C, Riedler J, Nowak D, von Mutius E (2004) Microbial exposure of rural school children, as assessed by levels of N-acetyl-muramic acid in mattress dust, and its association with respiratory health. J Allergy Clin Immunol 113(5):860–867

Vogel K, Blumer N, Korthals M, Mittelstadt J, Garn H, Ege M, von Mutius E, Gatermann S, Bufe A, Goldmann T, Schwaiger K, Renz H, Brandau S, Bauer J, Heine H, Holst O (2008) Animal shed Bacillus licheniformis spores possess allergy-protective as well as inflammatory properties. J Allergy Clin Immunol 122(2):307–312, 312 e301–308

Von Ehrenstein OS, Von Mutius E, Illi S, Baumann L, Bohm O, von Kries R (2000) Reduced risk of hay fever and asthma among children of farmers. Clin Exp Allergy 30(2):187–193

von Mutius E, Vercelli D (2010) Farm living: effects on childhood asthma and allergy. Nat Rev Immunol 10(12):861–868

Weiss R, Scheiblhofer S, Freund J, Ferreira F, Livey I, Thalhamer J (2002) Gene gun bombardment with gold particles displays a particular Th2-promoting signal that over-rules the Th1-inducing effect of immunostimulatory CpG motifs in DNA vaccines. Vaccine 20(25–26):3148–3154

Weiss R, Scheiblhofer S, Gabler M, Ferreira F, Leitner WW, Thalhamer J (2006) Is genetic vaccination against allergy possible? Int Arch Allergy Immunol 139(4):332–345

Weiss R, Scheiblhofer S, Roesler E, Ferreira F, Thalhamer J (2010) Prophylactic mRNA vaccination against allergy. Curr Opin Allergy Clin Immunol 10(6):567–574

Wolff JA, Malone RW, Williams P, Chong W, Acsadi G, Jani A, Felgner PL (1990) Direct gene transfer into mouse muscle in vivo. Science 247(4949 Pt 1):1465–1468

Approved Veterinary Vaccines: Paving the Way to Products for Human Health

13

Matthias Giese

Industrial production of veterinary vaccines started in the 1950s introducing the possibility to vaccinate millions of animals. In the meantime veterinary vaccines and mass vaccination became a necessary prerequisite for a modern livestock industry. Nearly all current veterinary vaccines worldwide are conventional vaccines, killed or modified live vaccines. Until now, the only animal infection eradicated by vaccination is rinderpest, and for numerous pathogens no effective and safe vaccine is available. There is an undisputed urgent need to develop novel vaccination strategies with improved efficacy.

Not only are veterinary vaccines a basis of an intensive livestock industry but also protect human health by preventing spread of zoonotic animal infections. They also protect consumers from associated risks such as the increase in antibiotic resistant pathogens, and consumption of pharmaceutical contaminates in food products.

DNA vaccines attracted attention in veterinary medicine as they harbor many advantages. Studies can be performed directly in the species of interest rather than using mouse models. Vaccine production is easy and flexible under good laboratory practice (GLP) guidelines. Furthermore, the features of gene vaccines enable humoral as well as cellular immune responses and vaccine cocktails containing genetic material from several pathogens can be employed. The range of application includes non-infectious diseases, such as allergy and cancer as well as fertility control. Additionally, gene vaccines are highly stable and no cold chain is required thus extending the field of application (wildlife animals, third world), and finally, gene vaccines are cheap and competitive products compared to conventional vaccines.

In this chapter the current status of gene vaccines licensed for veterinary used is summarized. These include the West Nile virus DNA vaccine for horses, a fish DNA

M. Giese
Institute for Molecular Vaccines (IMV) Heidelberg, Heidelberg, Germany
e-mail: info@imv-heidelberg.com

J. Thalhamer et al. (eds.), *Gene Vaccines*,
DOI 10.1007/978-3-7091-0439-2_13, © Springer-Verlag/Wien, 2012

265

vaccine against the Infectious Haematopoietic Necrosis virus, and the Canine Malignant Melanoma vaccine (ONCEPT™). Additionally, a vaccine against the Equine Arteritis Virus (EAV-THERA-VAC) used in clinical studies is discussed. Together these examples emphasize the broad applicability and clinical efficacy of the gene vaccine technology which will pave the way for future application in humans.

Cowpox Virus from Cattle Was the First Human Vaccine

The success story of vaccination started in 1798 with Edward Jenner immunizing a child by using bovine cowpox to induce protection against human smallpox. At this time, neither the immune system nor its functions were discovered, thus Jenner did not know anything about cross reactions and the relationship between animal and human viruses.

It was also Jenner, who called his approach 'vaccination' from the Latin term 'vacca,' meaning cow, and in a literal sense, he also can be considered as the originator of the empiric and science-based vaccine research. Till today the term 'vaccination' is still used in addition to the term immunization.

Industrial production of veterinary vaccines started in the 1950s and opened the possibility to vaccinate millions of animals. However, up to now the only animal infection which could be eradicated by worldwide vaccination is rinderpest (Roeder and Taylor 2002). Nevertheless, veterinary vaccines and mass vaccination represent a basis of modern livestock industry, but there is still an urgent need for developing novel and improved vaccines due to the following reasons:

1. For numerous pathogens no effective and safe vaccine exists.
2. Veterinary vaccines can protect human health by preventing zoonotic animal infections.
3. Veterinary vaccines can protect consumers from risks associated with spread of antibiotic resistances and pharmaceutical contaminates in food producing animals.
4. Veterinary vaccines can increase the efficiency of food production and thus contribute to improve the food supply for a growing world population.

In contrast to human medicine, where vaccines comprise only 2% of all pharmaceutical products, 28% of pharmaceuticals sold in veterinary medicine are vaccines, with an annual growth rate of 7%. This increase in animal vaccination has a major impact on animal health and welfare, but due to the aspects mentioned above, it also greatly influences public health (Redding and Weiner 2009).

The discrepancy between the absolute figures of veterinary and human vaccines is based on the fact that the major focus in human medicine lies on curative treatments whereas the most cost-effective intervention for controlling disease and reducing economic losses in veterinary medicine are protective approaches. But in contrast to human vaccines, the return of investment for animal vaccines is smaller, due to lower sales prices and smaller markets. This results in limited investment of pharmaceutical companies in research and development of animal vaccines.

Moreover, the principal scientific requirements and developmental costs of animal vaccines are similar to those of human vaccines. Taken together, this may explain the lack of commitment of pharmaceutical companies to invest in animal vaccine research.

Current Status of Veterinary Vaccines

The vast majority of animal vaccines worldwide are conventional vaccines, killed or modified live vaccines (Meeusen et al. 2007).

Killed vaccines display a high biological safety profile. The pathogen is inactivated by physical or chemical procedures and thus unable to proliferate and exert its infectious and pathogenic functions. However, most methods of inactivation can destroy important antigenic structures. Therefore, most killed vaccines only induce humoral but no cellular immune responses. In order to increase the immunogenicity of killed vaccines, they must be adjuvanted by chemical compounds which for their part can induce various side effects.

Modified live vaccines (MLV) are able to induce a complete immune response, production of neutralizing antibodies and activation of CD8+ T-cells. In contrast to killed vaccines, they also provoke superior protection. But the price for this excellent protection is high, as biological safety is not guaranteed. A MLV contains an active pathogen, is still infective and able to replicate. Potential safety risks include reversion to virulence and recombination with homologous environmental pathogens. Such an event took place in 1996 in Denmark during a vaccination program against a porcine viral infection (Mortensen et al. 2002).

Porcine reproductive and respiratory syndrome virus, PRRSV, is a small RNA virus, member of the Arteriviridae family of the Nidovirales order. There is high sequence variation between European and North American isolates. The identity at the nucleotide level is only 55–80%. PRRSV infection can cause severe reproductive damage in pregnant sows and respiratory distress in young and old pigs. PRRSV is the most important pathogen in countries with intensive pork industry and responsible for approximately US \$600 million in losses each year to U.S. producers. Similar losses also occur in Europe and Asia, here especially in China (Lunney et al. 2010).

Danish pigs were vaccinated by a licensed MLV PRRSV vaccine, based on the American virus strain. But at the same time the European PRSSV strain was present in the herds. Genetic recombination between these two related virus strains was the consequence. At the end of the day the vaccine had caused the PRRSV epidemic instead of preventing it.

The criteria for a successful vaccination in veterinary medicine can differ from human medicine. According to their specific requirements, veterinary vaccines can be grouped into three categories:

1. Companion animals. Health and welfare of the animal has the highest priority for the veterinarian. The benchmarks in human and veterinary medicine are similar.

2. Livestock animals. These animals are food-producing animals such as pigs, cattle, poultry, and fish. These animals live together in high numbers on limited space. The main objective of livestock vaccines is to improve overall production. Not the health and immunity of the individual animal, but overall herd immunity is the main concern. Vaccinations should prevent spreading of infectious diseases within the herd.
3. Wildlife animals. These animals can transmit important pathogens to humans, such as rabies, influenza, borrelia, or west nile virus. 61% of all known pathogens are zoonotic and affect humans. Zoonotic diseases must be combated at their source, namely in animals.

Over the next decades veterinary medicine will gain more and more public interest. Due to the constant growth in world population and economic growth in emerging countries such as China and India there will be an increasing demand of meat, milk and fish. The WHO expects a growth in world population from around 6.5 billion people now to more than nine billion people in 2,050 with a concomitant increase in meat consumption from 229 million tons of meat to 460 million tons of meat per year. Similarly, yearly milk consumption will rise from 580 to 1,200 million tons. Simultaneously, the amount of farmland and grassland needed for animal husbandry will remain unchanged or even decrease due to progressing urbanization.

As a consequence, livestock farming will be intensified without increasing the grassland for animals, thereby increasing the risk of infectious diseases. Only a consequent mass vaccination approach could prevent such diseases and warrant human health, as healthy livestock forms the basis for safe animal products for the consumer. Therefore veterinary vaccines are also an essential and inseparable part of public health.

Approved DNA Vaccines in Veterinary Medicine

Progress in the understanding of the molecular mechanisms underlying the immunogenicity of vaccines and technological progress will spur the development of novel veterinary vaccines. Killed vaccines with their limited immunogenicity could be replaced step-by-step with recombinant subunit vaccines. Modified live vaccines with their limited biological safety could be replaced with vector-driven but also DNA or RNA-based gene vaccines. While vector vaccines are an elegant solution, their efficacy is limited by the immune response raised against the vector. After multiple applications neutralizing antibodies against the vector will prevent efficient boosting of the vaccine.

DNA vaccines are of special interest for the veterinary medicine. One of the most important advantages is that experimental studies can be conducted directly in the species of interest and no mouse model is necessary (Giese 1998). Additionally, DNA vaccines harbour many other advantages including the following:
1. The construction is easy and flexible under GLP guidelines.
2. Induction of a complete, humoral and cellular immune response.

3. Construction of cocktails including various pathogens.
4. New developments for old unmet needs.
5. New indications (allergy, cancer, fertility control).
6. No dangerous pathogens in the laboratory.
7. Automatic fermenter production under GMP conditions.
8. High biological safety.
9. High chemical safety.
10. New application routes (needle-free injection).
11. No cold chain (wildlife animals, third world).
12. Cheap and competitive products.

However, greater efforts have to be undertaken to overcome some bottlenecks of gene vaccines. The antigen expression level depends on several factors such as the nature of the antigen, co-stimulatory signals, or the application route and is a critical factor for vaccine efficacy. The immunogenicity of the antigen has to be optimized, for example by employing fusion constructs as demonstrated for the West Nile Virus vaccine discussed in section "West Nile Virus: A severe zoonotic infection". A broad overview on such strategies is given in Chap. 2 of this book. DNA vaccines can only compete with MLV vaccines in the market if the DNA vaccine is equally efficient, of best quality, and affordable.

The first veterinary DNA vaccines were developed for horses for West Nile virus (Davis et al. 2001) and Equine Arteritis virus (Giese et al. 2002). Today the number of ongoing clinical trials worldwide regarding veterinary DNA vaccines is exhaustive and includes all relevant livestock species.

The objective of the following sections is to discuss approved veterinary DNA vaccines and their impact on human medicine and public health.

West Nile Virus: A Severe Zoonotic Infection

The Virus
West Nile virus (WNV) is a mosquito-borne member of the family Flaviviridae, genus flavivirus and was first identified 1937 in Uganda, Africa. It is a positive-sense, single stranded RNA virus, of about 11 kb that encodes a single polyprotein with seven non-structural proteins and three structural proteins (Fig. 13.1). The RNA strand is held within a nucleocapsid. WNV replicates in the cytoplasm of infected cells. Its structure is similar to the dengue fever virus (Murray et al. 2010).

Transmission
WNV is a zoonotic virus. The primary reservoir hosts are birds which has a significant impact on spreading the infection across countries and continents. More than 170 different species are described as carrier of this virus. WNV is spread from bird to bird by mosquitoes when they bite and take a blood meal. Depending on the species, birds will get ill and die or show no clinical signs at all. Mosquitoes are also capable of spreading the virus to diverse species such as horses, dogs, cats, mice, and alligators and also to humans.

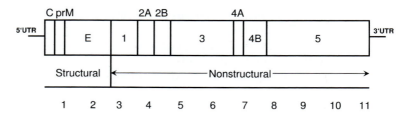

Fig. 13.1 Genomic organization of the WNV genome (Brault 2009). Three structural proteins (C, prM, E) and seven nonstructural proteins (NS1, 2A, 2B, 3, 4A, 4B and 5) are translated as a single polyprotein directly from the 11 kb positive-sense RNA genome (Kindly provided by Aaron C. Brault, Division of Vector-Borne Infectious Diseases Centers for Disease Control & Prevention Fort Collins, CO)

Disease

One third of all horses bitten by infected mosquitoes develop disease and die or have to be euthanized. Incubation time ranges from 3 to 14 days. Horses that do become ill vary in symptoms, including muscle trembling, skin twitching, ataxia, sleepiness, dullness, and listlessness. WNV may cross the placenta from mother to gestating foal. Horses cannot spread the disease to humans.

In humans, WNV displays a different progression and outcome of disease. Symptoms are similar to influenza and include fever, headaches, chills, diaphoresis, weakness, swollen lymph nodes, drowsiness, and pain in the joints. More severe neuroinvasive infections also may cause meningitis and encephalitis.

Special Characteristics

The virus, imported from Israel, was first encountered in the USA in 1999 in New York City and since then has spread nationwide within only 5 years. Meanwhile also Europe, Australia, and Asia are affected. The World Organization for Animal Health (OIE) reported a new outbreak of WNV in October 2010 in Portugal.

WNV-DNA Vaccine

The surface envelope protein E is the main target for the antibody response. There are more than 180 copies of the E protein in a mature WNV virion. Protein E is necessary for infection as it mediates interaction with cell surface and membrane fusion. During viral maturation, the pre-membrane protein prM gets processed into a smaller membrane M peptide. Expression of prM and E protein results in the formation of virus-like particles (VLP). These VLP share many of the antigenic and structural properties of fully mature viruses and are of special interest for vaccine development (Fig. 13.2).

The expression plasmid used for immunization of horses contains the human cytomegalovirus early gene promoter, signal sequences from Japanese Encephalitis Virus, and a fusion gene of prM and E. The WNV DNA vaccine induces stable and long lasting (12 months) cellular and humoral immune responses and is safe in horses.

The vaccine was approved for veterinary use by USDA in July, 2005 and released to public in December 2008 (USDA-APHIS-VS-CVB 2008). This vaccine was the first licensed DNA vaccine in the world and therefore represents a milestone not only for the development of veterinary DNA vaccines but also DNA vaccines in general.

Fig. 13.2 Map of the recombinant WN virus plasmid pCBWN (Davis et al. 2001). The transcription unit contains the human cytomegalovirus early gene promoter (CMV), JE virus signal sequence, WN virus prM and E gene region, and bovine growth hormone poly(A) signal (BGH) (Kindly provided by Gwong-Jen J. Chang, Division of Vector-Borne Infectious Diseases NCEID, CDC Fort Collins, CO)

The WNV DNA vaccine was also successfully tested in birds, as these are the primary reservoir hosts (Bunning et al. 2007). This data suggest that the vaccine is probably suitable for a broad range of animal species.

Impact for Human Medicine
- A Phase I clinical trial in humans demonstrated that the WNV-DNA vaccine induces neutralizing antibodies against prM and E protein and also measurable cellular responses (NCT00106769 2008).
- This DNA vaccine is safe and well tolerated in animals and humans.
- This DNA platform can be used both for veterinary and human vaccines without species-specific modifications.
- Simultaneous development of vaccines for veterinary as well as clinical use is cost-efficient but also time-saving. This is of high importance since about two-thirds of all known 1,400 pathogens transmitted by animals are zoonotic pathogens.

Equine Arteritis Virus: A Therapeutic Vaccine Against a Chronic Infection

Virus

Equine arteritis virus (EAV) is a member of the family Arteriviridae, genus Arterivirus. EAV is characterized by a small (60–65 nm) enveloped particle, containing an icosahedral capsid. The virus contains a positive-sense, single stranded RNA of about 12 kb that encodes for 9 ORFs (Fig. 13.3). EAV replicates in the cytoplasm of infected cells (Tobiasch et al. 2001). Its structure is similar to the porcine reproductive and respiratory syndrome virus (PRRSV), another member of the Arteriviridae, with enormous economical impact on the global pork industry.

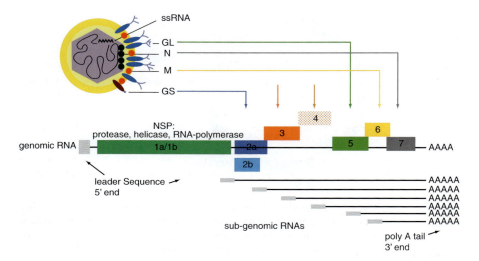

Fig. 13.3 Genome organization and transcriptional strategy of EAV (Giese et al. 2002; Tobiasch et al. 2001). Overlapping open reading frames (ORFs). ORF 1a/1b encodes the viral replicase and ORFs 2–7 encode structural proteins

Transmission

EAV is commonly found in breeding herds of horses worldwide. EAV is horizontally transmitted by the respiratory route with an incubation time of 3–5 days, or vertically by venereal secretion with an incubation period of several weeks via infected carrier stallions.

Disease

Clinical signs during the acute phase vary widely and can comprise fever, edema, nasal and ocular discharge, conjunctivitis, cough, diarrhoea, depression, and lethargy. The most severe form of EAV infection may cause abortions in 40–80% of infected mares during the second to eleventh month of pregnancy.

Special Characteristics

Infected mares, but not stallions, are able to lose the virus within some months. Lung cells are the first target cells for EAV. In stallions, EAV replicates in the testes, probably in accessory genital glands, and is continuously shed via semen.

EAV-DNA Vaccine

DNA vaccination against EAV was employed to treat chronically infected stallions with the aim to cure the animals without affecting the reproductive organs and to change the quality and quantity of sperm production. Such an approach has never before been studied in horses.

The challenge was to develop a dual vaccine with prophylactic as well as therapeutic activity. The DNA vaccine, called EAV-THERA-VAC, encodes the viral proteins of ORFs 2, 5, and 7 and is administered as three individual plasmids. This vaccine was the first vaccine that provided protection against EAV through both, a sustained cellular and humoral immune response in vaccinated horses.

Important Genes for the Vaccine Development
- **ORF 2** encodes two minor structural and highly conserved membrane proteins: Structural protein **E'** (encoded by ORF 2a) – a 7–8 kDa protein – is reported as indispensable for the generation of infectious virus particles and is membrane-associated. Structural protein $\mathbf{G_S}$' (encoded by ORF 2b) – a 25 kDa protein – is also needed for infection.
- **ORF 5** encodes for structural protein '$\mathbf{G_L}$,' one of two major EAV envelope proteins (30–44 kDa). ORF 5 protein is a powerful immunogen, but known for its high variability due to mutations.
- **ORF 7** encodes for the highly conserved 14 kD structural protein '**N**,' the only nucleocapsid protein. Together with the proteins encoded by ORFs 5 and 6 (namely structural proteins G_L and M), protein N is a major structural EAV protein. The nucleocapsid protects the EAV RNA genome and is shelled by an envelope consisting of a lipid bilayer and structural proteins.

Rational Vaccine Design
EAV-THERA-VAC development was the first reported rational vaccine design in veterinary medicine. Rational vaccine design means:

To fully appreciate the complex nature of all different steps of the viral infection process and to use molecular biotechnology to provide an intelligent vaccine design where all necessary components of the immune system are activated in the correct temporal sequence to thereby achieve a maximum immunoprotective effect.

To this end, one has to study the biology of the virus, its strategy of infection, its immune escape mechanisms, and the possibility to reactivate immune pathways that may have been inhibited by the virus. Tailor-made DNA vaccines can easily be designed to meet these requirements.

EAV's Molecular Immune Escape Mechanisms
We found small amounts of neutralizing antibodies against the G_L protein in chronically infected stallions. However, these antibodies were not able to clear the persistent infection. The reason for this could be the genetic instability of ORF5 under immune pressure. Indeed, ORF5 is known for its high mutation frequency. Furthermore, we observed that shortly after infection, EAV down regulates MHC I expression and thereby reduces antigen presentation to CD8+ T-cells and cellular immunity. We could also demonstrate virus induced down regulation of the TAP system. This intracellular *transporter associated with antigen presentation* directs antigenic peptides derived from proteasomal degradation into the MHC I pathway. The next puzzle was to elucidate the regulation of these EAV induced immune evasion mechanisms. Using DNA-chips we found that at least 12 interferon (IFN) related genes are up-regulated and at least two genes are down-regulated. One of these genes is Ifi 30 (also known as GILT), the IFN-gamma inducible protein 30,

suggesting that the virus interferes with IFN-gamma expression which is important for the regulation of the proteasome and MHC I expression.

In summary, we were able to identify some of the molecular mechanisms EAV employs to escape the immune system during persistent infection. Although not all details are known yet, we decided to develop a multigene DNA vaccine including ORFs 2, 5, and 7. While ORF5 is known for its mutations, ORF2 is a highly conserved envelope antigen and also able to induce neutralizing antibodies. ORF7 was demonstrated to provoke a very strong cellular immune response necessary for clearance of EAV in persistently infected stallions.

The results with this DNA vaccine are impressive. For the first time immunotolerance in chronically infected stallions could be broken:

1. All vaccinated animals developed only moderate antibody responses but strong cellular responses. The latter are necessary for viral clearance.
2. 6/10 chronically infected stallions proved to be EAV-free after completed therapy (horses with a moderate virus titer at the start of intervention). 1/10 showed a clearance of 90%. 3/10 did not respond to the vaccine (horses with a high virus titer at the beginning of therapy).
3. The viral load influences therapy outcome. Obviously, immune reactions induced by vaccination were not sufficient to overcome the virus infection in highly afflicted horses, and vaccine potency has to be further enhanced.
4. The libido as well as the quality and the quantity of the sperm production was never influenced by the DNA vaccination (Figs. 13.4 and 13.5, Claudia Dziomba, Veterinarian for Horses, University of Leipzig, Clinic for Large Animals, Prof. Dr. Dipl. ECEIM G.F. Schusser). These investigations were the first studies worldwide on the influence of DNA vaccination on sperm.

Impact for Human Medicine

- A DNA vaccine is able to break the immunotolerance in chronically infected patients and to induce a strong cellular immune response.
- A DNA vaccine can be used for prophylactic and therapeutic treatment.
- A DNA vaccine can clear all viruses from the patient, depending on the initial viral load.
- There are no detectable negative influences on the male germ line. The libido, sperm quality and quantity are comparable to the untreated control. The vaccine is biologically safe and well tolerated.
- To fully appreciate the complex nature of all different steps of the viral infection process and to use molecular biotechnology to provide an intelligent vaccine design where all necessary components of the immune system are activated in the correct temporal sequence to thereby achieve a maximum immunoprotective effect.

Salmon and the First Commercial DNA Fish Vaccine

Part of the fishing industry is aquaculture, also known as aquafarming which stands in contrast to commercial fishing, which is the harvesting of wild fish. Aquaculture

13 Approved Veterinary Vaccines: Paving the Way to Products for Human Health

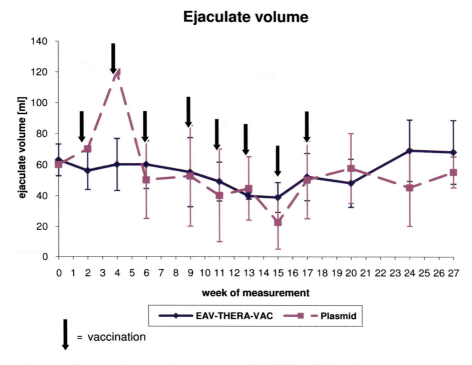

Fig. 13.4 Ejaculate volume in mL of vaccinated (EAV-THERA-VAC) and non-vaccinated (plasmid) stallions (study II/06). Data are shown as means ± SEM (Kindly provided by Claudia Dziomba, Vet. Faculty, University of Leipzig)

involves cultivating freshwater and saltwater fish and other seafood (shrimp, oyster) under controlled conditions.

Salmon is the major economic contributor to the world production of farmed fish, representing over U$1 billion annually in the USA. Salmon farming is also very big in Norway, Scotland, Canada, and Chile and is the source for most salmon consumed in America and Europe.

Like all other animals also fish is threatened by viruses, bacteria and parasites. One major problem for salmons is the Infectious Haematopoietic Necrosis (IHN) virus (Saksida 2006).

Virus

Infectious Haematopoietic Necrosis (IHN) virus is a common viral pathogen of both wild and farmed salmonids, in particular Pacific salmonids, rainbow trout, and Atlantic salmon. IHN virus is enzootic to the Pacific Northwest, however it has varying effects on different Pacific salmonids. It is a negative-sense single-stranded RNA virus that is a member of the Rhabdoviridae family, genus Novirhabdovirus. The RNA genome is 11,133 nucleotides long and contains leader (L) and trailer (T) sequences at its 3′-end and 5′-end, respectively. The coding regions are N, P, M, G,

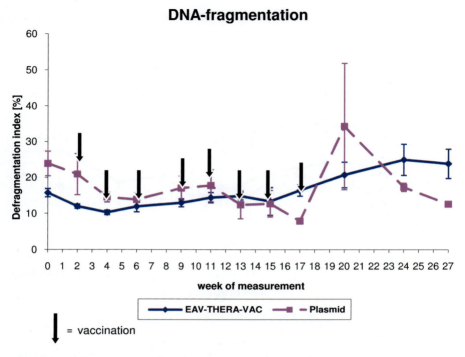

Fig. 13.5 DNA-fragmentation in sperm of vaccinated (EAV-THERA-VAC) and non-vaccinated (plasmid) stallions (study II/06). Data are shown as means of% defragmentation index ± SEM (Kindly provided by Claudia Dziomba, Vet. Faculty, University of Leipzig)

NV and L genes. G encodes the surface glycoprotein, forming the so-called spikes, the main target for the immune response.

Transmission
IHNV is transmitted following shedding of the virus in the feces, urine, sexual fluids, and external mucus and by direct contact or close contact with surrounding contaminated water. The virus gains entry into fish at the base of the fins. Salmons are carnivorous and are currently fed a meal produced from catching other wild fish and other marine organisms – a permanent origin of possible infections with IHNV.

Disease
Clinical signs of infection with IHNV include anemia, skin darkening, bulging of the eyes, fading of the gills, and abdominal distension. Infected fish commonly hemorrhage in several areas, such as the mouth, the pectoral fins, the muscles near the anus, and the yolk sac of fry. Diseased fish weaken and eventually float on the surface of the water. Necrosis is common in the kidney and spleen, and sometimes in the liver. Mortality rates in older fish (2–3 kg) tend to range from 10% to 20%, in

13 Approved Veterinary Vaccines: Paving the Way to Products for Human Health

smolts the mortality rate often exceeds 85%. The average cumulative mortality following an outbreak is estimated at 47%.

Special Characteristics
Salmon is one of the main foods producing fish in the world. A DNA vaccine for fish must not only be safe for the animal but especially safe for the fish consumer.

IHNV-DNA Vaccine
The major antigen is the viral surface glycoprotein (G) which is capable of eliciting neutralizing antibodies and the induction of a protective immune response. Significantly, the vaccine employs a fusion protein derived from two components on a single plasmid. The first part of the fusion protein is encoded by the G gene, which was cloned into a eukaryotic expression vector. The second part is derived from other fish pathogens such as ISAV, IPNV, iridovirus, NNV, SPDV, SVCV, VHSV, and koi herpesvirus (US Patent 7,501,128,B2m March 10, 2009). The rationale behind this design is that the presence of the IHNV G protein boosts the immune response against the second protein, resulting in an additional protective effect against the other pathogen. The vaccine is given intramuscularly with a dosage of only 10 µg in 50 µL on the left dorsal flank, in the area just below the dorsal fin (Traxler et al. 1999; Garver et al. 2005).

This first DNA fish vaccine was licensed in 2005 in Canada by Veterinary Biologics Section (VBS), Animal Health and Production Division, Canadian Food Inspection Agency (CFIA) and is also used in studies in Norway now (Canadian food inspection agency – VBS File # 870VV/I4.0/A8 2005).

Impact for Human Medicine
- This vaccine is a fusion of two antigens derived from two non-related viruses
- More than 6.6 million vaccine doses were used to vaccinate farmed Atlantic salmon. No adverse events in the farmed salmon were reported.
- Human safety risk factors associated with the use of this vaccine include consumption of food products derived from vaccinated fish and, in rare instances, self-injection of the vaccine by vaccinators. CFIA confirmed that the vaccine holds no safety risk for humans.
- The widespread use of the vaccine is not expected to have any significant effects on public health. Adverse effects on the environment are considered negligible. The vaccine is not shed from vaccinated fish.

Melanoma: A Life-Threatening Cancer Also for Animals

One of the most exciting fields in modern vaccinology is the development of therapeutic vaccines against cancer. This is completely different to the newly launched HPV-vaccines for cervix carcinoma. The HPV-vaccines (there are two commercial products on the market) are classical antiviral vaccines against the HPV subtypes 16 and 18. However, these HPV-vaccines can only be used prophylactically and not for the treatment of an established cervix carcinoma (Nieto et al. 2010). In contrast, novel DNA vaccine strategies for therapeutic intervention against HPV-induce cervix carcinoma are intensely studied (discussed in Chap. 2 of this book). Long before any HPV study investigated the correlation between the induction of cervix carcinoma and viral infections it was known that Epstein Barr could cause Burkitt Lymphoma (Burkitt 1958).

In many patients, solid tumours such as breast cancer, bladder cancer or malignant melanoma are only slowly developing. It seems that our immune system is able to control at least in part growth in these tumours. In 1863 Rudolf Virchow could find activated leucocytes in tumour tissues, and it was Paul Ehrlich in 1909 who postulated a 'body's own protection system' against tumour cells. 'The immune surveillance hypothesis' was born and elaborated in the 1950s and 1960s proposing that T-cell-mediated immunity evolved as a specific defense against cancer cells and that T cells constantly patrol the body, searching for abnormal body cells (Bowern et al. 1984; Ostrand-Rosenberg 2008).

Until now there are many clinical data demonstrating the impact of the immune system on the development of tumours: spontaneous remission of colon carcinoma, acute myeloid leukaemia, or remission of lung and liver metastases of non small cell lung cancer have been described. Consequently, there is clear evidence that immune suppression can promote tumour growth. For example immune dysfunctions or HIV infections have been associated with tumour development. But also modification of T-cells, such as T-cell anergy, reduced expression of molecules of signalling pathways, or reduced cytokine production can influence the development of cancer.

One of the most intensively studied cancers is melanoma, a malignancy of melanocytes, pigment-producing cells located predominantly in the skin, but also found in the eyes, ears, and internal organs. Melanoma causes the greatest number of skin cancer–related deaths worldwide. According to a WHO report about 48,000 melanoma related deaths occur worldwide per year (van Kempen et al. 2007).

Immunotherapy of Tumours

The findings that various cells of the immune system are able to fight against tumour cells led to different strategies for immunotherapies against cancer diseases. It is not in the focus of this chapter to discuss all these interesting approaches (for review see Kanduc (2009), Shindo and Yoshida (2010)).

Reseach on tumour immunology in humans was mostly done in melanoma patients and subsequently in related animal models because melanoma is a highly immunogenic cancer. Most vaccine strategies were thus investigated in melanoma models and thereafter in clinical trials (Alexandrescu et al. 2010; Neagu et al. 2010). The author himself was member of a development team in Vienna in 1994 when the first virus-vector based recombinant vaccine against melanoma started the phase I clinical trial (Stingl et al. 1996).

Canine Malignant Melanoma

Canine Malignant Melanoma (CMM) typically origins in the mouth or around the toes, and can spread within the body to the heart, lungs, intestines and other organs.

Fig. 13.6 Dog with oral melanoma. A golden retriever, named Olympus, diagnosed with malignant melanoma at the age of 9 years. This dog was involved in a melanoma vaccine study at the University of Florida/USA (Kindly provided by Jessica Tan, Florida/USA – in memoriam Olympus)

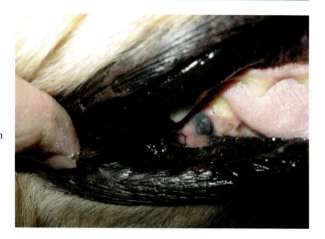

Canine malignant melanoma is known for being one of the most aggressive cancers in dogs with a high mortality rate. CMM is most commonly seen in golden retrievers (Fig. 13.6), scottish terriers, dachshunds, labradors and poodles (Bergman 2007; Shoieb et al. 2009).

Metastases of the tumours will be found very often in distant parts of the body. The overall biology of CMM is similar to the biology of human melanoma. However, depending on breed and other factors, melanomas in dogs can significantly divert in their biological characteristics. Standard treatment such as surgery, radiation, and chemotherapy are also commonly used to fight canine malignant melanoma. However, these traditional tools have only afforded minimal to modest clinical benefit depending on the stage of disease.

The Canine Melanoma DNA Vaccine

This vaccine (ONCEPT™) consists of a plasmid containing the cDNA encoding human tyrosinase (huTyr), a tumour-associated antigen (TAA). huTyr is a non-mutated differentiation antigen and specifically expressed in melanocytes. Tyrosinase is a glycoprotein and essential in melanin synthesis. Like other TAAs tyrosinase is overexpressed in tumour cells and therefore represents an ideal target for cancer therapy. Normally there is no strong immune reaction against this autologous protein. However, by using xenogeneic huTyr cDNA for immunization of dogs it was possible to break the immune tolerance against this self antigen and induce antibody and cytotoxic T-cell responses against melanoma cells (Bergman et al. 2006; Bergman and Wolchok 2008; Liao et al. 2006). Tyrosinase is highly conserved between species as different as mice, men, and dogs (Fig. 13.7).

In a recent clinical trial with 58 dogs diagnosed with stage II and III canine oral melanoma the safety and efficacy of the xenogeneic DNA vaccine was investigated (D.A. Grosenbaugh et al. 2010). Dogs received four therapeutic immunization series following surgical removal of the primary tumour and radiotherapy in cases with positive surgical margins or positive regional lymph nodes. One dose contained

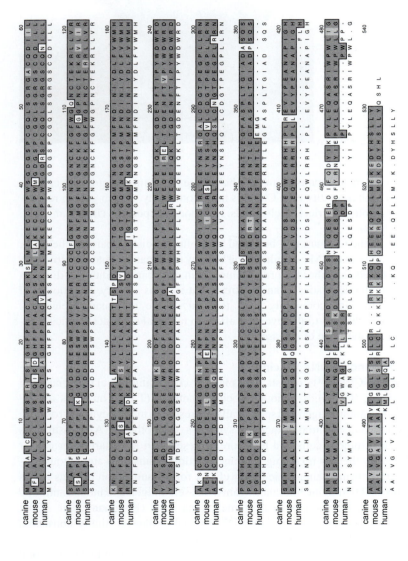

Fig. 13.7 Tyrosinase is highly conserved between species. Sequence comparison of tyrosinase from dog, mouse, and human shows a high degree of homology at the amino acid level. The calculated sequence identity between canine tyrosinase and that of mouse and human is 84.4% and 87.5%, respectively, indicating evolutionary conservation of this protein. Dark gray highlights identical residues and light gray highlights conservative amino acid changes (Kindly provided by Phil Bergman, BrightHeart Veterinary Centers, Armonk, NY, USA)

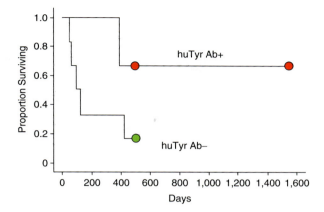

Fig. 13.8 Kaplan-Meier survival curves for canine patients with (huTyr Ab+; $n=3$) and without (huTyr Ab−; $n=6$) positive humoral responses to the xenogeneic huTyr DNA vaccination. Dots denote patients that were omitted from analysis. The difference in survival time between the two groups was not statistically significant ($P=0.148$; log-rank analysis), possibly due to the small patient group size (Kindly provided by Phil Bergman, BrightHeart Veterinary Centers, Armonk, NY, USA)

102 µg DNA given in a volume of 0.4 mL by the transdermal route via a needle-free vaccination device. Booster immunizations were given at 6-month intervals. In March 2007, the manufacturing company Merial received a conditional licence for ONCEPT™ from the USDA, and a full licence in 2010 (USDA 2010).

The results of the xenogeneic immunization of dogs with huTyr cDNA as an adjunct therapy for CMM demonstrate a significant increase of survival time compared to the control group (Fig. 13.8). None of the dogs developed systemic adverse reactions, no toxicity was seen. The overall safety of this DNA vaccine was confirmed. This vaccine development represents a tremendous milestone for gene vaccine technology.

Impact for Human Medicine
- The immune surveillance hypothesis is strengthened by successful immunotherapy in dogs.
- Xenogeneic DNA cancer vaccines can overcome the immune tolerance against self antigens.
- The transdermal application of DNA delivers the encoded antigens directly to professional antigen presenting cells of the skin.
- The overall biological safety and tolerability of this DNA vaccine as an adjunct therapy in cancer patients after surgery and radiation therapy has been confirmed.

References

Alexandrescu DT, Ichim TE, Riordan NH, Marincola FM, Di Nardo A, Kabigting FD, Dasanu CA (2010) Immunotherapy for melanoma: current status and perspectives. J Immunother 33(6):570–590

Bergman PJ (2007) Canine oral melanoma. Clin Tech Small Anim Pract 22(2):55–60

Bergman PJ, Wolchok JD (2008) Of mice and men (and dogs): development of a xenogeneic DNA vaccine for canine oral malignant melanoma. Cancer Ther 6:817–826

Bergman PJ, Camps-Palau MA, McKnight JA, Leibman NF, Craft DM, Leung C, Liao J, Riviere I, Sadelain M, Hohenhaus AE, Gregor P, Houghton AN, Perales MA, Wolchok JD (2006) Development of a xenogeneic DNA vaccine program for canine malignant melanoma at the animal medical center. Vaccine 24(21):4582–4585

Bowern N, Ramshaw IA, Badenoch-Jones P, Doherty PC (1984) Effect of an iron-chelating agent on lymphocyte proliferation. Aust J Exp Biol Med Sci 62(Pt 6 (6241825)):743–754

Brault AC (2009) Changing patterns of West Nile virus transmission: altered vector competence and host susceptibility. Vet Res 40(2):43

Bunning ML, Fox PE, Bowen RA, Komar N, Chang GJ, Speaker TJ, Stephens MR, Nemeth N, Panella NA, Langevin SA, Gordy P, Teehee M, Bright PR, Turell MJ (2007) DNA vaccination of the American crow (*Corvus brachyrhynchos*) provides partial protection against lethal challenge with West Nile virus. Avian Dis 51(2):573–577

Burkitt D (1958) A sarcoma involving the jaws in African children. Br J Surg 46(197):218–223

Canadian food inspection agency – VBS File # 870VV/I4.0/A8 (2005) Environmental assessment for licensing infectious haematopoietic necrosis virus vaccine, DNA vaccine in Canada. http://www.inspection.gc.ca/english/anima/vetbio/eaee/vbeaihnve.shtml. Accessed 25th september 2007

Davis BS, Chang GJ, Cropp B, Roehrig JT, Martin DA, Mitchell CJ, Bowen R, Bunning ML (2001) West Nile virus recombinant DNA vaccine protects mouse and horse from virus challenge and expresses in vitro a noninfectious recombinant antigen that can be used in enzyme-linked immunosorbent assays. J Virol 75(9):4040–4047

D.A. Grosenbaugh et al. 2010 Multicenter clinical trial with a xenogeneic DNA vaccine administered as an adjunct treatment for canine oral malignant melanoma following surgical excision of the primary tumor. Am J Vet Res (submitted)

Garver KA, Conway CM, Elliott DG, Kurath G (2005) Analysis of DNA-vaccinated fish reveals viral antigen in muscle, kidney and thymus, and transient histopathologic changes. Mar Biotechnol NY 7(5):540–553

Giese M (1998) DNA-antiviral vaccines: new developments and approaches – a review. Virus Genes 17(3):219–232

Giese M, Bahr U, Jakob NJ, Kehm R, Handermann M, Muller H, Vahlenkamp TH, Spiess C, Schneider TH, Schusse G, Darai G (2002) Stable and long-lasting immune response in horses after DNA vaccination against equine arteritis virus. Virus Genes 25(2):159–167

Kanduc D (2009) "Self-nonself" peptides in the design of vaccines. Curr Pharm Des 15(28): 3283–3289

Liao JC, Gregor P, Wolchok JD, Orlandi F, Craft D, Leung C, Houghton AN, Bergman PJ (2006) Vaccination with human tyrosinase DNA induces antibody responses in dogs with advanced melanoma. Cancer Immun 6:8

Lunney JK, Benfield DA, Rowland RR (2010) Porcine reproductive and respiratory syndrome virus: an update on an emerging and re-emerging viral disease of swine. Virus Res 154(1–2):1–6

Meeusen EN, Walker J, Peters A, Pastoret PP, Jungersen G (2007) Current status of veterinary vaccines. Clin Microbiol Rev 20(3):489–510; table of contents

Mortensen S, Stryhn H, Sogaard R, Boklund A, Stark KD, Christensen J, Willeberg P (2002) Risk factors for infection of sow herds with porcine reproductive and respiratory syndrome (PRRS) virus. Prev Vet Med 53(1–2):83–101

13 Approved Veterinary Vaccines: Paving the Way to Products for Human Health 283

Murray KO, Mertens E, Despres P (2010) West Nile virus and its emergence in the United States of America. Vet Res 41(6):67

NCT00106769 (2008) Vaccine to prevent West Nile virus disease. http://www.clinicaltrials.gov/ct2/show/NCT00106769

Neagu M, Constantin C, Tanase C (2010) Immune-related biomarkers for diagnosis/prognosis and therapy monitoring of cutaneous melanoma. Expert Rev Mol Diagn 10(7):897–919

Nieto K, Gissmann L, Schädlich L (2010) Human papillomavirus-specific immune therapy: failure and hope. Antivir Ther 15(7):951–957

Ostrand-Rosenberg S (2008) Immune surveillance: a balance between protumor and antitumor immunity. Curr Opin Genet Dev 18(1):11–18

Redding L, Weiner DB (2009) DNA vaccines in veterinary use. Expert Rev Vaccin 8(9):1251–1276

Roeder PL, Taylor WP (2002) Rinderpest. Vet Clin North Am Food Anim Pract 18(3):515–547, ix

Saksida SM (2006) Infectious haematopoietic necrosis epidemic (2001 to 2003) in farmed Atlantic salmon Salmo salar in British Columbia. Dis Aquat Organ 72(3):213–223

Shindo M, Yoshida Y (2010) Regulatory T cells and skin tumors. Recent Pat Inflamm Allergy Drug Discov 4(3):249–254

Shoieb AM, Donnell RL, Seaman R (2009) Oral malignant squamo-melanocytic tumor in a dog. J Vet Dent 26(4):234–237

Stingl G, Brocker EB, Mertelsmann R, Wolff K, Schreiber S, Kampgen E, Schneeberger A, Dummer W, Brennscheid U, Veelken H, Birnstiel ML, Zatloukal K, Schmidt W, Maass G, Wagner E, Baschle M, Giese M, Kempe ER, Weber HA, Voigt T (1996) Phase I study to the immunotherapy of metastatic malignant melanoma by a cancer vaccine consisting of autologous cancer cells transfected with the human IL-2 gene. Hum Gene Ther 7(8800750):551–563

Tobiasch E, Kehm R, Bahr U, Tidona CA, Jakob NJ, Handermann M, Darai G, Giese M (2001) Large envelope glycoprotein and nucleocapsid protein of equine arteritis virus (EAV) induce an immune response in Balb/c mice by DNA vaccination; strategy for developing a DNA-vaccine against EAV-infection. Virus Genes 22(2):187–199

Traxler GS, Anderson E, LaPatra SE, Richard J, Shewmaker B, Kurath G (1999) Naked DNA vaccination of Atlantic salmon Salmo salar against IHNV. Dis Aquat Organ 38(3):183–190

USDA (2010) USDA licenses DNA vaccine for treatment of melanoma in dogs. J Am Vet Med Assoc 236(5):495

USDA-APHIS-VS-CVB (2008) Veterinary biological products licensees and permittees. http://www.aphis.usda.gov/animal_health/vet_biologics/publications/CurrentProdCodeBook.pdf Accessed 25th september 2007

van Kempen LC, van Muijen GN, Ruiter DJ (2007) Melanoma progression in a changing environment. Eur J Cell Biol 86(2):65–67

Current Status of Regulations for DNA Vaccines

14

Bettina Klug, Jens Reinhardt, and James Robertson

DNA vaccines combine the biotechnological manufacturing aspects of a subset of gene therapeutic medicinal products with the mode of action of a classical vaccine. Due to this hybrid state, the regulation of DNA vaccines requires the expertise from both gene therapy and vaccine experts. This chapter will provide an overview of the regulatory status and requirements for DNA vaccines intended for human use. We first introduce the regulatory process in Europe and in the USA and then highlight the most relevant aspects of the already existing guidance documents for DNA vaccines.

Introduction

For almost two decades scientists have pursued the development of DNA vaccines, targeting a variety of infectious diseases. DNA vaccines are defined as purified bacterial plasmid preparations containing one or more DNA sequences that express a protein antigen capable of inducing an immune response. Expression plasmids consist in general of an antigen expression cassette and structural elements required for plasmid propagation in bacterial cells. The expression cassette typically contains the gene of interest flanked by a eukaryotic promoter/enhancer and a transcription termination/polyadenylation sequence to promote gene expression in vaccine recipients.

To date four DNA medicinal products based upon plasmid DNA have been authorised for veterinary use. Three vaccines, one against West Nile virus in horses, one against infectious haematopoetic necrosis virus in farmed salmon, one for treatment of melanoma in dogs and a growth hormone releasing hormone (GHRH)

B. Klug (✉)
Paul-Ehrlich Institut, Langen, Germany
e-mail: klube@pei.de

J. Thalhamer et al. (eds.), *Gene Vaccines*,
DOI 10.1007/978-3-7091-0439-2_14, © Springer-Verlag/Wien, 2012

product for foetal loss in swine (Kutzler and Weiner 2008). Detailed information on these veterinary DNA-based vaccines is given in Chap. 13 in this book.

To date, no human DNA vaccine has been authorised; however, many are under clinical investigation worldwide, including plasmids expressing malarial, HIV, influenza, tuberculosis (TB) and Ebola virus antigens.

Scientists in academia whose research is the backbone of the development of a new vaccine or approach to vaccination may not always be fully aware of the regulatory process by which a successful candidate vaccine becomes an authorised medicinal product. It is useful for research scientists to be aware of these processes as the development of a novel vaccine starts in the research laboratory and an exhaustive amount of data to support a marketing authorisation application is gained from these early studies. This chapter will provide an overview of the regulatory status and requirements for DNA vaccines intended for human use.

The Regulatory Status of DNA Vaccines

DNA vaccines combine the biotechnological manufacturing aspects of a subset of gene therapeutic medicinal products with the mode of action of a classical vaccine. Due to this hybrid state, the regulation of DNA vaccines requires the expertise from both gene therapy and vaccine experts. The regulatory authorities in Europe and in the USA have established slightly different regulatory pathways for plasmid DNA vaccines for prophylaxis against infectious diseases versus for therapeutic use.

In the European Union, a therapeutic DNA (vaccine) is considered as a Gene Therapy Medicinal Product (GTMP), whereas vaccines against infectious diseases are explicitly excluded from GTMP definition (2001/83/EC). The centralised procedure for the marketing authorisation application is mandatory for DNA vaccines, whether they are used for therapeutic purposes or against infectious disease (726/2004/EC).

In the USA, the distinction between the alternative usage of plasmid DNA as a medicinal product is similarly recognised and impacts on their regulation. DNA vaccines against infectious diseases are regulated by the Center for Biologics Evaluation and Research's (CBER) Office of Vaccines Research and Review (OVRR) whilst DNA vaccines that are intended for non-infectious therapeutic indications fall under the responsibility of CBER's Office of Cellular, Tissue and Gene Therapies (OCTGT).

The Regulatory Process

Although the development of a novel medicinal product, from the first data derived in a research laboratory to a marketing authorisation, is likely to take a considerable number of years it is a well-defined process consisting of the following steps:
- Laboratory demonstration of the proof of concept
- Design and establishment of the manufacturing process
- Demonstration of adequate quality and non-clinical safety

14 Current Status of Regulations for DNA Vaccines

- Clinical trial approval
- Demonstration of clinical safety and efficacy
- Marketing authorisation application

The conduct of a clinical trial of a novel medicinal product typically has to be authorised by the national competent authority (NCA) (2001/20/EC). A pre-requisite of a clinical trial authorisation is a demonstration of the potential safety of the investigational compound supported by quality and non-clinical data as well as a proof-of-concept of the vaccine. Thus the submission of a clinical trial application is accompanied by extensive quality and non-clinical data as well as the study protocol of the proposed clinical trial.

Clinical development typically starts with a small Phase I study(ies) assessing the short term safety, local tolerance and immunogenicity in a limited number of volunteers. Based on the data generated in this study(ies), data on the dosage of the vaccine and the vaccination schedule are then generated in Phase II studies involving a larger number of subjects. The data on immunogenicity and safety obtained in Phase II determine whether or not to proceed to Phase III trial(s) during which the protective efficacy of the vaccine will be assessed in addition to increasing the size of the safety database. These Phase III trials typically involve a large number of subjects, involving up to several thousands of volunteers, depending on the prevalence of the condition under consideration.

Submitting a marketing authorisation application (MAA) fulfilling the dossier requirements as laid down in the Common Technical Document (CTD) to the competent authorities, e.g. EMA for centralised marketing applications in the European Union or FDA for applications in the United States, initiates the review process which may eventually result in a marketing authorisation. The CTD provides for a harmonised structure and format for new product applications in three regions, namely Europe, Japan and the United States (CTD05-2008).

Once a marketing authorisation is granted, safety and effectiveness data continue to be gathered in an increasing number of vaccine recipients (Phase IV studies). These data are usually required by the regulatory authorities and establish the true level of safety and the long term efficacy of a vaccine.

The first interaction between the manufacturer and the regulatory authority will be at minimum at the submission of an application for a clinical trial. However, it is very useful to seek informal and/or formal regulatory input in the earlier stages of product development.

Europe

Within the European Union the conduct of a clinical trial has to be authorised by the competent authority of the individual member states. However, if a clinical trial is going to be conducted in three or more member states a voluntary harmonisation procedure (VHP) by the NCAs is available.

In the case of a VHP, a single application will be evaluated in a single procedure jointly by the competent authorities of those member states where the clinical trial is planned to be carried out. Scientific questions on the protocol and the investigational medicinal product will thus be clarified together in one procedure. Subsequently, the clinical trial authorisation will be granted by each competent authority within a reduced time frame as compared to individual applications.

As for all medicinal products derived from a biotechnology process, DNA vaccines are subject to a centralised marketing authorisation procedure. Such a single MAA is submitted to the European Medicines Agency (EMA) for assessment.

In addition to medicinal products derived from biotechnology processes the centralised procedure is also mandatory for:

- Advanced-therapy medicinal products, such as gene-therapy, somatic cell-therapy or tissue-engineered medicines;
- Medicinal products intended for the treatment of HIV/Aids, cancer, diabetes, neurodegenerative disorders or autoimmune diseases and other immune dysfunctions;
- Orphan medicinal products.

For medicines that do not fall within these categories (the 'mandatory scope'), companies have the option of submitting an application for a centralised MAA to the Agency, as long as the medicine concerned is a significant therapeutic, scientific or technical innovation, or if its authorisation would be in the interest of public health.

The centralised MAA procedure, if successful, results in a single marketing authorisation which is valid in all member states of the European Community as well as in the EEA/EFTA states Iceland, Liechtenstein and Norway.

Following a strict timetable and a well defined review procedure, the appropriate Agency committee, the Committee for Medicinal Products for Human Use (CHMP) or the Committee for Medicinal Products for Veterinary Use (CVMP) must assess the quality, non-clinical and clinical data within 210 days; this process is interspersed with 'clock stops,' periods which provide applicants time to consider their responses to questions posed by the relevant Committee. At the end of the evaluation process, the Committee prepares a final assessment report on the quality, safety and efficacy of the medicinal product and provides an 'opinion' on granting the Marketing Authorisation. This opinion is transmitted to the European Commission which is the ultimate authority for granting marketing authorisations in the EU. Once a Marketing Authorisation has been granted, a centralised Marketing Authorisation is valid in all the EU/EEA States for 5 years on a renewable basis.

Whenever a Community marketing authorisation has been granted, the marketing-authorisation holder can begin to make the medicine available to patients and healthcare professionals in all EU countries.

FDA

The FDA's Center for Biologics Evaluation and Research (CBER) is responsible for regulating vaccines in the USA.

14 Current Status of Regulations for DNA Vaccines 289

Vaccine clinical development within the USA follows the same general pathway as for drugs and other biologics. A sponsor who wishes to begin clinical trials with a vaccine must submit an application for the conduct of a clinical trial (Investigational New Drug application (IND)) to FDA. The IND describes the vaccine, its method of manufacture, and quality control tests for release. Also included is information about the vaccine's safety and ability to elicit a protective immune response (immunogenicity) in non-clinical studies, as well as the proposed clinical protocol for studies in humans.

Following completion of a successful clinical development program, a submission of a Biologics License Application (BLA) can be made to the FDA. To be considered, the license application must provide the multidisciplinary FDA reviewer team (medical officers, microbiologists, chemists, biostatisticians, etc.) with the efficacy and safety information necessary to make a risk/benefit assessment and to recommend or oppose the approval of a vaccine.

Following the review of a license application for a new indication, the sponsor and the FDA may present their findings to the Vaccines and Related Biological Products Advisory Committee (VRBPAC). This non-FDA expert committee (consisting of scientists, physicians, biostatisticians and a consumer representative) provides advice to the Agency regarding the safety and efficacy of the vaccine for the proposed indication.

Guidelines

So far specific guidelines for DNA vaccines to support product development are available from the World Health Organisation (WHO) and the US Food and Drug Administration (FDA) (WHO Technical Report Series No. 941/20; FDA Vaccine Guidance Documents 2007).

In Europe, guidance for DNA vaccine development is provided in the CPMP note for guidance on the quality, preclinical and clinical aspects of gene transfer medicinal products (CPMP/BWP/3088/99), which came into effect in 2001. Whilst little has changed regarding quality aspects of plasmid DNA, considerable experience has accrued regarding their safety at both the non-clinical and clinical levels. Therefore the CHMP announced recently that a specific guideline on the development of DNA vaccines will be published in the near future (EMEA/CHMP/308136/2007).

In the following part, the most relevant aspects of the already existing guidance documents are summarised.

Quality Issues

General Requirements
As for all biological/biotechnology derived medicinal products, the general manufacturing requirements have to be taken into account. These include critical step analysis and implementation of adequate in-process controls as well as application of appropriated tests to characterise intermediate and final products.

In-process control is an invaluable tool used for decades to ascertain the quality and the consistency of biological/biotechnology derived products. It involves documenting the laboratory development of the product, ensuring the quality of the starting material, full description of the manufacturing process, and implementation of appropriate tests at various stages of the manufacturing process.

Many of the general test requirements for biological/biotechnology derived medicinal products, such as tests for potency, endotoxin, stability and sterility, also apply to DNA vaccines.

A further important tool to assure appropriate quality of a medicinal product is a manufacturing procedure in compliance with Good Manufacturing Practice (GMP) which involves a manufacturing process which has highly defined, carefully controlled and reproducible conditions.

Specific Requirements

A detailed description of the development of the DNA plasmid is an essential part of the quality documentation. Information on the origin of the gene(s) encoding the protein (or peptide) against which an immune response is sought should be detailed and include the identity of the microorganism or organism from which the gene was derived and the origin of the microorganism that will be used for expansion of the plasmid, including its species, subtype and passage history.

A description of the molecular cloning steps involved in constructing the DNA vaccine, sequence data of the gene and a restriction map, the source of distinct regions within the plasmid and the choice of selection marker should all be provided. The selection marker should be carefully chosen; the use of certain selection markers such as resistance to antibiotics, which might have an impact on public health, should be avoided.

The identity of the plasmid after transformation of the bacteria used for production and the phenotype of the transformed bacteria should be confirmed and data on the stability of the plasmid within the bacterial cell during fermentation generated. Production should be based upon a seed bank system which typically would involve the establishment of a highly characterised bank of the bacterial cells containing the plasmid vaccine.

The data generated are to be supported by the rational for the use of the gene(s), the rational for the choice of the host bacterial cells used for production of the plasmid and a rational for the selection marker. A discussion on the potential for chromosomal integration should be provided taking into account the route and method of administration.

Non-Clinical Issues

General Considerations on the Non-Clinical Safety Program

The scope of the non-clinical testing of a vaccine is to investigate the immunological properties of the vaccine and to determine whether the candidate vaccine has the potential to elicit safety signals in an appropriate animal model prior to its inoculation into humans. In many cases a disease model exists and protective efficacy can

14 Current Status of Regulations for DNA Vaccines 291

(and should) be demonstrated in such an animal model; this is the proof-of-concept. Relevant animal models should be used where possible, i.e. species/models whose immunogenic/biological response to the delivery system and expressed gene product would be expected to be similar to the response in humans.

In principle the non-clinical development program has to be in line with the general requirements for vaccines (CPMP/SWP/465/95). Further guidance can be found in the product specific guidelines.

Specific Requirements for DNA Vaccines

With the advent of DNA vaccines more than two decades ago, several potential safety issues associated with administering plasmid DNA into humans have been discussed, for example, integration of the plasmid DNA into the host's chromosomes, immunopathological reactions and risks related to expression of cytokines or co-stimulatory factors (Robertson and Griffiths 2006). These concerns, albeit hypothetical, require consideration in the development of the non-clinical safety program.

Biodistribution/Persistence

Biodistribution and persistence studies will be expected, unless substantial experience is already gained with an almost identical or similar product. Biodistribution and persistence should be investigated using e.g. sensitive nucleic acid detection techniques, and the justification for the chosen assays should be stated. Sensitivity, specificity, and the potential for tissue- or preparation-specific inhibitors should be established during the assay validation.

Publications resulting from the use of DNA vaccines in biodistribution studies indicate that intramuscular, subcutaneous, intradermal, or particle mediated delivery does not result in long-term persistence of plasmid at ectopic sites. At the site of injection, in some cases ≤30 copies of plasmid per 100,000 host cells persist after 60 days (Bureau et al. 2004; Kim et al. 2003; Pilling et al. 2002), while other studies have shown that plasmids can persist at the injection site at levels greater than 500 copies per 100,000 cells 6 months post-administration (Ledwith et al. 2000a). If ≤30 copies of plasmid DNA per 100,000 host cells persist after 60 days, then further integration assessment may not be necessary. As more experience is gained, this issue needs to be addressed further.

Integration

Several investigators have assessed the ability of their plasmid to integrate into the vaccine recipient's chromosomes in vivo using assays based on the association of plasmid DNA with genomic DNA after gel purification (Ledwith et al. 2000a; Ledwith et al. 2000b). In most cases negative results have been obtained at a level of detection of one potential plasmid integration event per microgram of host-cell DNA. However, alternative formulations or administration devices such as co-inoculation of a plasmid encoding a growth promoting factor, or electrostimulation, can lead to an enhanced potential for integration of plasmid DNA.

Thus, investigation of the potential integration of the plasmid DNA in vivo into the host's genome is an aspect of the non-clinical safety testing of a DNA vaccine.

Depending on the potential for integration and the proposed clinical indication, there may be a need for further studies to investigate integration directly, or eventually the potential for tumour formation or disruption of normal gene expression.

Tolerance Induction

Knowledge of the duration of expression of an antigen from injected DNA is limited although some reports suggest that expression could continue for many months. However, so far, tolerance has not been observed in non-clinical studies in adult animals. But tolerance can be induced in neonatal mice, which might be linked to the immature system at birth. Development of tolerance might be a concern for a specific product used in a specific age group such as neonates and very young children.

Autoimmunity

Non-clinical studies have revealed evidence that DNA vaccination can activate auto-reactive B cells to secrete IgG anti-DNA auto-antibodies. However, the magnitude and duration of this response appears to be insufficient to cause disease in healthy animals or accelerate disease in autoimmune-prone mice. These non-clinical studies suggest that systemic autoimmunity is unlikely to result from DNA vaccination although it cannot be excluded that DNA vaccines might idiosyncratically cause or worsen organ-specific autoimmunity by encoding antigens (including cryptic antigens) that cross-react with self.

Although, under existing knowledge, neither FDA nor WHO requires non-clinical studies to specifically assess the development of auto-antibodies, it is recommended that animals in non-clinical immunogenicity and toxicity studies continue to be carefully monitored.

In cases where an immune response is induced by a gene product encoding a self-antigen such as a cytokine, chemokine, surface receptor/ligand, or cryptic self-antigen, the potential cross-reactivity with the corresponding endogenous protein should be determined. If these studies reveal a persistent immune response against an endogenous protein, further non-clinical studies to evaluate potential adverse effects in a relevant animal model may be required.

Genotoxicity

As for most vaccines the standard battery of genotoxicity and conventional carcinogenicity studies are not applicable to DNA vaccines. However, genotoxicity studies may be required to address a concern about a specific impurity or novel chemical component, e.g. a complexing material that has not been tested previously.

Developmental and Reproductive Toxicity

Integration of a plasmid DNA into reproductive tissue could result in germline alteration. Reassurance regarding lack of germline alterations may be gained from investigating the presence and persistence of the plasmid DNA in gonadal tissue from both male and female animals, using for example, PCR technology. Persistence of plasmids in gonadal tissue over time would require further investigation, for example,

14 Current Status of Regulations for DNA Vaccines 293

of ova and sperm cells, and considerations regarding any effect on fertility and general reproductive function.

In addition, embryo-fetal and perinatal toxicity studies may be required if women of childbearing potential are to be exposed to the product, depending on the intended clinical use and target population.

Further Considerations

While candidate DNA vaccines have demonstrated immune responses in various animal models, and even in many cases protection from disease, these results have generally not been reproduced in humans. Thus, various approaches to enhance the human immune response by enhancing uptake, stabilising expression, modulating the immune response, or by use of an adjuvant are being pursued. Special safety concerns might be related to the above and to the following approaches and these should also be addressed in the non-clinical development program.

- Complexing the DNA with polymers
- Encapsulating the DNA on or within microparticles
- Optimization of the codon usage of the gene encoding the antigen of interest
- Encoding a variety of T cell epitopes either instead of or in addition to a full size protein antigen
- Optimizing administration, e.g. by particle-mediated delivery (gene gun) or electroporation
- Route of administration, e.g. mucosal vs. parenteral
- Boosting with viral vectors or protein antigen following an initial priming with plasmid DNA
- Co-administration of DNA encoding an immune stimulatory molecule

Clinical Issues

The EU Guideline on clinical evaluation of vaccines (EMEA/CHMP/VWP/164653/2005) provides a comprehensive overview of the clinical development of prophylactic vaccines for infectious disease and the clinical data that should accompany a MAA submitted to the EMA.

Pharmacokinetic studies are usually not required for vaccines. However, such studies might be applicable when new delivery systems are employed or when the vaccine contains novel adjuvants or excipients. Regulatory guidance is provided within the EU on the use of adjuvants (CHMP/VEG/134716/04; CHMP/VWP/244894/2006).

In the development of any new vaccine, adequate data on immunogenicity should be assembled during the clinical development programme. Some of the areas that should usually be covered include characterisation of the immune response, investigation of an appropriate dose and primary schedule, assessment of the persistence of detectable immunity and consideration of the need for and response to booster doses.

However, a demonstration of protective efficacy may not be necessary and/or may not be feasible for all vaccines as some will be influenced by the prevalence and characteristics of the infectious diseases that are to be prevented. Special attention should be paid to issues surrounding case definition and detection. Special consideration is needed for the clinical development of vaccines when protective efficacy studies are not feasible and when there is no established immunological correlate of protection.

Vaccine effectiveness reflects direct (vaccine induced) and indirect (population related) protection during routine use. Thus, the assessment of vaccine effectiveness can provide useful information in addition to any pre-authorisation estimates of protective efficacy. Even if it was not feasible to estimate the protective efficacy of a vaccine pre-authorisation it may be possible and highly desirable to assess vaccine effectiveness during the post-authorisation period.

References

2001/83/EC: Directive 2001/83/EC of the European Parliament and the Council of 13 November 2007 on the Community code relating to medicinal products for human use. Official Journal L 311, 28 November 2001, p 67 consolidated version 05/10/2009

2001/20/EC: Directive 2001/20/EC - on the approximation of the laws, regulations and administrative provisions of the Member States relating to the implementation of good clinical practice in the conduct of clinical trials on medicinal products for human use. Official Journal L 121, 1 May 2001, p 34

726/2004/EC: Regulation 726/2004/EC- authorisation and supervision of medicinal products for human and veterinary use and establishing a European Medicines Agency. Official Journal L 136, 30 April 2004, p 1

Bureau MF, Naimi S, Torero Ibad R, Seguin J, Georger C, Arnould E, Maton L, Blanche F, Delaere P, Scherman D (2004) Intramuscular plasmid DNA electrotransfer: biodistribution and degradation. Biochim Biophys Acta 1676(2):138–148

CHMP/VEG/134716/04 Adjuvants in vaccines for human use. http://www.ema.europa.eu/docs/en_GB/document_library/Scientific_guideline/2009/09/WC500003809.pdf. Accessed 7 july 2011

CHMP/VWP/244894/2006 Explanatory note on immunomodulators for the guideline on adjuvants in vaccines for human use. http://www.ema.europa.eu/docs/en_GB/document_library/Scientific_guideline/2009/09/WC500003810.pdf. Accessed 7 july 2011

CPMP/BWP/3088/99 Note for guidance on the qulity, preclinical and clinical aspects of gene transfer medicinal products. http://www.ema.europa.eu/docs/en_GB/document_library/Scientific_guideline/2009/10/WC500003987.pdf. Accessed 7 july 2011

CPMP/SWP/465/95 Note for guidance on preclinical pharmacological and toxicological testing of vaccines. http://www.ema.europa.eu/docs/en_GB/document_library/Scientific_guideline/2009/10/WC500004004.pdf. Accessed 7 july 2011

CTD05-2008 Notice to applicants medicinal products for human use – presentation and format of the dossier – Common Technical Document (CTD), vol. 2B. http://ec.europa.eu/health/files/eudralex/vol-2/b/update_200805/ctd_05-2008_en.pdf. Accessed 7 july 2011

EMEA/CHMP/308136/2007 Concept paper on guidance for DNA vaccines. http://www.ema.europa.eu/docs/en_GB/document_library/Scientific_guideline/2009/09/WC500003855.pdf. Accessed 7 july 2011

EMEA/CHMP/VWP/164653/2005 Guideline on clinical evaluation of new vaccines. http://www.ema.europa.eu/docs/en_GB/document_library/Scientific_guideline/2009/09/WC500003870.pdf. Accessed 7 july 2011

Kim B-M, Lee D-S, Choi J-H, Kim C-Y, Son M, Suh Y-S, Baek K-H, Park K-S, Sung Y-C, Kim W-B (2003) In vivo kinetics and biodistribution of a HIV-1 DNA vaccine after administration in mice. Arch Pharm Res 26(12877561):493–498

Kutzler MA, Weiner DB (2008) DNA vaccines: ready for prime time? Nat Rev Genet 9(18781156): 776–788

14 Current Status of Regulations for DNA Vaccines

Ledwith BJ, Manam S, Troilo PJ, Barnum AB, Pauley CJ, Griffiths TG 2nd, Harper LB, Beare CM, Bagdon WJ, Nichols WW (2000a) Plasmid DNA vaccines: investigation of integration into host cellular DNA following intramuscular injection in mice. Intervirology 43(4–6):258–272

Ledwith BJ, Manam S, Troilo PJ, Barnum AB, Pauley CJ, Griffiths TG 2nd, Harper LB, Schock HB, Zhang H, Faris JE, Way PA, Beare CM, Bagdon WJ, Nichols WW (2000b) Plasmid DNA vaccines: assay for integration into host genomic DNA. Dev Biol Basel 104:33–43

Pilling AM, Harman RM, Jones SA, McCormack NA, Lavender D, Haworth R (2002) The assessment of local tolerance, acute toxicity, and DNA biodistribution following particle-mediated delivery of a DNA vaccine to minipigs. Toxicol Pathol 30(3):298–305

Robertson JS, Griffiths E (2006) Assuring the quality, safety, and efficacy of DNA vaccines. Meth Mol Med 127:363–374

FDA Vaccine Guidance Documents (2007) Guidance for industry: considerations for plasmid DNA vaccines for infectious disease indications. http://www.fda.gov/BiologicsBloodVaccines/GuidanceComplianceRegulatoryInformation/Guidances/Vaccines/default.htm. Accessed 7 july 2011

WHO Technical Report Series No. 941/20 Guidelines for assuring the quality and nonclinical safety evaluation of DNA vaccines. http://www.who.int/biologicals/publications/trs/areas/vaccines/dna/Annex%201_DNA%20vaccines.pdf. Accessed 7 july 2011

Minicircle-DNA

15

Peter Mayrhofer and Michaela Iro

The use of plasmid DNA in clinical applications is anticipated to increase significantly in the years to come as DNA vaccines and non-viral gene therapies have entered phase three clinical trials and are already approved for use. Therefore, employing appropriate plasmids that are specifically suited for the production of DNA pharmaceuticals becomes an aspect of major importance. Especially safety issues have to be carefully reconsidered and adequately addressed. The presence of bacterial backbone sequences in conventional plasmids is one of the major drawbacks in this regard. These sequences reduce the overall efficiency of the DNA agent and, most important, they represent a biological safety risk in clinical applications. Typically, bacterial backbone sequences consist of an antibiotic selection marker, an origin of replication and unmethylated bacterial CpG motifs. This report gives a short introduction in problems and drawbacks associated with these elements and focuses on the production of plasmid derived DNA agents devoid of bacterial backbone sequences by site-specific recombination and subsequent purification by DNA interaction affinity chromatography (minicircle-DNA).

Introduction

Plasmid DNA (pDNA) expression vectors are fundamental to all forms of non-viral gene transfer. The major objective in this field is the development of safe and efficient vectors for the transfer of genetic information in eukaryotic cells. Although plasmid based systems are generally considered as safe when compared to the pathological

---

P. Mayrhofer (✉)
RBPS-Technologies e.U, Vienna, Austria

Department of Pathobiology, Institute of Bacteriology, Mycology and Hygiene,
University of Veterinary Medicine Vienna, Vienna, Austria
e-mail: Peter.Mayrhofer@rbps-technology.com

J. Thalhamer et al. (eds.), *Gene Vaccines*,
DOI 10.1007/978-3-7091-0439-2_15, © Springer-Verlag/Wien, 2012

risks associated with their viral counterparts, there is still need to improve the safety profile of conventional plasmid DNA. The safety, as well as the efficiency profile of conventional plasmid DNA can be improved by the removal of bacterial backbone DNA. Basically, plasmid DNA can be divided into two functional units namely the transcription unit and the bacterial backbone. For use in non-viral gene transfer the transcription unit usually carries the target gene or sequence along with necessary eukaryotic regulatory elements like a promoter sequence and a polyadenylation signal (Jechlinger 2006). The bacterial backbone includes elements which are required for plasmid selection and amplification in bacterial cells, that is, an antibiotic resistance gene and an origin of replication. Unmethylated CpG motifs and potential cryptic expression signals are further backbone elements of concern (Jechlinger 2006). Some of these elements are necessary for plasmid DNA production in bacteria but backbone sequences are completely dispensable and constitute a major safety concern when used for gene transfer purposes in clinical applications.

Pang et al. demonstrated that intra-muscular injection of plasmid-DNA without an eukaryotic promoter element leads to expression of bacterial sequences (Pang 1994). This result correlates well with the observation made in our group that the mRNA of the aminoglycoside 3′-phosphotransferase gene (KanR) can be detected by reverse transcriptase PCR after transfection of HeLa cells with a plasmid containing a eukaryotic GFP expression cassette and KanR (unpublished data). Additionally, Valera et al. showed that the expression of aminoglycoside 3′-phosphotransferase gene conferring resistance to antibiotics causes changes in metabolism and gene expression in eukaryotic cells (Valera et al. 1994).

Furthermore, bacterial backbone sequences have been shown to be responsible for transgene silencing (Chen et al. 2004). Chen and coworkers demonstrated that the covalent linkage of bacterial backbone DNA to a eukaryotic expression cassette leads to silencing of the transfected gene in vivo, whereas backbone sequences when co-applied without a covalent connection to the expression cassettes had a very minor effect on transgene expression (Chen et al. 2003, 2004). Riu et al. and Suzuki et al. proposed that this is due to the conversion of plasmid DNA into densely packed heterochromatic structures (Riu et al. 2007; Suzuki et al. 2006). The findings of Suzuki et al. suggest that the bacterial sequences are rapidly recognized by unknown host defense mechanisms and transcriptionally silenced by chromatin modification. Starting at bacterial backbone sequences heterochromatin formation is hypothesized to spread into the surrounding eukaryotic sequence elements leading to the down regulation of the eukaryotic promoter (Suzuki et al. 2006).

Unmethylated CpG motifs of bacterial DNA are known to activate the innate immune system by binding to the Toll-Like-Receptor 9 (TLR9) of antigen presenting cells (Klinman 2004; Krieg et al. 1995). The binding of CpG motifs to TLR9 leads to the maturation, differentiation and proliferation of natural killer cells (NK), macrophages and T-cells, which then secrete cytokines and thereby direct the immune system into a TH1 dominated response (Klinman 2004; Krieg et al. 1995). This adjuvant effect is certainly desirable for vaccination purposes, where the induction of an immune response is necessary for the protective effect. However, as the

TLR9 differs markedly between species (Hemmi et al. 2000; Rankin et al. 2001) the optimal immunogenic CpG motif is species specific too. Different CpG motifs and flanking sequences have been shown to activate different types of immune cells and cytokines when co-applied as oligonucleotides (Klinman 2004). Therefore, the use of specific CpG motifs stimulating the desired immune response has to be carefully considered. Consequently, rational DNA vaccine design is only possible if backbone sequences carrying an undefined set of CpG motifs are removed. In gene therapy applications, where an immune stimulation is not required, the effect of CpG motifs is clearly counterproductive.

On an average bacterial backbone sequences make up about 50% of conventional plasmid DNA. So the removal of backbone sequences results in significantly smaller molecules that are proposed to have better bioavailability characteristics than larger ones. A plasmid encoded gene has to cross several barriers before it can be expressed. For instance, it has to diffuse into the tissue, enter through the cell membrane, escape the endo/lysosome in case of internalization via endocytosis, diffuse into the cytoplasm and finally cross the nuclear membrane. As discussed in different reports, all these processes might be influenced by the size of the plasmid DNA (Darquet et al. 1999; Kreiss et al. 1999; Yin et al. 2005).

Summing up, the bacterial backbone of conventional plasmid DNA (1) consists of sequences associated with biosafety concerns (2) leads to inefficient and short-lived expression of the transgene in eukaryotic cells (3) contains motifs eliciting an inflammatory response in the host and (4) constitutes a significant portion of the plasmid DNA without a therapeutic effect ('junk' DNA) leading to a decreased bioavailability due to the increased size of the plasmid DNA. It is obvious that the removal of bacterial backbone DNA can significantly improve the safety and efficiency of plasmid DNA used for gene therapy and vaccination.

The minicircle-DNA technology was designed to remove these unwanted backbone sequences by a site-specific recombination process in *E. coli*. The so called parental plasmid used for minicircle production carries the eukaryotic expression cassette flanked by two recognition sequences of a site-specific recombinase. Expression of the respective recombinase in vivo results in the excision of the interjacent DNA sequences dividing the parental plasmid (PP) into two supercoiled molecules: (1) a replicative miniplasmid (MP) carrying the undesired backbone sequences and (2) a minicircle (MC) carrying the therapeutic expression unit. The main challenge in minicircle production is to achieve a high degree of recombination to efficiently remove the backbone sequences of the parental plasmid. The second problem that has to be addressed is the purification of the minicircle-DNA. Minicircle-DNA and miniplasmids are equally sized pDNA molecules with almost identical physicochemical properties like charge or hydrophobicity. Therefore, these molecules cannot be separated by conventional chromatographic techniques like anion exchange, hydrophobic interaction or size exclusion. Alternative methods like affinity based chromatography techniques or in vivo restriction digestion have been developed to overcome this problem.

This chapter focuses on the production of minicircle-DNA by site-specific recombination and affinity chromatography. Various technical approaches to achieve high recombination efficiencies as well as techniques for minicircle purification will be discussed.

Minicircle-DNA Production

The first step in minicircle production is the rearrangement of plasmid DNA by site-specific recombination. DNA rearrangements in bacteria may either occur by general recombination between homologous DNA sequences or by a variety of specialized events, such as site-specific recombination that is focused at specific sites in the genome. During site-specific recombination, four DNA strands are broken, exchanged and resealed at specific positions of two separate recombination sites. The outcome of a recombination event depends on the relative disposition of the two sites (Jayaram 1994; Landy 1993; Nash 1996; Stark et al. 1992). Intramolecular recombination between inverted or directly repeated sites will respectively invert or excise the intervening DNA segment. Recombination between sites on separate DNA molecules will integrate one molecule into the other (Hallet and Sherratt 1997). Important features of site-specific recombination are that (1) the recombination reaction may occur in the absence of replication, (2) energy co-factors (such as ATP) are not required, (3) and strand exchange is completed without any DNA synthesis or degradation (Hallet and Sherratt 1997; Nash 1996). The conservative nature of site-specific recombination refers to the inherent nature of strand exchange that occurs without any DNA synthesis or degradation, and thus, allows the reaction to be reversible (Hallet and Sherratt 1997).

The recombinases used so far for minicircle-DNA production were either derived from the λ integrase family (tyrosine recombinases) or the resolvase/invertase family (serine recombinases). The integrase of bacteriophage lambda, the Cre recombinase from bacteriophage P1 and the FLP recombinase of the yeast 2 μm plasmid which are members of the λ integrase family as well as the integrase of *Streptomyces* bacteriophage Phi31 or the ParA resolvase from the multimer resolution system of the broad host range plasmid RK2 or RP4 belonging to the resolvase/invertase family have been explored for this purpose (Bigger et al. 2001; Chen et al. 2003; Darquet et al. 1997; Jechlinger et al. 2004; Mayrhofer et al. 2008; Nehlsen et al. 2006). There are differences in the recombination events mediated by the various recombinases which are relevant for the production process of minicircle-DNA in *Escherichia coli*. Some of the recombinases possess a remarkable ability to sense the relative orientation of two recombination sites on the same molecule (Sadowski 1986). Resolvases, for example, carry out excisions between two directly orientated resolution sites but are unable to perform inversions if the sites are inverted (Krasnow and Cozzarelli 1983; Reed 1981). On the other hand, the P1 Cre protein and the yeast FLP protein carry out either excision or inversion provided that the sites are in the direct or inverse orientation, respectively (Abremski et al. 1983; Babineau et al. 1985; Gronostajski and Sadowski 1985; Vetter et al. 1983). Furthermore, recombinases vary in their capacity to promote intermolecular recombination. The resolvases and invertases perform only intramolecular recombination (Johnson and Simon

1985; Kahmann et al. 1985; Mertens et al. 1984; Reed 1981), whereas the λ Int system, the Cre protein and the FLP protein are able to carry out intermolecular recombination as well as intramolecular recombination (Abremski et al. 1983; Gronostajski and Sadowski 1985). Genetic crossovers created by the Cre recombinase (*lox*) and by the FLP recombinase (*FRT*) are reversible and act as potential substrates for intra- and intermolecular recombination events (Sadowski 1986; Gilbertson 2003). Therefore, besides the production of monomeric minicircle molecules, the bidirectionality of the Cre and FLP recombinases results in unwanted side products like the multimeric forms of the recombination products or the parental plasmids, as well as mixed concatemers (Bigger et al. 2001; Nehlsen et al. 2006). Thus, Bigger and coworkers constructed a parental plasmid with one *lox* site being mutated to prefer unidirectional recombination events (Bigger et al. 2001). However, even if the generation of monomeric minicircle molecules was improved, still a high amount of concatemerization was observed (Bigger et al. 2001). The lambda integrase on the other hand is supposed to favor unidirectional recombination events between *attB* and *attP* sites in the absence of the Xis protein (Sadowski 1986). The resulting molecules carrying *attL* and *attR* sites are recombined mainly in the presence of Xis. However, results obtained by Kreiss et al. showed that about 30% of minicircles produced with the lambda integrase system were present as dimers (Kreiss et al. 1998). To solve this problem, Kreiss et al. additionally integrated the multimer resolution system of broad host range plasmid RK4 into the parental plasmid thereby achieving resolution of the dimeric minicircles originally produced by the lambda integrase (Kreiss et al. 1998).

The integrase of bacteriophage Phi31, a member of the serine recombinases family, has been shown to be strictly unidirectional. This enzyme mediates recombination events between an *attP* and an *attB* site resulting in recombination products containing *attL* and *attR* sites (Thorpe and Smith 1998; Thorpe et al. 2000). The reverse reaction has neither been observed in *Escherichia coli* nor in vitro (Thorpe and Smith 1998; Thorpe et al. 2000). Thus, the minicircle production can be driven to a high percentage without unwanted side reactions (Chen et al. 2003). Likewise, the ParA resolvase of the multimer resolution system of the broad host range plasmids RK2 and RP4 mediates only intramolecular recombination events between the corresponding directly repeated resolution sites and is thus not able to revert excision events (Eberl et al. 1994; Smith and Thorpe 2002; Thomson and Ow 2006). It has been demonstrated by quantitative real time PCR analysis of the recombination products that using the ParA resolvase a recombination efficiency greater than 99.5% can be achieved (Mayrhofer et al. 2008). Furthermore, it has been shown in this study that the ParA resolvase is capable of completely converting the parental plasmid into the corresponding recombination products without the formation of unwanted side products (Mayrhofer et al. 2008).

Besides the appropriate catalytic activity of the enzyme, its ratio to the substrate also plays a crucial role. To achieve the required recombination efficiency, a high ratio of recombinase to parental plasmid is necessary as these enzymes seem to function stoichiometrically rather than catalytically (Sadowski 1986). Basically, this ratio is influenced by the copy number of the recombinase gene and the promoter

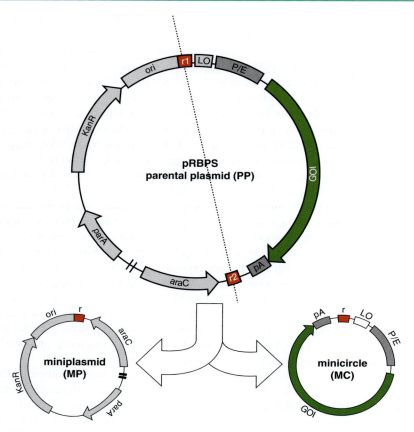

Fig. 15.1 Schematic representation of the RBPS-Technology parental plasmid and the resulting recombination products. The ParA resolvase is under the control of the arabinose promotor/operator system. Expression of the ParA resolvase is induced by addition of L-arabinose. Site specific recombination takes places between the resolution sites r1 and r2 (*red boxes*) of the parental plasmid resulting in the generation of a miniplasmid and a minicircle. *LO* tandem repeat of modified lactose operator sites separated by a spacer sequence, *P/E* eukaryotic promoter and enhancer sequences, *GOI* gene of interest, *pA* polyadenylation sequence, *r1*, *r2* ParA resolution sites, *r* resolution site resulting from ParA catalyzed recombination, *araC* gene encoding the repressor of the arabinose operon, *parA* parA resolvase gene, *KanR* kanamycin resistance gene, *ori* MB1 origin of replication

system used to regulate its expression. The copy number of the recombinase gene is determined by its localization, that is, chromosomal, on a separate compatible plasmid which may carry a low or high copy number origin, or on the parental plasmid itself which usually has a high copy number origin. Regarding the promoter system, stringent control of repression and expression of the site-specific recombinase in *E. coli* is of high importance. Tight repression prior to the induction of gene expression is necessary to avoid premature recombination that leads to displacement of the parental plasmid by the replicative miniplasmid. The temperature sensitive lambda

$cI857/p_R$ promoter (Darquet et al. 1997; Nehlsen et al. 2006) and the $P_{BAD}/araC$ arabinose expression system (Chen et al. 2003; Jechlinger et al. 2004; Bigger et al. 2001) have been successfully used to repress background expression of the recombinases. A high copy number of the recombinase gene is vital to achieve high recombination efficiency. *E. coli* minicircle production strains constructed via approaches that integrate single copies of respective recombinase genes under the control of the lambda or arabinose expression system in the chromosome led to overall low recombination efficiency ranging between 50% and 90% at the maximum (Bigger et al. 2001; Darquet et al. 1997, 1999; Kreiss et al. 1999; Nehlsen et al. 2006). Co-transformation of a compatible low copy number plasmid expressing the ParA resolvase and a high copy number plasmid containing the corresponding resolution sites in *E. coli* led to a recombination efficiency of only 50% (Jechlinger et al. 2004). However, the integration of recombinase expression systems into the parental plasmid containing the corresponding recombination sites led to a very high recombination efficiency of about 97% in the case of the Phi31 integrase (Chen et al. 2003) and to complete recombination when the ParA resolvase system was used (Jechlinger et al. 2004). By integrating the ParA resolvase in the bacterial backbone of the parental plasmid, Mayrhofer and Jechlinger developed the RBPS-Technology for minicircle production (Mayrhofer et al. 2008) (Fig. 15.1). The high recombination yields achieved with the RBPS-Technology in a scalable fermentation process, together with the high product homogeneity, constitute the basis of a minicircle production process that has been shown to be suitable for further scale-up in industrial manufacturing (Mayrhofer et al. 2008).

Minicircle-DNA Purification

Apart from unwanted side products, minicircle-DNA production in *E. coli* via site-specific recombination results in a mixture of three plasmid species, namely minicircles, miniplasmids, and depending on the recombination efficiency, residual amounts of parental plasmids. This leads to a major problem as the difference in the physico-chemical parameters of these three molecules is not significant enough to allow purification by standard methods for plasmid purification, such as ion exchange chromatography. Therefore, in the first studies describing recombination based minicircle production, the miniplasmids and the parental plasmids were linearized by restriction digestion in vitro, and subsequently the minicircles were purified via ultracentrifugation in cesium chloride gradients (Bigger et al. 2001; Darquet et al. 1997, 1999) or by agarose gel electrophoresis (Nehlsen et al. 2006). However, these methods are not only laborious and expensive but also not suitable for large-scale production.

Chen and coworkers developed a technique to degrade the remaining mini- and parental plasmid in vivo by the co-expression of a restriction enzyme (Chen et al. 2005). The homing endonuclease used in this procedure (I-*Sce*I) and the Phi31 recombinase are located on the parental plasmid. Both genes are under the control of a $P_{BAD}/araC$ arabinose promoter. Thus, addition of the inducer L-arabinose results in the simultaneous transcription of two mRNAs. Expression of the recombinase generates minicircle-DNA and miniplasmids by site-specific recombination and the I-*Sce*I endonuclease recognizes a 18 bp sequence which is neither present in the *E. coli* genome nor in the transcription unit, but incorporated in the backbone sequence of the parental plasmid DNA (Chen et al. 2005). However, even after 240 min induction of the recombinase and the endonuclease expression, contaminating miniplasmid and unrecombined parental plasmid still made up 3% of the total plasmid DNA (Chen et al. 2005). Another potential problem of this system is that the simultaneous expression of both enzymes destroys the parental plasmid through the action of the endonuclease before the minicircle can be formed by recombination thereby reducing the minicircle yield. Various measures were necessary to minimize premature degradation of the parental plasmid (Chen et al. 2005). First, an additional copy of the recombinase gene was inserted into the system to accelerate the recombination process. Second, the cultivation temperature was increased from 32°C for recombination to 37°C for I-*Sec*I endonuclease activity as the recombination event is favored at the lower temperature. Third, recombination was performed at a lower pH than the restriction reaction as I-*Sec*I activity is known to be optimal at higher pH values (Monteilhet et al. 1990). For I-*Sec*I mediated pDNA degradation the pH of the culture broth was increased by adding one half-volume of fresh LB broth with pH 8.0. Although the concept of in vivo restriction is a promising approach, the results achieved so far do not demonstrate the suitability of the currently available system for large scale minicircle-DNA production.

Affinity based purification of minicircle-DNA has been hampered for a long time by (1) the problem of inefficient recombination and (2) the lack of a high performance affinity chromatography system for DNA purification. For affinity based purification strategies, a short recognition sequence is integrated into the parental plasmid at a position that is located on the minicircle after the recombination process. Thus, an almost 100% efficient separation of the parental plasmid is required because only plasmids carrying the recognition sequence are separated from plasmids without it, that is, unrecombined parental plasmid will always co-purify. Provided that the parental plasmid can be efficiently converted into the recombination products, affinity based chromatography is the method of choice for large scale minicircle-DNA purification.

Affinity chromatography systems for the isolation of plasmid-DNA described so far are either based on DNA/DNA interaction (Schluep and Cooney 1998; Wils et al. 1997) or on protein/DNA interaction (Darby et al. 2007; Darby and Hine 2005; Forde et al. 2006; Ghose et al. 2004; Woodgate et al. 2002). The DNA/DNA interaction based system described by Wils et al. captures plasmid-DNA by triple-helix formation between a polypurine dsDNA sequence on the plasmid $(GAA)_{17}$ and a single stranded oligonucletide $(CTT)_7$ covalently bound to a chromatographic matrix (Wils et al. 1997). The pyrimidine oligonucleotide, which is immobilized on the matrix, binds in the major groove of the duplex DNA through the formation of Hoogsteen hydrogen bonds: thymine (T) specifically recognizes adenine (A) to form a TA-T triple helix, and protonated cytosine (C^+) can specifically recognize guanine (G) to form CG-C^+ triplexes. Stable triple-helix formation was reported at acidic pH (4.5) and high ionic strength (2 M NaCl) and elution of bound plasmid-DNA was performed with alkaline buffer (1 M Tris, pH 9.0) without NaCl. Under these conditions efficient binding of a plasmid carrying the polypurine recognition sequence was achieved with incubation times above 1 h whereas shorter incubation significantly lowered the yield of bound DNA (Wils et al. 1997). To explore the selectivity of the system, a mixture of a non-binding plasmid (75%) and a binding plasmid containing the polypurine sequence (25%) was applied to the column. The plasmid DNA that was recovered in the elution step as well as plasmid DNA eluted during the washing step was used to transform competent *E. coli* cells. Clones bearing the binding plasmid formed white colonies on medium supplemented with X-gal whereas clones harboring the non-binding plasmid formed blue colonies. While DNA eluted during the washing step gave both white and blue colonies, DNA recovered with the alkaline elution buffer gave only white colonies (Wils et al. 1997). Although this data suggests sufficient selectivity, so far no report has been published to describe the use of triple helix chromatography in minicircle-DNA purification. The binding capacity of the triple-helix based systems was reported to be 23–49 μg per mL affinity matrix (Wils et al. 1997) and 28 μg/mL (Schluep and Cooney 1998), respectively, in studies performed with purified plasmid-DNA. The economical value of this purification system is limited by the poor capacity of the support, the slow kinetics of triple helix formation and by the low reduction of the endotoxin level (Ferreira et al. 2001; Schluep and Cooney 1998; Wils et al. 1997).

The first example of a protein/DNA interaction system was described by Woodgate et al. and Ghose et al. (Ghose et al. 2004; Woodgate et al. 2002). This system is based on the interaction of a zinc finger DNA-binding protein fused to glutathione S-transferase (GST) and a plasmid carrying the corresponding recognition sequence. The strategy was first established in batch adsorption experiments by incubating the purified zinc finger fusion protein with clarified cell lysate containing the plasmid-DNA (Woodgate et al. 2002). The resulting protein/DNA complex was isolated by affinity capture using a glutathione Sepharose matrix (Woodgate et al. 2002). Ghose et al. immobilized this GST-zinc finger DNA binding protein ligand on different adsorbents with covalently bound glutathione to perform a packed bed chromatography (Ghose et al. 2004). Recovery of the protein/DNA complex was achieved by competitive elution with reduced glutathione, albeit yields of 23–27% of the bound DNA were relatively low (Ghose et al. 2004). No attempt was described by Woodgate et al. or Ghose et al. to release the plasmid-DNA from the protein/DNA complex (Ghose et al. 2004; Woodgate et al. 2002). A different strategy exploiting the interaction between the repressor of the lactose operon (LacI) and the corresponding operator sequence has been reported by Darby et al. (Darby et al. 2007; Darby and Hine 2005), Hasche and Voss (2005) and Forde et al. (2006). Darby and coworkers constructed a DNA binding protein by fusing the LacI repressor to a His-tag sequence and the green fluorescent protein (NH_2-LacI-His_6-GFP-COOH) to capture plasmid-DNA carrying the $lacO_3$/lacOs operators. The protein/DNA complex was established by mixing two crude cell lysates, one containing the plasmid and the other containing the protein affinity ligand. After complex formation, the mixture was absorbed onto a polyhistidine-tag specific immobilized metal ion affinity chromatography (IMAC) resin (TALON™) for washing and subsequent elution with NaCl/IPTG buffer (10 mM Tris pH 7.4, 1 mM IPTG and 500 mM NaCl) (Darby et al. 2007; Darby and Hine 2005). According to data from these studies, approximately 100 µg of plasmid-DNA can be purified from 200 mL *E. coli* culture using 250 pmol affinity ligand (LacI-His$_6$-GFP) and 5 mL chromatography matrix (Darby et al. 2007). A C-terminal His-tagged lactose repressor protein was used by Hasche and Voss (2005) for selective capturing of plasmid DNA (pQE30 from QIAGEN) carrying the lactose operator. The purified LacI fusion protein was non-covalently immobilized on different polyhistidine-tag specific IMAC matrices. However, low DNA binding capacities of the constructed chromatographic matrices were reported (for example, 42 µg/mL for Ni-Sepharose as solid phase) (Hasche and Voss 2005). Forde et al. (2006) used a 64mer synthetic peptide representing helix II of the DNA-binding domain of the lactose repressor. The peptide was covalently immobilized to a solid chromatography support to capture pUC19 plasmid-DNA carrying the lacO$_3$/lacOs operator sequences. Plasmid-DNA bound to this matrix was eluted with alkaline buffer (up to pH 12.0) as this truncated LacI protein lacks the core domain necessary for IPTG elution. Capacity in terms of eluted DNA was reported to be 39.8 ± 2.8 µg per mL affinity matrix in packed bed adsorption of pure pUC19$_{lacO3/lacOs}$ (Forde et al. 2006). In a follow-up study the same peptide was immobilized on a monolith matrix (Han and Forde 2008). Again, plasmid pUC19 carrying the lacO$_3$/lacOs operator sequences was used to assay selective binding to the affinity adsorbent. In this approach, the plasmid DNA was eluted with 0.01 M PBS buffer containing 1 M NaCl resulting in the recovery of $80.1 \pm 5.5\%$ of the bound DNA. The capacity was reported to be $21.6 \pm 4.5\%$ µg pUC19 per milliliter monolith matrix (Han and Forde 2008).

Up to now there is no report that one of the mentioned protein/DNA affinity chromatography systems was used for minicircle-DNA purification. The first protein/DNA interaction based affinity chromatography system that was described for this purpose is the RBPS-Chromatography system developed by Mayrhofer and Jechlinger (Mayrhofer et al. 2008) (Fig. 15.2). The RBPS-Technology exploits the interaction of immobilized lactose repressor with dual lacOs sites. The lacOs sequence is a symmetric version of the wild type lactose operator sequence with a tenfold higher affinity to the LacI repressor (Sadler et al. 1983). For immobilization on the affinity matrix a biotinylated version of lactose repressor was constructed. Modification was achieved by the C-terminal fusion of an in vivo biotinylation sequence (ivb) consisting of 15 amino acids (Beckett et al. 1999) to the LacI protein. Consequently, a biotin molecule was covalently attached to the resulting LacI-ivb fusion protein in a post translational modification reaction. The RBPS affinity matrix was established by applying the purified LacI-ivb protein to sepharose carrying covalently bound tetrameric streptavidin (Mayrhofer et al. 2008).

Binding studies revealed that the selective affinity for plasmid DNA carrying dual lacOs sites (that is, minicircle-DNA) depends on the ionic strength of the buffer. Although the material captured unspecific plasmid-DNA (without lacOs sites) at low salt concentrations, plasmid DNA lacking lacOs sites was removed by increasing the NaCl concentration in the washing buffer. Using a buffer with

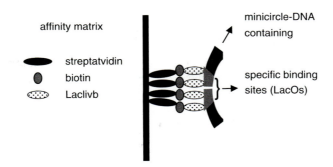

Fig. 15.2 Set-up of the RBPS-Chromatography matrix. The DNA binding protein (LacI) is immobilized via biotin/streptavidin interaction on a chromatography resin carrying covalently bound tetrameric streptavdin. The minicircle-DNA binds to the chromatography matrix via a tandem repeat of a symmetric version of the lactose operator sites (LacOs). The LacI protein, the repressor of the lactose operon, used in this set-up is biotinylated in a post-translational modification reaction. A single biotin molecule is attached to a defined lysine residue of the in vivo biotinylation (ivb) sequence which is C-terminally fused to the LacI protein

400 mM NaCl for sample application prevented non-specific binding of plasmid-DNA lacking the lacOs sites (miniplasmids) but did not interfere with capturing minicircle-DNA. Elution was achieved with buffer containing 5 mM isopropyl-β-D-thiogalactopyranosid (IPTG) and 500 mM NaCl. To regenerate the affinity matrix for further runs, IPTG was removed by a simple washing step with buffer. The average capacity determined for three different batches of RBPS-Chromatography affinity matrix was 184 ± 45 μg minicircle-DNA per milliliter matrix, which is far more than it has been reported for comparable attempts made by other groups (see above). The capacity varied with the sample concentration applied for purification with a maximum value of 238 μg minicircle-DNA per milliliter matrix (Mayrhofer et al. 2008). The composition of the eluate was analyzed by quantitative real time PCR. Comparing the molar amounts, the eluted DNA consisted of 98.8% minicircle-DNA, 1% miniplasmid and 0.2% parental plasmid after a single purification step with the RBPS affinity matrix (Mayrhofer et al. 2008). The RBPS-Chromatography set-up provides several advantages. Firstly, the biotinylated LacI-ivb protein can be efficiently produced in *E. coli* and large amounts can be purified to a high degree by just two simple chromatographic steps. Secondly, column set-up is easy to do by simply applying the purified protein to commercially available matrices carrying covalently immobilized tetrameric streptavidin. Moreover, leaching of the column can be excluded due to the exploitation of the high affinity between biotin and tetrameric streptavidin. Finally, LacI tetramer formation that is necessary for the binding of two lacOs sites (Oehler et al. 1994) is predetermined due to the linkage to tetrameric streptavidin.

Taken together, ever since the first studies were published (Darquet et al. 1997), the production of minicircle-DNA has been hampered by low recombination yields, a high percentage of unwanted side products and lack of appropriate purification strategies. A technology overcoming these problems was described by Mayrhofer and Jechlinger who developed a production process for this improved non-viral vectors, which is feasible for further scale-up in industrial large-scale manufacturing (Mayrhofer et al. 2008).

References

Abremski K, Hoess R, Sternberg N (1983) Studies on the properties of P1 site-specific recombination: evidence for topologically unlinked products following recombination. Cell 32(4):1301–1311

Babineau D, Vetter D, Andrews BJ, Gronostajski RM, Proteau GA, Beatty LG, Sadowski PD (1985) The FLP protein of the 2-micron plasmid of yeast. Purification of the protein from *Escherichia coli* cells expressing the cloned FLP gene. J Biol Chem 260(22):12313–12319

Beckett D, Kovaleva E, Schatz PJ (1999) A minimal peptide substrate in biotin holoenzyme synthetase-catalyzed biotinylation. Protein Sci 8(4):921–929

Bigger BW, Tolmachov O, Collombet JM, Fragkos M, Palaszewski I, Coutelle C (2001) An *araC*-controlled bacterial cre expression system to produce DNA minicircle vectors for nuclear and mitochondrial gene therapy. J Biol Chem 276(25):23018–23027

Chen ZY, He CY, Ehrhardt A, Kay MA (2003) Minicircle DNA vectors devoid of bacterial DNA result in persistent and high-level transgene expression in vivo. Mol Ther 8(3):495–500

Chen ZY, He CY, Meuse L, Kay MA (2004) Silencing of episomal transgene expression by plasmid bacterial DNA elements in vivo. Gene Ther 11(10):856–864

Chen ZY, He CY, Kay MA (2005) Improved production and purification of minicircle DNA vector free of plasmid bacterial sequences and capable of persistent transgene expression in vivo. Hum Gene Ther 16(1):126–131

Darby RA, Hine AV (2005) LacI-mediated sequence-specific affinity purification of plasmid DNA for therapeutic applications. FASEB J 19(7):801–803

Darby RA, Forde GM, Slater NK, Hine AV (2007) Affinity purification of plasmid DNA directly from crude bacterial cell lysates. Biotechnol Bioeng 98(5):1103–1108

Darquet AM, Cameron B, Wils P, Scherman D, Crouzet J (1997) A new DNA vehicle for nonviral gene delivery: supercoiled minicircle. Gene Ther 4(12):1341–1349

Darquet AM, Rangara R, Kreiss P, Schwartz B, Naimi S, Delaere P, Crouzet J, Scherman D (1999) Minicircle: an improved DNA molecule for in vitro and in vivo gene transfer. Gene Ther 6(2):209–218

Eberl L, Kristensen CS, Givskov M, Grohmann E, Gerlitz M, Schwab H (1994) Analysis of the multimer resolution system encoded by the *parCBA* operon of broad-host-range plasmid RP4. Mol Microbiol 12(1):131–141

Ferreira GN, Prazeres DM, Cabral JM, Schleef M (2001) Plasmid manufacturing – an overview. In: Schleef M (ed) Plasmids for therapy and vaccination. Wiley-VCH Verlag GmbH, KGaA, Weinheim, pp 193–236

Forde GM, Ghose S, Slater NK, Hine AV, Darby RA, Hitchcock AG (2006) LacO-lacI interaction in affinity adsorption of plasmid DNA. Biotechnol Bioeng 91(1):67–75

Ghose S, Forde GM, Slater NK (2004) Affinity adsorption of plasmid DNA. Biotechnol Prog 20(3):841–850

Gilbertson L (2003) Cre-lox recombination: creative tools for plant biotechnology. Trends Biotechnol 21(12):550–555

Gronostajski RM, Sadowski PD (1985) The FLP protein of the 2-micron plasmid of yeast. Inter- and intramolecular reactions. J Biol Chem 260(22):12328–12335

Hallet B, Sherratt DJ (1997) Transposition and site-specific recombination: adapting DNA cut-and-paste mechanisms to a variety of genetic rearrangements. FEMS Microbiol Rev 21(2):157–178

Han Y, Forde GM (2008) Single step purification of plasmid DNA using peptide ligand affinity chromatography. J Chromatogr B Analyt Technol Biomed Life Sci 874(1–2):21–26

Hasche A, Voss C (2005) Immobilisation of a repressor protein for binding of plasmid DNA. J Chromatogr A 1080(1):76–82

Hemmi H, Takeuchi O, Kawai T, Kaisho T, Sato S, Sanjo H, Matsumoto M, Hoshino K, Wagner H, Takeda K, Akira S (2000) A toll-like receptor recognizes bacterial DNA. Nature 408(6813):740–745

Jayaram M (1994) Phosphoryl transfer in Flp recombination: a template for strand transfer mechanisms. Trends Biochem Sci 19(2):78–82

Jechlinger W (2006) Optimization and delivery of plasmid DNA for vaccination. Expert Rev Vaccines 5(6):803–825

Jechlinger W, Azimpour Tabrizi C, Lubitz W, Mayrhofer P (2004) Minicircle DNA immobilized in bacterial ghosts: in vivo production of safe non-viral DNA delivery vehicles. J Mol Microbiol Biotechnol 8(4):222–231

Johnson RC, Simon MI (1985) Hin-mediated site-specific recombination requires two 26 bp recombination sites and a 60 bp recombinational enhancer. Cell 41(3):781–791

Kahmann R, Rudt F, Koch C, Mertens G (1985) G inversion in bacteriophage Mu DNA is stimulated by a site within the invertase gene and a host factor. Cell 41(3):771–780

Klinman DM (2004) Immunotherapeutic uses of CpG oligodeoxynucleotides. Nat Rev Immunol 4(4):249–258

Krasnow MA, Cozzarelli NR (1983) Site-specific relaxation and recombination by the Tn3 resolvase: recognition of the DNA path between oriented res sites. Cell 32(4):1313–1324

Kreiss P, Cameron B, Darquet AM, Scherman D, Crouzet J (1998) Production of a new DNA vehicle for gene transfer using site-specific recombination. Appl Microbiol Biotechnol 49(5):560–567

Kreiss P, Cameron B, Rangara R, Mailhe P, Aguerre-Charriol O, Airiau M, Scherman D, Crouzet J, Pitard B (1999) Plasmid DNA size does not affect the physicochemical properties of lipoplexes but modulates gene transfer efficiency. Nucleic Acids Res 27(19):3792–3798

Krieg AM, Yi AK, Matson S, Waldschmidt TJ, Bishop GA, Teasdale R, Koretzky GA, Klinman DM (1995) CpG motifs in bacterial DNA trigger direct B-cell activation. Nature 374(6522):546–549

Landy A (1993) Mechanistic and structural complexity in the site-specific recombination pathways of Int and FLP. Curr Opin Genet Dev 3(5):699–707

Mayrhofer P, Blaesen M, Schleef M, Jechlinger W (2008) Minicircle-DNA production by site specific recombination and protein-DNA interaction chromatography. J Gene Med 10(11):1253–1269

Mertens G, Hoffmann A, Blocker H, Frank R, Kahmann R (1984) Gin-mediated site-specific recombination in bacteriophage Mu DNA: overproduction of the protein and inversion in vitro. EMBO J 3(10):2415–2421

Monteilhet C, Perrin A, Thierry A, Colleaux L, Dujon B (1990) Purification and characterization of the in vitro activity of I-Sce I, a novel and highly specific endonuclease encoded by a group I intron. Nucleic Acids Res 18(6):1407–1413

Nash HA (1996) Site-specific recombination: integration, excision, resolution and inversion of defined DNA segments. In: Neidhardt FC (ed) *Escherichia coli* and salmonella. ASM Press, Washington DC, pp 2363–2376

Nehlsen K, Broll S, Bode J (2006) Replicating minicircles: generation of nonviral episomes for the efficient modification of dividing cells. Gene Ther Mol Biol 10:233–244

Oehler S, Amouyal M, Kolkhof P, von Wilcken-Bergmann B, Muller-Hill B (1994) Quality and position of the three lac operators of *E. coli* define efficiency of repression. EMBO J 13(14):3348–3355

Pang AS (1994) Production of antibodies against *Bacillus thuringiensis* delta-endotoxin by injecting its plasmids. Biochem Biophys Res Commun 202(3):1227–1234

Rankin R, Pontarollo R, Ioannou X, Krieg AM, Hecker R, Babiuk LA, Drunen Littel-van den Hurk S (2001) CpG motif identification for veterinary and laboratory species demonstrates that sequence recognition is highly conserved. Antisense Nucleic Acid Drug Dev 11(5):333–340

Reed RR (1981) Transposon-mediated site-specific recombination: a defined in vitro system. Cell 25(3):713–719

Riu E, Chen ZY, Xu H, He CY, Kay MA (2007) Histone modifications are associated with the persistence or silencing of vector-mediated transgene expression in vivo. Mol Ther 15(7):1348–1355

Sadler JR, Sasmor H, Betz JL (1983) A perfectly symmetric lac operator binds the lac repressor very tightly. Proc Natl Acad Sci USA 80(22):6785–6789

Sadowski P (1986) Site-specific recombinases: changing partners and doing the twist. J Bacteriol 165(2):341–347

Schluep T, Cooney CL (1998) Purification of plasmids by triplex affinity interaction. Nucleic Acids Res 26(19):4524–4528

Smith MC, Thorpe HM (2002) Diversity in the serine recombinases. Mol Microbiol 44(2):299–307

Stark WM, Boocock MR, Sherratt DJ (1992) Catalysis by site-specific recombinases. Trends Genet 8(12):432–439

Suzuki M, Kasai K, Saeki Y (2006) Plasmid DNA sequences present in conventional herpes simplex virus amplicon vectors cause rapid transgene silencing by forming inactive chromatin. J Virol 80(7):3293–3300

Thomson JG, Ow DW (2006) Site-specific recombination systems for the genetic manipulation of eukaryotic genomes. Genesis 44(10):465–476

Thorpe HM, Smith MC (1998) In vitro site-specific integration of bacteriophage DNA catalyzed by a recombinase of the resolvase/invertase family. Proc Natl Acad Sci USA 95(10):5505–5510

Thorpe HM, Wilson SE, Smith MC (2000) Control of directionality in the site-specific recombination system of the Streptomyces phage phiC31. Mol Microbiol 38(2):232–241

Valera A, Perales JC, Hatzoglou M, Bosch F (1994) Expression of the neomycin-resistance (neo) gene induces alterations in gene expression and metabolism. Hum Gene Ther 5(4):449–456

Vetter D, Andrews BJ, Roberts-Beatty L, Sadowski PD (1983) Site-specific recombination of yeast 2-micron DNA in vitro. Proc Natl Acad Sci USA 80(23):7284–7288

Wils P, Escriou V, Warnery A, Lacroix F, Lagneaux D, Ollivier M, Crouzet J, Mayaux JF, Scherman D (1997) Efficient purification of plasmid DNA for gene transfer using triple-helix affinity chromatography. Gene Ther 4(4):323–330

Woodgate J, Palfrey D, Nagel DA, Hine AV, Slater NK (2002) Protein-mediated isolation of plasmid DNA by a zinc finger-glutathione S-transferase affinity linker. Biotechnol Bioeng 79(4):450–456

Yin W, Xiang P, Li Q (2005) Investigations of the effect of DNA size in transient transfection assay using dual luciferase system. Anal Biochem 346(2):289–294

Industrial Manufacturing of Plasmid-DNA Products for Gene Vaccination and Therapy

16

Jochen Urthaler, Hermann Schuchnigg, Patrick Garidel, and Hans Huber

Although today only a few DNA vaccine products have gained market approval for veterinary applications, still numerous human clinical trials are performed. Clinical progress in the field of DNA vaccination and gene therapy has led to an increased demand of pharmaceutical-grade plasmid DNA (pDNA), manufactured under the conditions of current Good Manufacturing Practices (cGMP). Consequently, significant progress in process science and manufacturing technology of plasmid DNA has been made during the past years. In upstream processing (vector design, host strain, fermentation process), significant achievements have been made, resulting in steadily increasing pDNA fermentation titers. In general, the downstream processing steps such as cell lysis and chromatographic purification still often represent engineering challenges in view of high product scales. This article summarizes the state of the art in industrial plasmid manufacturing and discusses bottlenecks and pitfalls to be avoided in order to obtain pDNA products of high and reproducible quantity and quality.

General Aspects of Plasmid DNA Manufacturing

As a consequence of intensive process development and engineering, a number of pDNA manufacturing processes have been established and applied (reviewed in Cai et al. (2009), Ongkudon et al. (2010)). This is also indicated by a number of patents and patent applications in the field of plasmid upstream and downstream processing (Carnes and Williams 2007; Tejeda-Mansir and Montesinos 2008). Despite the remarkably big variety of different production approaches, most pDNA

J. Urthaler (✉)
Boehringer Ingelheim RCV GmbH & Co KG,
Vienna, Austria
e-mail: Jochen.Urthaler@boehringer-ingelheim.com

J. Thalhamer et al. (eds.), *Gene Vaccines*,
DOI 10.1007/978-3-7091-0439-2_16, © Springer-Verlag/Wien, 2012

manufacturing processes are characterized by the following common features: (i) the bacterial host *Escherichia coli* is used, and the corresponding *E. coli* replicons are utilized for propagation of host and plasmid in a bioreactor, (ii) alkaline lysis is applied in order to release the plasmid from the bacterial cells, and (iii) the plasmid is predominantly purified by chromatographic techniques and (ultra)filtration steps. As a representative example, a general pDNA manufacturing flow chart is shown in Fig. 16.1.

In contrast to recombinant proteins, advanced downstream processing concepts for industrially manufactured plasmid DNA are characterized by their generic applicability. This means that once established for a particular plasmid, a certain manufacturing process may be adapted to other plasmids with only few or minor process changes. Generic pDNA processes offer a number of benefits such as a short project lead time and reduced process development efforts for every new plasmid, as well as a straight-forward process validation timeline for mature projects. Another advantage of generic processes is that they are easily transferable between different sites and facilities. For the manufacturer's client (i.e. the clinical sponsor) it is important to limit the number and degree of process changes over the course of clinical development, in order to save costs and time. In this context, the threat of pandemic diseases have led to considerations how plasmid DNA process engineering could contribute to the supply of kilogram-scale amounts of DNA vaccines in a short period of time (Hoare et al. 2005). To address this scale issue, technology cooperations between small- and large-scale contract manufacturing organizations (CMOs) is becoming increasingly common. By applying the same generic manufacturing process, technology transfer from one manufacturing company, site or facility to another is thereby considerably simplified without any major process change or loss of product quality.

Plasmid Design and its Implication on Manufacturing

For manufacturing of plasmid DNA, Good Manufacturing Practice begins with prudent vector design (for reviews, see Gill et al. (2009), Prather et al. (2003), Tolmachov (2009), Williams et al. (2009a)). All elements, features, and characteristics of the vector backbone must be evaluated in view of process robustness and product quality. Many elements of plasmid vaccine vectors primarily affect the eukaryotic expression of the target gene (promoter, gene of interest, transcription terminator, polyadenylation signal) or the immunogenicity of the plasmid (e.g. unmethylated, immunostimulatory CpG sequences). Other vector elements however, are functionally necessary only in the prokaryotic production host and directly influence progress and outcome of the manufacturing process. The most important prokaryotic vector elements of a DNA vector are the origin of replication and the selection marker.

The plasmid's *origin of replication* (*ori*) is essential to propagate it as an extrachromosomal DNA element in the *E. coli* host cell. Therefore, the choice of the plasmid *ori* is critical. In order to maximize the manufacturing yield and minimize the cost

16 Industrial Manufacturing of Plasmid-DNA Products for Gene Vaccination   313

Fig. 16.1 Flow chart of an industrial production process for manufacturing of cGMP-grade plasmid DNA (Boehringer Ingelheim RCV)

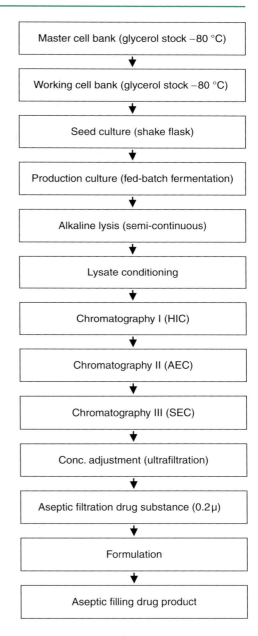

of goods, a high-copy-number *ori* is employed for most therapeutic plasmids. The vast majority of pharmaceutical plasmids currently in development contain a pUC origin, which is a high-copy-number derivative of the pMB1/ColE1 replicon. The principle of the pMB1/ColE1 *ori* is based on the hybridization of two plasmid-encoded antisense RNA transcripts, namely RNA II and RNA I. RNA II acts as a pre-primer for the host encoded DNA polymerase I thereby enhancing the replication rate. In contrast, RNA I controls (reduces) plasmid replication by forming an RNA I:RNA II hybrid thereby reducing the replication rate. In contrast to the original pMB1/ColE1 replicon, the high copy number pUC *ori* has a deletion in the plasmid-encoded protein repressor of primer (Rop) and a second mutation altering the RNAI/II interaction. The reproducibly high replication rate and the good plasmid yield obtained from pUC derived vectors have led to their broad industrial and academic application. Other plasmid *oris* have been suggested for therapeutic plasmids (Prather et al. 2003; Williams et al. 2009a), but have not found wide-spread clinical application.

The *selection marker* of the plasmid is another factor to be taken into account. Commonly, plasmids code for an antibiotic-resistance gene to allow selection of plasmid-carrying bacterial clones. While beta-lactam antibiotic markers (like ampicillin resistance) should be avoided and are considered critical by regulatory authorities due to safety issues, many therapeutic plasmids today contain a less critical aminoglycosid marker like kanamycin resistance. However in general, the therapeutic co-administration of a prokaryotic antibiotic resistance gene and the use of the corresponding antibiotics during manufacturing are becoming increasingly problematic from a regulatory point of view.

Therefore, a number of innovative concepts for antibiotic-free plasmid selection have been developed in the past years. Such alternative selection systems may be for instance based on the selection with biocides which are bacteria-toxic but not classified as antibiotics (Goh and Good 2008), auxotrophic complementation of an essential gene (Soubrier et al. 1999, 2005; Vidal et al. 2008), operator-repressor titration (Cranenburgh et al. 2001) or plasmid-borne antisense RNAs controlling a cell-toxic gene (Luke et al. 2009). Despite those alternative selection systems avoiding the use of antibiotics, all of them rely on the action of foreign plasmid-borne DNAs, RNAs or proteins, which may contain problematic immuno-stimulatory sequences and unnecessarily increase the vector's size.

In order to avoid the drawbacks of additional plasmid-borne selection sequences, a host-vector system for antibiotic free plasmid selection based on the natural ColE1/pUC *ori* was developed (Mairhofer et al. 2008, 2010). This system utilizes the natural RNA I from the plasmid replication origin in order to silence a host-encoded repressor gene. This inhibition of the repressor by RNA antisense hybridization allows the expression of an essential *E. coli* gene, which enables growth and propagation of the plasmid-carrying cells. The key advantage of this concept is the complete avoidance of additional selection sequences on the plasmid and the generation of minimized plasmids containing only the eukaryotic expression cassette and the inevitable replication origin.

A completely different and innovative plasmid selection approach is pursued with the production of CpG free minicircle DNA by the application of recombination-based plasmid selection ("RBPS-Technology" (Mayrhofer et al. 2008, 2009)). The RBPS concept utilizes the action of the *parA* resolvase which is present on the parental plasmid. Upon induction and expression, *parA* mediates the *in vivo* recombination and division of the parental plasmid into (i) a minicircle containing essentially the expression cassette, and (ii) a miniplasmid which contains all other sequences not necessary for therapeutic action (replication origin, antibiotic selection marker, *parA* resolvase, etc.). Minicircle and miniplasmid are then separated by application of DNA/protein affinity chromatography, utilizing a minicircle borne *lac* operator sequence and recombinant *LacI* protein as an affinity ligand. For more details about this technology, see Chap. 15 in this book.

A generally important factor for vector design is the *size* of the plasmid. From a regulatory, manufacturing, and therapeutic point of view, it is evident that all unnecessary DNA sequences should be removed from the vector. As a general rule, the plasmid should be designed to be as small as possible. Since a large plasmid exerts a metabolic load on the *E. coli* host, it will reduce the cell's resources for plasmid replication, leading to a decreased pDNA yield. From a therapeutic point of view, a small plasmid should penetrate the eukaryotic cells more efficiently and should show increased expression rates. The size of the plasmid, however, may be predetermined by the therapeutic approach. Plasmids coding for one gene (monocistronic) typically have about 3–5 kbp, while such coding for multiple genes (polycistronic) may have 7–15 kbp or larger.

Selection of Host Strain (Cell Line)

The *E. coli* production host significantly affects the yield and quality of the produced pDNA. Careful selection of an efficient and suitable host strain is therefore a critical factor right at the beginning of a pDNA process development project. Currently, mainly *E. coli* K-12 strains are used for pDNA manufacturing as they are non-pathogenic, well-known, regulatory accepted, environmentally non-persistent and simply cultivated in bioreactors. However, selection of the right pDNA host out of the hundreds of existing K-12 derivatives is not a simple and straightforward task. Although a number of systematic investigations on the performance of host strains have been made (Huber et al. 2005a; Singer et al. 2009; Yau et al. 2008), it is at the moment hardly possible to deduct the processing behaviour of a certain strain (pDNA yield and quality) from its genotype. Examples for *E. coli* hosts successfully used in an industrial or pharmaceutical pDNA manufacturing setting include the strains DH5-alpha (Carnes et al. 2006; Williams et al. 2009b), DH5 (Listner et al. 2006), DH10B (Cai et al. 2010), JM109 (Yang et al. 2009) and XL-1 Blue (Przybylowski et al. 2007). Excellent experience was made with *E. coli* JM108 as pDNA host for successful high-cell-density cultivation. It was found that *E. coli* JM108 consistently showed superior performance in small- and large-scale cGMP manufacturing fermentations (Huber et al. 2005a, 2008; Urthaler et al. 2005a).

Although many host features are generic, specific plasmid-host combinations may show unexpected effects, therefore a systematic case-by-case host screening program is recommended. From the manufacturer's point of view, the most important criteria a host should fulfill – and which therefore should be addressed during host screening – are (i) an efficient growth behaviour, (ii) a high plasmid yield (volumetric and specific), and (iii) a high plasmid DNA quality (high percentage of supercoiled form, no recombination products).

In order to avoid drawbacks of "off-the-shelf" strains, a number of attempts have been made for genetic engineering of *E. coli* strains for plasmid production, as reviewed by Bower and Prather (Bower and Prather 2009). Host engineering approaches may target towards improved pDNA sequence stability by the avoidance of insertion sequence (IS) transposed into the plasmid. As shown by Posfai et al. (2006), IS-mediated genetic instability can be addressed by the construction of multiple-deletion series strains of reduced genome *E. coli* which showed no detectable transposon activity. Other host engineering approaches may aim at improved safety, for instance to avoid antibiotic selection markers. Mairhofer et al. (2010) engineered *E. coli* JM108 to control the expression of an essential host gene by the presence of antisense RNA I which is a "natural" control element of the *ori* of ColE1 plasmids, thereby achieving the propagation of minimized and CpG-reduced plasmids without any external selection marker.

The K-12 group of *E. coli* strains is not the only host option as shown recently: *endA* and *recA* mutants of the B strain *E. coli* BL21 showed superior specific and volumetric pDNA yield compared to the conventional *E. coli* K-12 DH5-alpha (Phue et al. 2008).

Cell Bank Establishment

In order to obtain a fermentation inoculum of reproducible quality, the generation, characterization and maintenance of a standardized cryo-conserved cell bank (glycerol stock) is mandatory. After transformation of the plasmid into an *E. coli* host strain and subsequent clone screening, a cGMP manufactured Master Cell Bank (MCB) should be established. From one MCB vial, usually a Working Cell Bank (WCB) is derived. Usually, one vial of WCB serves as starting inoculum for each individual GMP plasmid manufacturing batch. Both the MCB and WCB shall be specified, characterized, release tested, stored and maintained under controlled conditions. Typical acceptance criteria for pDNA cell banks include: plasmid identity and integrity (sequencing, restriction mapping), segregational plasmid stability/plasmid retention, plasmid productivity, host strain identity, host viability and growth performance and absence of contamination (bacteria, yeasts, bacteriophages).

Fermentation

Fermentation (cultivation) of the plasmid-bearing *E. coli* cells is the first essential processing step in pDNA manufacturing. Commonly, the cultivation process is initiated by the inoculation of a thawed WCB into a shake flask as pre-culture (seed culture) step, followed by the transfer into a bioreactor (fermenter) and therein the performance of the main culture (production culture) step. Although batch-mode fermentation (low cell density cultivation) would be still an option for plasmid DNA

16 Industrial Manufacturing of Plasmid-DNA Products for Gene Vaccination 317

manufacturing due to its simple execution and short duration, high-cell-density cultivation (HCDC) by applying a fed-batch process mode is meanwhile well established and state of the art (Carnes et al. 2006; Huber et al. 2005b; Listner et al. 2006; Rozkov et al. 2006, 2008; Tejeda-Mansir and Montesinos 2008).

The fundamental principle of high-cell-density cultivation is based on the assumption that the plasmid yield is maximized by the increase of cell density (*E. coli* biomass), measured by optical density units (e.g. OD_{600}) or dry or wet cell mass per unit culture volume. Typical final optical density values of plasmid fermentations range between $OD_{600} = 100–200$, corresponding to a dry cell mass of ~30–60 g/L. One key feature of high-cell-density cultivation is a well-balanced culture medium that supports predictable substrate conversion into plasmid containing biomass. This is efficiently achieved by the application of a synthetically defined culture medium without using complex medium compounds like yeast extract or soy peptone, thereby avoiding drawbacks as varying quality, undefined chemical composition and problematic handling due to foaming, dusting or clumping.

In fed-batch cultivation, a feeding medium with concentrated substrate (glucose or glycerol) is fed into the fermenter according to a certain feeding regime, thereby (i) controlling (pre-defining) the specific growth rate μ of the culture at its optimum level, and (ii) limiting the residual substrate concentration in the culture broth. Fed-batch cultivation employing an exponential feeding regime is the most efficient mode for controlling μ at a defined and constant level in order to support enrichment of plasmid DNA in the biomass. The stringent control of the feeding rate on a pre-defined time-scale basis, the absence of an operator influence and the prevention of a non-robust feedback-control mechanism are the key benefits of exponential and pre-defined nutrient feeding. Examples for exponential-mode fed-batch processes for pDNA productions are provided in Huber et al. (2005b) and Rozkov et al. (2008). Exponential feeding in combination with a temperature up-shift can induce the plasmid replication rate in order to obtain high pDNA titers, as shown by Carnes et al. (Carnes et al. 2006). Furthermore, linear-increasing combined with linear-constant feeding can be successfully applied as well (Listner et al. 2006).

During the recent years, steadily increasing volumetric plasmid yields (titers) were achieved by means of process engineering. Today, a final plasmid titer beyond 1 g/L can be regarded as state of the art (1.5 g/L in Carnes et al. (2006), 1.6 g/L in Listner et al. (2006), 2 g/L in Phue et al. (2008), 2.2 g/L in Williams et al. (2009a), and can increase beyond 3 g/L, as shown in Fig. 16.2.

It must be noted that the plasmid titer alone is not the only important fermentation criterion. The achievement of a high specific plasmid yield (i.e., pDNA per biomass unit) is particularly important for the subsequent alkaline lysis step. A specific pDNA yield of 20–60 mg pDNA/g dry cell weight has already been achieved (Fig. 16.2; Listner et al. 2006; Phue et al. 2008).

Finally, the definition of the optimum harvesting time point (end of cultivation) is critical in order to prevent the deterioration of pDNA quality. The maintenance of the pDNA homogeneity at >80% supercoiled form at the end of the cultivation should be the target. Technically, biomass harvest is usually performed by applying tubular bowl centrifuges or disc stack separators.

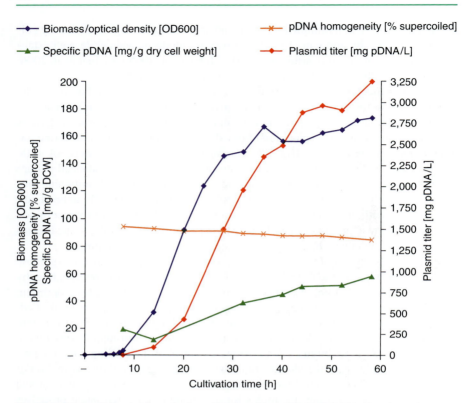

Fig. 16.2 High cell density fermentation of *Escherichia coli* K-12 JM108 harbouring a therapeutic plasmid (~5 kb, pUC/ColE1 ori). The culture was operated in exponential fed-batch mode with a synthetically defined culture medium and without the use of antibiotics (Boehringer Ingelheim RCV) dry cell weight (DCW), optical density (OD)

Cell-Disintegration by Alkaline Lysis

The treatment of the bacterial cells with a strong alkaline solution containing a detergent is still – almost 40 years after publishing of this procedure (Birnboim and Doly 1979) – the method of choice for disintegrating the cells in order to release plasmid DNA. High pressure homogenization or other techniques applying high shear stress cannot be performed for pDNA due to its mechanical sensitivity (Levy et al. 1999; Urthaler et al. 2007). Enzymatic methods may be applied at the bench-scale but are economically unfavourable for industrial production and problematic from a regulatory point of view. Another approach is heat induced lysis, which could be an alternative for the industrial scale, if the issue of low yield can be overcome (Hoare et al. 2005; Lee and Sagar 1996).

For alkaline lysis, most commonly sodium hydroxide (NaOH) at pH 12 in combination with sodium dodecylsulfate (SDS) is used for lysis of the cell walls, while potassium acetate is applied for subsequent neutralisation. During this step, a voluminous flock-like precipitate containing cell debris, chromosomal DNA and

16 Industrial Manufacturing of Plasmid-DNA Products for Gene Vaccination

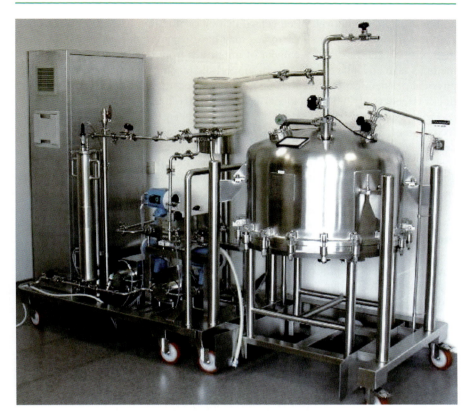

Fig. 16.3 Example for an automated facility for alkaline lysis of plasmid containing cells, realized under industrial GMP conditions. The qualified and validated system combines alkaline lysis, neutralization and precipitate removal in a continuous way (Urthaler et al. 2007). It is predominantly constructed of stainless steel and is hygienically designed in order to enable cleaning in place (CIP)

host proteins is generated. There are four major points to be considered for alkaline lysis and neutralization: (i) as the DNA is released, viscosity of the lysate strongly increases, significantly impacting the mixing characteristics, (ii) the pH value and the residence time have to be accurately controlled in order to irreversibly denature chromosomal DNA but to avoid degradation of the plasmid, (iii) mixing procedures have to be optimized with respect to homogeneity, the avoidance of local pH extremes, and the reduction of shear forces, (iv) a significant precipitate amount must be separated. Therefore, alkaline lysis was the processing bottleneck at industrial scale plasmid production for years.

Meanwhile, plasmid DNA manufacturers have individually designed and optimized automated continuous systems for alkaline lysis, neutralization and precipitate removal (preferably directly combined) as shown for example in Fig. 16.3 (Urthaler et al. 2007). Such systems work accurately with minimal manual handling and reproducible results.

For precipitate removal, often centrifugation or filtration is used (Ferreira et al. 1999). While for the first shear forces may have negative impact on pDNA, both methods bear the risk of detachment of impurities from retained flocks. Advanced methods take advantage and actively support the tendency of the flocks to float by physical or chemical treatment as an improved procedure for the separation of the flocks (Hebel et al. 2004; Hucklenbroich and Müller 2003; Urthaler et al. 2009).

From a production-related and an economic perspective, the main goal is to recover more than 80% of the cells plasmid DNA in the clarified lysate without decrease of the supercoiled form and an already significantly reduced level of impurities (Urthaler et al. 2007). The devices used and the corresponding methods (predominantely covered by patents) have to be scaleable while meeting all regulatory and GMP requirements.

Purification

The objective of plasmid purification is to separate the plasmid from impurities related to the host strain (proteins, endotoxins, RNA, chromosomal DNA), from undesired plasmid forms (open circular, linearized and di-/oligomers and size variants), and from process related additives (e.g. detergents). State of the art plasmid DNA purification at the industrial scale differs significantly from the methods applied at the bench scale (Hoare et al. 2005; Kelly 2003). For analytical or research purposes often enzymes like RNAse, organic solvents and detergents are applied (Hoare et al. 2005; Prather et al. 2003). Omitting these and other problematic substances is an economic prerequisite for the regulatory compliant production of a safe pharmaceutical grade DNA drug (FDA 2007).

Although a few processes without chromatography steps have been reported (see e.g. Hayashizaki (1997)), purification processes for plasmid DNA still predominantly consist of different chromatographic steps. It is important to vary the chromatography-principles and/or -parameters in a way that removal of the different impurities is achieved (Kitamura and Nakatani 2002; Urthaler et al. 2005b). A well balanced combination is crucial to meet the specifications and acceptance criteria for purity and homogeneity of pharmaceutical-grade plasmid DNA (FDA 2007). A brief overview on suitable chromatography supports is given in Stadler et al. (2004).

For conventional bead-based chromatography supports, the limited plasmid binding capacity has to be considered, with rather large columns as a consequence. In contrast to proteins, only the binding sites at the outer bead surface are accessible for the plasmids since these molecules are too large to penetrate the beads. Scaleable pre-packed monolithic chromatography supports (Convective Interaction Media, CIM®) are alternatives to particulate media. Due to much larger pores/channels and a high porosity of more than 50% their dynamic plasmid DNA binding capacity (up to 10 g/L) is up to an order of magnitude higher compared to many particulate media. A further advantage is that monoliths are not diffusion limited, enable significantly higher flow rates at moderate back-pressure and therefore reduce processing time (Smrekar et al. 2010; Urthaler et al. 2005c).

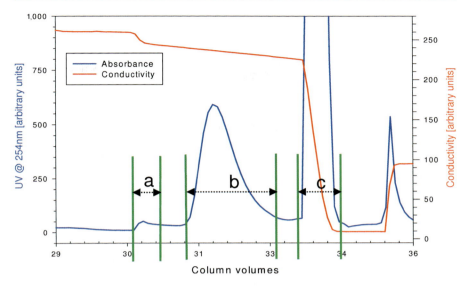

Fig. 16.4 Typical elution-profile of a preparative capture step for plasmid production carried out by hydrophobic interaction chromatography (HIC). Feed solution: clarified and conditioned alkaline lysate. Baseline separation of (**a**) the undesired open circular plasmid DNA, (**b**) the required supercoiled plasmid DNA and (**c**) host-related impurities like proteins and RNA is achieved, providing high product recovery rates in this process step (Urthaler et al. 2005b)

Although there have been some attempts to establish very specialized chromatography techniques such as e.g. triple-helix affinity chromatography (Wils et al. 1997), predominantly traditional methods used for decades in biopharmaceutical production are still the chromatographic principles of choice. Salt promoted binding can be carried out by hydrophobic interaction chromatography (HIC) or the so called thiophilic aromatic chromatography (Stadler et al. 2004); both are often used as the first purification step (capture step) (Stadler et al. 2004; Urthaler et al. 2005a, b). Optimization of the binding and elution conditions for HIC enables reduction of endotoxins, RNA, and chromosomal DNA levels and allows baseline separation of the supercoiled plasmid from open circular form (Fig. 16.4; Urthaler et al. 2005b). Due to the high salt concentrations (up to 3 M ammonium sulphate) the issue of bed swelling or shrinking must be addressed.

Based on its negative charge, plasmid DNA is pre-destined for purification by anion exchange chromatography (AEC). This technique is suitable especially for endotoxin removal and to significantly increase the pDNA bulk concentration.

Size exclusion chromatography (SEC) is a well suited method for the separation of the large plasmid DNA molecules from low molecular weight impurities and salts. Plasmid DNA leaves the column within the void volume while the other components follow much later. The loading volume in pDNA purification therefore may be up to 35% of the column volume before peaks start to overlap. As the final column step, SEC is appropriate for buffer exchange and to obtain the desired bulk formulation. Alternatively, ultra/diafiltration (UF/DF) using hollow-fiber cartridges or cassette modules can be applied for this purpose. Main optimization potential lies in the selection of the ideal cut-off (30–300 kD for plasmid DNA) and the trans-membrane pressure. Beside application for buffer exchange, ultrafiltration systems may be also applied to increase the plasmid concentration. Viscosity-related technical challenges have to be considered at possible final concentrations of up to 10 g/L (Urthaler et al. 2005b).

With respect to plasmid yield, plasmid manufacturers skilled and experienced in industrial production meanwhile reproducibly reach overall downstream yields (from biomass to pharmaceutical-grade drug substance) in the range of 40–60%, potentially even up to 70% (Urthaler et al. 2005b).

Formulation and Pharmaceutical Technology

The final step in pDNA manufacturing for pharmaceutical and medical applications is formulation and drug product manufacturing (Garidel and Peschka-Süss 2006; Gill et al. 2009). Besides the application of naked plasmid DNA, usually the process step "formulation" has two main objectives: (i) the development of a plasmid delivery system in order to achieve a sufficiently high transfection level into the target tissue and (ii) the stabilisation of the drug product. Today, formulation strategies as well as implemented pharmaceutical processes are available which allow manufacturing under aseptic conditions.

To increase the transfection efficiency of naked plasmid DNA, various physical application devices were developed (e.g. electroporation catheter) (Seidler et al. 2005) or gene gun systems (Dufour 2001; Mahvi et al. 1997). For detailed information about delivery of gene vaccines by electroporation or via gene gun, see Chaps. 1, 2, 7, and 8 in this book. Main challenges using naked pDNA are related to in vivo degradation by deoxyribonuclease attack as well as to the high bio-barriers encountered in biological systems. These facts strongly reduce effective immunisation (Bodles-Brakhop and Draghia-Akli 2008; Liu 2010; Tyagi et al. 2008).

Besides the physical approach, chemical drug delivery systems like lipids or polymers are of relevance as shown by different proof of concept studies (Kiefer et al. 2004; Kodama et al. 2006; Li and Huang 2006; Morille et al. 2008; Muhs et al. 2004; Ogris and Wagner 2002a). A number of tested non-viral delivery systems are positively charged (Wagner 2004; Wagner and Kloeckner 2006) (Fig. 16.5a). The polycations used include natural DNA binding proteins (e.g. histones), or synthetic amino acid polymers (e.g. polylysine), or polytheylenimines (PEI), cationic dendrimer, carbohydrate-based polymers (chitosan) or lipids (Morille et al. 2008; O'Rorke et al. 2010; Schaffert and Wagner 2008; Wagner 2004). Approaches based on (cationic) polymers, cationic lipids, combinations of these two and their in vivo performance are discussed in detail in Chaps. 5 and 6 in this book. Currently, by using higher concentration of non-viral complex particles, the most potent polymer-DNA-complex formulations have reached transfection efficiencies similar to that observed with viral vectors (Wagner 2004).

16 Industrial Manufacturing of Plasmid-DNA Products for Gene Vaccination

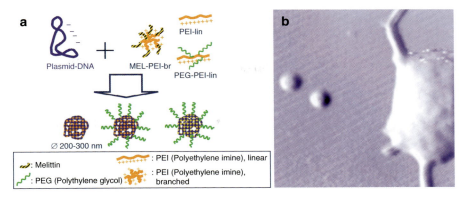

Fig. 16.5 (**a**) Schematic representation of the formation and composition of different polymer-DNA-complexes (polyplexes). (**b**) AFM (atomic force microscopy) images of liposomes, DNA embedded lipid and lipid-DNA-complex (lipoplex)

In order to achieve such high transfection efficiencies, non-viral delivery systems like polymers have to combine different requirements. First of all, these systems are positively charged allowing a strong plasmid DNA compaction into small particles of virus-like dimensions. This is especially the case for polymers (Ogris and Wagner 2002b), whereas with lipids, the formed lipid-DNA complexes (lipoplexes) have sizes from ~100–1,000 nm (Clement et al. 2005) (Fig. 16.5b). However, larger polyplexes have also successfully been used (Lenter et al. 2004). In a next step, the formed complex can migrate to and into the target cells (polyplex), or fuse with the cell membrane of the target cell (lipoplex). In these complexed structures, the DNA is protected from nuclease degradation and shielded against undesired interactions of the components of the biological fluids. Furthermore, functionalization (e.g. the presence of cell binding ligands, fusogenic amphiphiles, membrane active peptides like melittin, protecting polymers like polyethylene glycol (see Fig. 16.5a)) of the used polymers, respectively lipids can enhance cell binding and intracellular delivery into the cytoplasm and nucleus (Tan et al. 2005; van den Berg et al. 2010). Targeted delivery is an additional strategy to enhance local transfection efficiency (Moffatt and Cristiano 2006; Wagner et al. 2005). Also the structure of the polymer itself, i.e. linear PEI versus branched PEI is of relevance (Fig. 16.5a).

Stability of the formed complexes is also influenced by the microenvironment like (i) the ionic strength of the solution, (ii) the concentration of the used excipients, (iii) the positive/negative charge ratios of non-viral transfection agent and DNA, (iv) and the pharmaceutical mixing and manufacturing technology. Especially the order of mixing and complexation, concentration, mixing ratio, etc. of non-viral transfection agents with DNA is crucial for the structure and stability of the formed complexes (i.e. kinetically versus thermodynamically controlled process) (Clement et al. 2005; Wagner and Kloeckner 2006). It is also recommended to investigate the stability of the DNA complexes in physiologically relevant fluids (e.g. serum, blood), because the interaction of the DNA complex with the components of such fluids largely dictate the stability and thus transfection efficiency of the DNA-complex.

The complexing of cationic lipids with DNA induces the formation of various lipoplex phases. Lamellar versus non-lamellar (so-called hexagonal) phases have been reported with different transfection efficiencies (de la Torre et al. 2009; Garidel and Funari 2006; Zantl et al. 1999). Various studies have shown that the fusogenic activity of lipoplexes forming a hexagonal phase is higher compared to lamellar lipid-DNA complexes, thus increasing transfection efficiency (Barteau et al. 2008; Koynova et al. 2008; Tenchov et al. 2008).

Clement et al. (2005) have proposed a process for the large scale preparation of lipoplexes under aseptic conditions. The drug product is a one-vial approach (ready to use lipoplexes) presented as a lyophilised product, compared to another applied approach which uses two vials (one vial of lyophilised DNA and one vial of lyophilised lipids or polymers). These two vials have to be re-suspended and freshly mixed at the "bed-side" of the patient. The two-vial approach often lacks of reproducibility. The formed lipoplexes, stored at 2–8 °C, as presented by Clement et al. (2005), were stable for at least 18 months.

Pharmaceutical requirements for the development of lipoplexes have been described by Garidel and Peschka-Süss (2006). One main problem in the field of non-viral gene therapy is the limited correlation between in vitro and in vivo transfection efficiencies, the reason of which is not fully clear (McNeil et al. 2010). However, for the evaluation of the quality of manufactured DNA complex batches, in vitro transfection assays can be used.

Analytical Plasmid Characterization and GMP Quality Control

Bulk plasmid preparations purified from *E. coli* fermentation contain predominantly supercoiled (ccc) form, with varying levels of recombination products, open-circular (oc) and linear isoforms, which arise through single-strand and double-strand nicks, respectively. Oligomeric forms, such as concatemers and cantenanes which exist in different isoforms as well, may also be present in crude plasmid preparations (Schleef and Blaesen 2009; Schleef and Schmidt 2004; Ulmer 2001; Urthaler et al. 2005a). Since open circular and linear forms are randomly damaged at different locations, promoter or coding regions may be disrupted, making these isoforms inefficient. The compact supercoiled pDNA isoform is hence considered to be the intact and undamaged plasmid form with a transfection efficiency of up to four times higher than that of the oc isoform (Quaak et al. 2009) and thus most appropriate for therapeutic applications.

Analysis and quality control of plasmid DNA for pharmaceutical applications is regulated by several regulatory guidelines (FDA 2007). The U.S. Food and Drug Administration (FDA) requests that for bulk and drug product release testing, standard assays of adequate specificity and sensitivity should be used. In addition to bulk and final product release testing, in-process control (IPC) is recommended to ensure manufacturing consistency and product safety. Furthermore, stability testing should be initiated prior to Phase I clinical studies.

16 Industrial Manufacturing of Plasmid-DNA Products for Gene Vaccination   325

Table 16.1 Recommended analytical parameters for in-process control and release testing, possible analytical methods and suggested specifications

Parameter	Method	Suggested specifications
DNA concentration	UV-absorption (260 nm)	Depending on product specifications
General purity	UV-scan (220–320 nm) or A_{260}/A_{280}	>1.75
Homogeneity (ccc content)	AEC-HPLC, CGE, AGE	> 90%[a]
Appearance	Visible inspection	Clear, colorless
Residual genomic DNA	AGE, quantitative PCR, Southern blot	<1%
Residual RNA	AGE, quantitative PCR, fluorescence assays	Undetectable in AGE
Residual host cell proteins	BCA, ELISA	<1%
Endotoxi6n LPS)	LAL test	£1 EU/mg pDNA[b]
Purity (microorganisms)	Bioburden test and/or sterility test	<1 CFU
Identity (vector structure)	AGE, Bioanalyzer	Restriction fragments conform
Identity (sequence)	Sequencing	Conforms
pH	–	Depending on product specifications

[a]>80 % suggested by US FDA (2007)
[b]≤40 EU/mg suggested by US FDA (2007)

Typically, the bulk release criteria (see also Table 16.1) will include tests for visual appearance and plasmid concentration. Fraction of plasmid in supercoiled conformation (covalently closed circular/ccc) should be included in the bulk release criteria with a recommended minimum specification of ccc > 80% (FDA 2007).

While plasmid DNA topology and stability is commonly analyzed by agarose gel electrophoresis (AGE) or anion exchange HPLC (Diogo et al. 2001; Quaak et al. 2009; Smith et al. 2007), the latter provides a higher degree of sensitivity, precision and accuracy (Ulmer 2001), allowing the quantitative analysis of different pDNA topologies. Thus, both homogeneity and pDNA concentration can be determined (Urthaler et al. 2005a). An example of the analysis of *E. coli* lysate compared to purified product on anion exchange HPLC is depicted in Fig. 16.6. Other assays with comparable methodical features include analytical hydrophobic interaction chromatography (Cai et al. 2010) and capillary gel electrophoresis (Schleef and Blaesen 2009; Schleef and Schmidt 2004; Voss 2007).

Plasmid preparations should be evaluated for presence of host cell proteins (HCPs) as well as genomic DNA (gDNA) and RNA. Host cell protein content is commonly quantified with either a colorimetric assay such as BCA or Bradford (Cai et al. 2010; Schleef and Schmidt 2004; Urthaler et al. 2005a) or ELISA. Applicable analytical assays for genomic DNA include Southern slot blot analysis (Diogo et al. 2000; Urthaler et al. 2005a) and the highly sensitive quantitative polymerase chain reaction (PCR) (Cai et al. 2010; Schleef and Schmidt 2004; Urthaler et al. 2005a). The quantification of RNA can be achieved by fluorescence assays (Ribogreen), AGE (Urthaler et al. 2005a), or with PCR. Endotoxins (lipopolysaccharides) from the *E. coli* cell

Fig. 16.6 Plasmid analysis: chromatograms of analytical anion exchange high performance liquid chromatography/AEC-HPLC of crude *E. coli* alkaline lysate (**a**) and purified drug substance bulk samples (**b**)

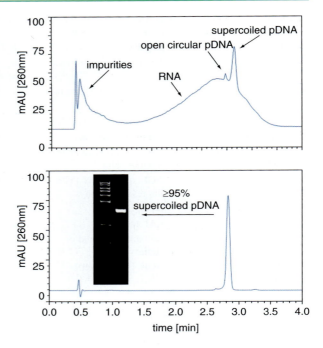

wall are critical impurities in drug products due to their pyrogenic effect. In purified pDNA solutions, the endotoxin content is analyzed by the *Limulus* amoebocyte lysate (LAL) gel clotting assay (Cai et al. 2010; FDA 2007; Urthaler et al. 2005a).

The formulated final drug product furthermore has to be tested for general safety (21 CFR section 610.11) and purity, quantity, identity and sterility (FDA 2007). Analysis of DNA concentration/quantity and general purity is commonly done by UV/VIS spectrophotometry (Cai et al. 2010; Russel and Sambrook 2001). Plasmid identity testing can be accomplished by AGE after restriction digest (restriction mapping). The resulting fragments have to conform with either the theoretical size or a reference standard (Schleef and Schmidt 2004). Bioburden of plasmid drug substance and sterility of drug product are tested by cultivating drug samples on culture media. Furthermore, a potency assay must be developed and applied in order to confirm the eukaryotic expression of the target gene (FDA 2007). In cases, the plasmid DNA is complexed with e.g. polymers of lipids, the formed drug product complex and dosage form has to be characterized, including the used excipients (Garidel and Peschka-Süss 2006).

References

Barteau B, Chevre R, Letrou-Bonneval E, Labas R, Lambert O, Pitard B (2008) Physicochemical parameters of non-viral vectors that govern transfection efficiency. Curr Gene Ther 8(5):313–323

Birnboim HC, Doly J (1979) A rapid alkaline extraction procedure for screening recombinant plasmid DNA. Nucleic Acids Res 7(6):1513–1523

Bodles-Brakhop AM, Draghia-Akli R (2008) DNA vaccination and gene therapy: optimization and delivery for cancer therapy. Expert Rev Vaccines 7(7):1085–1101

Bower DM, Prather KL (2009) Engineering of bacterial strains and vectors for the production of plasmid DNA. Appl Microbiol Biotechnol 82(5):805–813

Cai Y, Rodriguez S, Hebel H (2009) DNA vaccine manufacture: scale and quality. Expert Rev Vaccines 8(9):1277–1291

Cai Y, Rodriguez S, Rameswaran R, Draghia-Akli R, Juba RJ Jr, Hebel H (2010) Production of pharmaceutical-grade plasmids at high concentration and high supercoiled percentage. Vaccine 28(8):2046–2052

Carnes AE, Williams JA (2007) Plasmid DNA manufacturing technology. Recent Pat Biotechnol 1(2):151–166

Carnes AE, Hodgson CP, Williams JA (2006) Inducible *Escherichia coli* fermentation for increased plasmid DNA production. Biotechnol Appl Biochem 45(Pt 3):155–166

Clement J, Kiefer K, Kimpfler A, Garidel P, Peschka-Süss R (2005) Large-scale production of lipoplexes with long shelf-life. Eur J Pharm Biopharm 59(1):35–43

Cranenburgh RM, Hanak JA, Williams SG, Sherratt DJ (2001) *Escherichia coli* strains that allow antibiotic-free plasmid selection and maintenance by repressor titration. Nucleic Acids Res 29(5):E26

de la Torre LG, Rosada RS, Trombone AP, Frantz FG, Coelho-Castelo AA, Silva CL, Santana MH (2009) The synergy between structural stability and DNA-binding controls the antibody production in EPC/DOTAP/DOPE liposomes and DOTAP/DOPE lipoplexes. Colloids Surf B Biointerfaces 73(2):175–184

Diogo MM, Queiroz JA, Monteiro GA, Martins SA, Ferreira GN, Prazeres DM (2000) Purification of a cystic fibrosis plasmid vector for gene therapy using hydrophobic interaction chromatography. Biotechnol Bioeng 68(5):576–583

Diogo MM, Ribeiro SC, Queiroz JA, Monteiro GA, Tordo N, Perrin P, Prazeres DM (2001) Production, purification and analysis of an experimental DNA vaccine against rabies. J Gene Med 3(6):577–584

Dufour V (2001) DNA vaccines: new applications for veterinary medicine. Vet Sci Tom 2:1–26

FDA (2007) Guidance for industry: considerations for plasmid DNA vaccines for infectious disease indications. Accessed on Dec 20th, 2010 http://www.fda.gov/BiologicsBloodVaccines/GuidanceComplianceRegulatoryInformation/Guidances/Vaccines/default.htm

Ferreira GN, Cabral JM, Prazeres DM (1999) Development of process flow sheets for the purification of supercoiled plasmids for gene therapy applications. Biotechnol Prog 15(4):725–731

Garidel P, Funari SS (2006) Lipid to plasmid ratio influences the supramolecular structure of lipoplexes: a SAXS study. HASYLAB Annu Rep 1:1299–1300

Garidel P, Peschka-Süss R (2006) Lipoplexes in gene therapy under the considerations of scaling up, stability issues, and pharmaceutical requirements. In: Gregoriadis G (ed) Liposome Technology, 3rd edn. CRC Press, New York, pp 97–138

Gill DR, Pringle IA, Hyde SC (2009) Progress and prospects: the design and production of plasmid vectors. Gene Ther 16(2):165–171

Goh S, Good L (2008) Plasmid selection in *Escherichia coli* using an endogenous essential gene marker. BMC Biotechnol 8:61

Hayashizaki Y (1997) Method for purification of DNA. CA 1997/2207852

Hebel H, Ramakrishnan S, Gonzalez H, Darnell J (2004) Devices and methods for biomaterial production. WO 2004/108260

Hoare M, Levy MS, Bracewell DG, Doig SD, Kong S, Titchener-Hooker N, Ward JM, Dunnill P (2005) Bioprocess engineering issues that would be faced in producing a DNA vaccine at up to 100 m^3 fermentation scale for an influenza pandemic. Biotechnol Prog 21(6):1577–1592

Huber H, Kollmann F, Reinisch C, Pacher C, Necina R (2005a) Method for producing plasmid DNA on a manufacturing scale by fermentation of the *Escherichia coli* K-12 strain JM108. WO2005098002

Huber H, Weigl G, Buchinger W (2005b) Fed-batch fermentation process and culture medium for the production of plasmid DNA in *E. coli* on a manufacturing scale. WO2005097990

Huber H, Buchinger W, Diewok J, Ganja R, Keller D, Urthaler J, Necina R (2008) Industrial manufacturing of plasmid DNA. Genet Eng Biotechn NY 28(4):44–45

Hucklenbroich J, Müller M (2003) Methods for coarse purification of cell digests from microorganism. WO 2003/070942

Kelly WJ (2003) Perspectives on plasmid-based gene therapy: challenges for the product and the process. Biotechnol Appl Biochem 37(Pt 3):219–223

Kiefer K, Clement J, Garidel P, Peschka-Süss R (2004) Transfection efficiency and cytotoxicity of nonviral gene transfer reagents in human smooth muscle and endothelial cells. Pharm Res 21(6):1009–1017

Kitamura T, Nakatani S (2002) Separating plasmids from contaminants using hydrophobic or haydrophobic and ion exchange chromatography. US 6441160

Kodama K, Katayama Y, Shoji Y, Nakashima H (2006) The features and shortcomings for gene delivery of current non-viral carriers. Curr Med Chem 13(18):2155–2161

Koynova R, Wang L, Macdonald RC (2008) Cationic phospholipids forming cubic phases: lipoplex structure and transfection efficiency. Mol Pharm 5(5):739–744

Lee A, Sagar S (1996) A method for large scale plasmid purification. WO 96/36706

Lenter MC, Garidel P, Pelisek J, Wagner E, Ogris M (2004) Stabilized nonviral formulations for the delivery of MCP-1 gene into cells of the vasculoendothelial system. Pharm Res 21(4):683–691

Levy MS, Collins IJ, Yim SS, Ward JM, Titchener-Hooker N, Shamlou PA, Dunnill P (1999) Effect of shear on plasmid DNA in solution. Bioprocess Eng 20(1):7–13

Li SD, Huang L (2006) Gene therapy progress and prospects: non-viral gene therapy by systemic delivery. Gene Ther 13(18):1313–1319

Listner K, Bentley L, Okonkowski J, Kistler C, Wnek R, Caparoni A, Junker B, Robinson D, Salmon P, Chartrain M (2006) Development of a highly productive and scalable plasmid DNA production platform. Biotechnol Prog 22(5):1335–1345

Liu MA (2010) Gene-based vaccines: recent developments. Curr Opin Mol Ther 12(1):86–93

Luke J, Carnes AE, Hodgson CP, Williams JA (2009) Improved antibiotic-free DNA vaccine vectors utilizing a novel RNA based plasmid selection system. Vaccine 27(46):6454–6459

Mahvi DM, Sheehy MJ, Yang NS (1997) DNA cancer vaccines: a gene gun approach. Immunol Cell Biol 75(5):456–460

Mairhofer J, Pfaffenzeller I, Merz D, Grabherr R (2008) A novel antibiotic free plasmid selection system: advances in safe and efficient DNA therapy. Biotechnol J 3(1):83–89

Mairhofer J, Cserjan-Puschmann M, Striedner G, Nobauer K, Razzazi-Fazeli E, Grabherr R (2010) Marker-free plasmids for gene therapeutic applications – lack of antibiotic resistance gene substantially improves the manufacturing process. J Biotechnol 146(3):130–137

Mayrhofer P, Blaesen M, Schleef M, Jechlinger W (2008) Minicircle-DNA production by site specific recombination and protein-DNA interaction chromatography. J Gene Med 10(11):1253–1269

Mayrhofer P, Schleef M, Jechlinger W (2009) Use of minicircle plasmids for gene therapy. Methods Mol Biol 542:87–104

McNeil SE, Vangala A, Bramwell VW, Hanson PJ, Perrie Y (2010) Lipoplexes formulation and optimisation: in vitro transfection studies reveal no correlation with in vivo vaccination studies. Curr Drug Deliv 7(2):175–187

Moffatt S, Cristiano RJ (2006) Uptake characteristics of NGR-coupled stealth PEI/pDNA nanoparticles loaded with PLGA-PEG-PLGA tri-block copolymer for targeted delivery to human monocyte-derived dendritic cells. Int J Pharm 321(1–2):143–154

Morille M, Passirani C, Vonarbourg A, Clavreul A, Benoit JP (2008) Progress in developing cationic vectors for non-viral systemic gene therapy against cancer. Biomaterials 29(24–25):3477–3496

Muhs A, Lenter MC, Seidler RW, Zweigerdt R, Kirchengast M, Weser R, Ruediger M, Guth B (2004) Nonviral monocyte chemoattractant protein-1 gene transfer improves arteriogenesis after femoral artery occlusion. Gene Ther 11(23):1685–1693

O'Rorke S, Keeney M, Pandit A (2010) Non-viral polyplexes: Scaffold mediated delivery for gene therapy. Prog Polym Sci 35(4):441–458

Ogris M, Wagner E (2002a) Targeting tumors with non-viral gene delivery systems. Drug Discov Today 7(8):479–485

Ogris M, Wagner E (2002b) Tumor-targeted gene transfer with DNA polyplexes. Somat Cell Mol Genet 27(1–6):85–95

16 Industrial Manufacturing of Plasmid-DNA Products for Gene Vaccination 329

Ongkudon CM, Ho J, Danquah MK (2010) Mitigating the looming vaccine crisis: production and delivery of plasmid-based vaccines. Crit Rev Biotechnol 31(1), 32–52

Phue JN, Lee SJ, Trinh L, Shiloach J (2008) Modified *Escherichia coli* B (BL21), a superior producer of plasmid DNA compared with *Escherichia coli* K (DH5alpha). Biotechnol Bioeng 101(4):831–836

Posfai G, Plunkett G 3rd, Feher T, Frisch D, Keil GM, Umenhoffer K, Kolisnychenko V, Stahl B, Sharma SS, de Arruda M, Burland V, Harcum SW, Blattner FR (2006) Emergent properties of reduced-genome *Escherichia coli*. Science 312(5776):1044–1046

Prather KJ, Sagar S, Murphy J, Chartrain M (2003) Industrial scale production of plasmid DNA for vaccine and gene therapy: plasmid design, production, and purification. Enzyme Microb Technol 33(7):865–883

Przybylowski M, Bartido S, Borquez-Ojeda O, Sadelain M, Riviere I (2007) Production of clinical-grade plasmid DNA for human Phase I clinical trials and large animal clinical studies. Vaccine 25(27):5013–5024

Quaak SG, van den Berg JH, Oosterhuis K, Beijnen JH, Haanen JB, Nuijen B (2009) DNA tattoo vaccination: effect on plasmid purity and transfection efficiency of different topoisoforms. J Control Release 139(2):153–159

Rozkov A, Avignone-Rossa CA, Ertl PF, Jones P, O'Kennedy RD, Smith JJ, Dale JW, Bushell ME (2006) Fed batch culture with declining specific growth rate for high-yielding production of a plasmid containing a gene therapy sequence in *Escherichia coli* DH1. Enzyme Microb Technol 39(1):47–50

Rozkov A, Larsson B, Gillstrom S, Bjornestedt R, Schmidt SR (2008) Large-scale production of endotoxin-free plasmids for transient expression in mammalian cell culture. Biotechnol Bioeng 99(3):557–566

Russel D, Sambrook J (2001) Molecular Cloning: A Laboratory Manual. Cold Spring Harbor Laboratory Press, Cold Spring Harbor

Schaffert D, Wagner E (2008) Gene therapy progress and prospects: synthetic polymer-based systems. Gene Ther 15(16):1131–1138

Schleef M, Blaesen M (2009) Production of plasmid DNA as a pharmaceutical. In: Walther WaUSS (ed) Methods in molecular biology, gene therapy of cancer, vol 542. Humana Press, New York, pp 471–495

Schleef M, Schmidt T (2004) Animal-free production of ccc-supercoiled plasmids for research and clinical applications. J Gene Med 6(Suppl 1):S45–S53

Seidler RW, Allgauer S, Ailinger S, Sterner A, Dev N, Rabussay D, Doods H, Lenter MC (2005) In vivo human MCP-1 transfection in porcine arteries by intravascular electroporation. Pharm Res 22(10):1685–1691

Singer A, Eiteman MA, Altman E (2009) DNA plasmid production in different host strains of *Escherichia coli*. J Ind Microbiol Biotechnol 36(4):521–530

Smith CR, DePrince RB, Dackor J, Weigl D, Griffith J, Persmark M (2007) Separation of topological forms of plasmid DNA by anion-exchange HPLC: shifts in elution order of linear DNA. J Chromatogr B Analyt Technol Biomed Life Sci 854(1–2):121–127

Smrekar F, Podgornik A, Ciringer M, Kontrec S, Raspor P, Strancar A, Peterka M (2010) Preparation of pharmaceutical-grade plasmid DNA using methacrylate monolithic columns. Vaccine 28(8):2039–2045

Soubrier F, Cameron B, Manse B, Somarriba S, Dubertret C, Jaslin G, Jung G, Caer CL, Dang D, Mouvault JM, Scherman D, Mayaux JF, Crouzet J (1999) pCOR: a new design of plasmid vectors for nonviral gene therapy. Gene Ther 6(8):1482–1488

Soubrier F, Laborderie B, Cameron B (2005) Improvement of pCOR plasmid copy number for pharmaceutical applications. Appl Microbiol Biotechnol 66(6):683–688

Stadler J, Lemmens R, Nyhammar T (2004) Plasmid DNA purification. J Gene Med 6(Suppl 1):S54–S66

Tan PH, Beutelspacher SC, Wang YH, McClure MO, Ritter MA, Lombardi G, George AJ (2005) Immunolipoplexes: an efficient, nonviral alternative for transfection of human dendritic cells with potential for clinical vaccination. Mol Ther 11(5):790–800

Tejeda-Mansir A, Montesinos RM (2008) Upstream processing of plasmid DNA for vaccine and gene therapy applications. Recent Pat Biotechnol 2(3):156–172

Tenchov BG, Wang L, Koynova R, MacDonald RC (2008) Modulation of a membrane lipid lamellar-nonlamellar phase transition by cationic lipids: a measure for transfection efficiency. Biochim Biophys Acta 1778(10):2405–2412

Tolmachov O (2009) Designing plasmid vectors. In: Walther WaUSS (ed) Methods in molecular biology, gene therapy of cancer, vol 542. 2009/07/02 edn. Humana Press, New York, pp 117–129

Tyagi RK, Sharma PK, Vyas SP, Mehta A (2008) Various carrier system(s)-mediated genetic vaccination strategies against malaria. Expert Rev Vaccines 7(4):499–520

Ulmer JB (2001) An update on the state of the art of DNA vaccines. Curr Opin Drug Discov Dev 4(2):192–197

Urthaler J, Buchinger W, Necina R (2005a) Improved downstream process for the production of plasmid DNA for gene therapy. Acta Biochim Pol 52(3):703–711

Urthaler J, Buchinger W, Necina R (2005b) Industrial scale cGMP purification of pharmaceutical grade plasmid-DNA. Chem Eng Technol 28(11):1408–1420

Urthaler J, Schlegl R, Podgornik A, Strancar A, Jungbauer A, Necina R (2005c) Application of monoliths for plasmid DNA purification development and transfer to production. J Chromatogr A 1065(1):93–106

Urthaler J, Ascher C, Wohrer H, Necina R (2007) Automated alkaline lysis for industrial scale cGMP production of pharmaceutical grade plasmid-DNA. J Biotechnol 128(1):132–149

Urthaler J, Ascher C, Bucheli D (2009) Methods and devices for producing biomolecules. WO 2009/098284

van den Berg JH, Oosterhuis K, Hennink WE, Storm G, van der Aa LJ, Engbersen JF, Haanen JB, Beijnen JH, Schumacher TN, Nuijen B (2010) Shielding the cationic charge of nanoparticle-formulated dermal DNA vaccines is essential for antigen expression and immunogenicity. J Control Release 141(2):234–240

Vidal L, Pinsach J, Striedner G, Caminal G, Ferrer P (2008) Development of an antibiotic-free plasmid selection system based on glycine auxotrophy for recombinant protein overproduction in *Escherichia coli*. J Biotechnol 134(1–2):127–136

Voss C (2007) Production of plasmid DNA for pharmaceutical use. Biotechnol Annu Rev 13:201–222

Wagner E (2004) Strategies to improve DNA polyplexes for in vivo gene transfer: will "artificial viruses" be the answer? Pharm Res 21(1):8–14

Wagner E, Kloeckner J (2006) Gene delivery using polymer therapeutics. Adv Polym Sci 192:135–173

Wagner E, Culmsee C, Boeckle S (2005) Targeting of polyplexes: toward synthetic virus vector systems. Adv Genet 53:333–354

Williams JA, Carnes AE, Hodgson CP (2009a) Plasmid DNA vaccine vector design: impact on efficacy, safety and upstream production. Biotechnol Adv 27(4):353–370

Williams JA, Luke J, Langtry S, Anderson S, Hodgson CP, Carnes AE (2009b) Generic plasmid DNA production platform incorporating low metabolic burden seed-stock and fed-batch fermentation processes. Biotechnol Bioeng 103(6):1129–1143

Wils P, Escriou V, Warnery A, Lacroix F, Lagneaux D, Ollivier M, Crouzet J, Mayaux JF, Scherman D (1997) Efficient purification of plasmid DNA for gene transfer using triple-helix affinity chromatography. Gene Ther 4(4):323–330

Yang YP, Li YH, Zhang AH, Bi L, Fan MW (2009) Good manufacturing practices production and analysis of a DNA vaccine against dental caries. Acta Pharmacol Sin 30(11):1513–1521

Yau SY, Keshavarz-Moore E, Ward J (2008) Host strain influences on supercoiled plasmid DNA production in *Escherichia coli*: implications for efficient design of large-scale processes. Biotechnol Bioeng 101(3):529–544

Zantl R, Baicu L, Artzner F, Sprenger I, Rapp G, Radler JO (1999) Thermotropic phase behavior of cationic lipid-DNA complexes compared to binary lipid mixtures. J Phys Chem B 103(46):10300–10310

Printing: Ten Brink, Meppel, The Netherlands
Binding: Stürtz, Würzburg, Germany